ETHICS CODES IN MEDICINE

Ethics Codes in Medicine

Foundations and achievements of codification since 1947

Edited by Ulrich Tröhler and Stella Reiter-Theil
in cooperation with Eckhard Herych

Center for Ethics and Law in Medicine
University Hospital Freiburg, Germany
Elsaesser Strasse 2m, Haus 1a
D - 79110 Freiberg, Germany

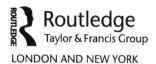

Routledge
Taylor & Francis Group

LONDON AND NEW YORK

First published 1998 by Ashgate Publishing

Reissued 2018 by Routledge
2 Park Square, Milton Park, Abingdon, Oxon, OX14 4RN
711 Third Avenue, New York, NY 10017, USA

Routledge is an imprint of the Taylor & Francis Group, an informa business

Publisher's Note
The publisher has gone to great lengths to ensure the quality of this reprint but points out that some imperfections in the original copies may be apparent.

Disclaimer
The publisher has made every effort to trace copyright holders and welcomes correspondence from those they have been unable to contact.

A Library of Congress record exists under LC control number: 98072798

ISBN 13: 978-1-138-33482-3 (hbk)
ISBN 13: 978-1-138-33483-0 (pbk)
ISBN 13: 978-1-138-33484-7 (ebk)

Contents

THE PARADIGM SHIFT IN MEDICAL ETHICS: PATIENTS' RIGHTS, EDUCATION, INSTITUTIONS

ETHICS AND MEDICINE FOR THE 21st CENTURY: THE QUEST FOR NEW CODES

APPENDIX

Preface

Jürgen Rüttgers

Drawn up some 50 years ago in an effort to confront the crimes committed by the National Socialists in their experiments on human beings, the Nuremberg Code has proved to be an important set of basic ethical guidelines for research. These historic events will always be part of the present, especially in Germany. However, many new ethical grey areas have become evident from new scientific possibilities since the Nuremberg Code was drawn up. The scientific advances made in research on DNA have raised questions about the appropriateness of our influence on procreation, on unborn life and generations to come. The importance of such questions for the future of mankind are obvious.

I myself was therefore quick to support global efforts to prohibit the application of cloning techniques used on the sheep "Dolly" onto human beings. The G8 recently spoke out against such practices at their recent summit, and a positive response to a veto on human cloning was also reached during the talks on the *Convention for the Protection of Human Rights and Dignity of the Human Being with Regard to the Application of Biology and Medicine: Convention of Human Rights and Medicine* of the Council of Europe and on the draft of a "General Declaration of UNESCO on the Human Genome and Human Rights". All of this bodes well for future cooperation on an international level.

In other respects, the consensus between nations remains to be established on norms and principles. The very concept of human dignity can lead to various national discrepancies. Ethical considerations are never free from the various cultural and religious traditions of respective nations. The quest for international agreements thus always entails compromises.

Despite all of the difficulties, the attempt to reach international conventions on ethical codes is the right way. The universality of fundamental ethical principles and their legal realizations, not to mention the striving of researchers toward "internationality", makes such international conventions necessary; this is also all a challenge to national governments and international organizations. And yet, these national laws and international conventions are not enough: those involved in such fields must constantly redefine their roles, their personal responsibility, and the guidelines within the profession, as such people know their fields best and can react quickly to the ever-changing scientific possibilities. The development of a supra-national legal context for science must be accompanied by a universal ethical understanding of the role of science within the profession, regard-less of country.

Fifty years after the Nuremberg Trials, the discussions about form and content of ethical principles in medicine and biotechnology are as lively as ever. This makes me feel optimistic. The ongoing debates about grey areas sharpen our view for the fundamentals to be upheld. Unlike the many cul-tural pessimists who distrust medicine and biotechnology, I am convinced that human's sense of ethics can keep pace with the advances of science. The Nuremberg Code is one sign of that and is simultaneously a challenge to researchers to look for consent on ethical categories themselves above and beyond national borders.

Foreword

Hans-Konrat Wellmer and Dietrich von Engelhardt

Fifty years have passed since the Nuremberg Doctors' Trials and their rulings and the guidelines they resulted in. And yet, the need for ethical rules of law for medical research and therapy has not decreased at all. New ethical responses to scientific advances in theory and practice have to be found again and again.

From October 12th to 15th, 1997, the Freiburg Center for Ethics and Law in Medicine of the Albert-Ludwigs University (ZERM), organized the First World Conference *Ethics Codes in Medicine and Biotechnology* in the name of the German Academy for Ethics in Medicine (AEM). The present volume contains contributions from two preparatory European Workshops leading up to this conference which were held in Freiburg in 1996. There, discussions revolved around the requirements for and consequences of the Nuremberg Doctors' Trials in their socio-cultural context. Along with efforts to gain historical knowledge, the focus will remain on the guidelines from the past few decades in the humanization of medicine as well as on the question of which conclusions are to be drawn and which initiatives seem meaningful and necessary.·

As a general forum for ethical reflection and communication, the Academy for Ethics in Medicine knows first-hand that codes in medicine not only depend on ethical theory and legislation, but also on the force and will of individuals - doctors, nurses, family members, as well as patients.

May these observations, analyses, and appeals collected in this volume from various countries further these aims.

Introduction of the Editors

Ulrich Tröhler and Stella Reiter-Theil

Ethics, being the science of morals, is one of the three basic disciplines of philosophy. Comprehensive treatises on ethical questions have been in existence ever since antiquity. Besides those, one can also find short versions, reduced to the enumeration of rules. Concerning medical practice, such rules have existed in the form of oaths, covenants, and prayers since antiquity, as ecclesiastic dogmas and laws since the Middle Ages, and as professional rules since the 19th century. For some time now, the concept of "ethics codes" has been established to name these shortened documents. Their number has increased enormously since the Nuremberg Code (1947), especially over the last two decades, since they were considered to provide the means of orientation and ideal self-representation.

In terms of their content, these codes typically thematize the qualities of a "good doctor", the healer- or physician-patient-relationship, and basic questions of medical practice at the beginning and at the end of life (abortion, euthanasia). More recently, they deal with questions of research (animal and human experimentation), and specific forms of patient care (transplantation, gene therapy, reproduction techniques). Time and again, the contents of such documents are intra- and inter-professional issues, e.g. the relationship among members of the various health professions and paramedical groups, as well as vis-à-vis society and the state.

Some codes facilitate a general medical or health care *ethos*, i.e. the moral attitude for professionals to live by, while upholding specific values, particularly those related to the individual conscience. Other documents contain guidelines, founded in the wider framework and principles of medical *ethics,* which focus on a specific problem. The content of the majority of codes is a combination of both types.

In general, the codification of ethics has been consented to by professionals, in public, however, it has often raised criticism. In our times of democracy, documents drafted by members of a profession are sometimes considered as representing tendencies towards securing a monopoly, reinforcing its own ends and its claims for self-regulation. At the same time, the quest for ideals which usually characterizes these codes is dismissed as being too vague. Similarly, there is regret that philosophical and religious value systems are replaced by a professional and secularized organization of medical ethics. Nonetheless, this modern type of ethics is being developed by people who themselves are influenced by the predominant values of a society. A good example is the decline of traditional paternalism hitherto determining the doctor-patient relationship. Today, models of mutual consensus predominate: the phenomenon is not only reflected by the majority of codes but can equally be found in many domains of the everyday-life: at home, at work, and in public.

The development, the explosion, of codification of medical ethos and medical ethics over the last decades raises fundamental questions in a situation, in which the potential of medicine has obviously grown more rapidly than the capacity to cope with it: Who will put the multiple facets of codification in an order? Who will be responsible to decide what an ethically correct action is? Does the drafting of ethics guidelines fall within the domain of medical and/or health care professions, the churches, philosophy, lay groups, or rather the general public which includes all of them via parliament and legislation? How can differing value systems be related and adapted to one another in the light of globalization? By no means have all domains and problematic situations in medicine and biotechnology been regulated by ethics codes, let alone by the less flexible law. Therefore, every health professional still has a great responsibility that is challenging his or her conscience and character against the backdrop of the general moral standards of society. This fact also holds true for those responsible in industry, insurance, politics, and the media: One really has to wonder to what extent the polymorphic wave of codification has been and is being perceived and put into practice. These are the questions addressed in this volume.

The following contributions have their origine in two international workshops which the editors organized together with an European scientific panel in April and May of 1996 in Freiburg (Germany). The goal of these workshops was to sketch, in English and French, respectively, the *state of the art* in the discussion about the codification of medical ethics, given the actual challenges to the health care system. This made it possible to present central themes of present-day debates in the light of history and from various national and/or (inter-) disciplinary perspectives. The German edition was scheduled to be ready for the First World Conference on Ethics Codes in Medicine and Biotechnology, also to be held in Freiburg, in October of 1997.

Thirty-two authors from 15 countries have studied the complex operations of codification related to the phenomenon of ethics in medicine. The book sets about with the historical roots. Two contributions study the preconditions of ethical conduct in medicine from antiquity to 1947 (Leven, Lepicard). The ever-present relationship between science, myths, and medicine before and after 1947 is thematized (Moulin, de Wachter, von Engelhardt). The inception of the codification wave is the year 1947 with the Nuremberg Code, which is shown to be a historically significant event

(Rothman). A shocking testimony on the medical experiments in Nazi concentration camps has to be given (Kanovitch), before it is possible to describe the mechanisms by which the Nuremberg Trials attempted to constructively overcome the abuse of human beings in research (Deutsch) and the formulation of rules of international law (Sprumont and Arnold). But what about respecting inherent ethical norms throughout the world following the Nuremberg Trials? This is still a question of great relevance, as is exemplified by the more or rather less complete adoption of the 10 Nuremberg preconditions for ethically acceptable human experiments into ethics codes since 1947 in an international comparison (Herranz). This relevance is also illustrated by the latest discoveries on the use of scientific data, obtained by unethical research (Kimura). The relationship between a code of ethics and the law during the last 50 years also needs an evaluation from the ethical and legal perspective (Winslade and Krause). The idea of a code as "soft" law, i.e. an alternative to, or a preliminary step towards a law, confronts us with the problem of legitimacy, particularly with questions of democratic legitimacy (Mathieu, Honigman). The example of the human genome project viewed from the perspective of coping with the future, makes this topic very clear (Levi and Plantholz). The question of paradigm shift in critical fields of medicine leads from an analysis of the experiences with the Nuremberg Code an evaluation of the present-day situation in medical ethics: patient rights, teaching and training as well as institutions are presented by authors from the United States (Carson), France (Michaud), Great Britain (Horner), Italy (Spagnolo), Germany (Reiter-Theil) and from the perspective of international organizations (Douraki). Relative to coping with the problems we are facing, these discussions unveil more or less critical conclusions.

The search for new ethics codes is an ambivalent venture, for there are too many unsolved questions on the side of science, as it is shown in the contribution on predictive medicine and genetic testing (Archer) as well as in those on the allocation of scarce resources (Hermerén; Mattéi, Moatti and Rauch). Furthermore, one has to question, whether concepts of ethics, codes, and human rights are universally valid. Probing the depths of these questions are the perspectives on a transcultural form of ethics (Baker) and of human rights in South America (Riquelme).

This volume could not have been made possible without the generous funding for the 1996 workshops and the 1997 First World Conference by the Federal Ministry of Education, Science, Research and Technology (BMBF), the German Research Association (DFG), and the Robert Bosch Foundation. Finally, the authors deserve thanks and recognition for readily entering into the interdisciplinary and international debate and for openly and courageously facing the moral and political challenges of the scientific issues of our times.

Ethics Codes in Medicine: Historical, Legal and Philosophical Aspects

1 The Invention of Hippocrates: Oath, Letters and Hippocratic Corpus

Karl-Heinz Leven

In 1948, the *World Medical Association*, which had been founded two years before in London, was given an ethical code[1] called the "Declaration of Geneva", which was formulated in both English and French. Its subtitle in French, "Serment d'Hippocrate, formule de Genève", clearly shows the intent to have it associated with the Hippocratic Oath in terms of form and content. The myth of Hippocrates had proved once again to be an integral element of the image that doctors had of themselves. The idealized vision of Hippocrates that is behind all this goes back to antiquity, as will be demonstrated below. During the first half of the 20th century, a historical critique on the philological aspects of Hippocratic medicine and a nostalgic view of history both led to the formulation of rather unusual misunderstandings which have an impact on the ethical discourse still today.

Hippocrates in Geneva and Nuremberg

The "Declaration of Geneva" was expressed in the Hippocratic tradition partly to show that the Hippocratic Oath, when formulated in modern terms, could serve as the basis for medical ethics in the 20th century. This was held to be all the more true since the Nuremberg trials against Nazi doctors (1946-47) had shown what ethical crimes modern medicine was capable of.[2] These trials dealt with the cruel and often deadly experiments that German doctors had conducted on prisoners of war and inmates of concentration camps - acts held by the tribunal to constitute murder and crimes against humanity. The defense tried to relativize and play down the atrocities perpetrated by the defendants by citing cases in the international medical literature that were ostensibly comparable. The prosecution and the tribunal thus were faced with the unexpected difficulty of finding a generally acceptable standard with which to judge the crimes of the Nazi doctors. At the same time, the judges realized that ethical guidelines had to be drawn up for regulating and keeping in check any future medical research. The Nuremberg tribunal met both of these needs, but not by

3

applying the Hippocratic Oath. Instead, it created a new ethical guideline, the Nuremberg Code (1947).

Although the prosecution had initially accused all of the Nazi doctors of having violated the Hippocratic Oath, which they had sworn to uphold, it did not quote any parts of the Oath.[3] Later, two witnesses for the prosecution who served as experts on medical ethics, the German medical historian Werner Leibbrand (1896-1974) and the American physiologist Andrew C. Ivy (1893-1978), did make reference to the Oath. When cross-examined by the defense, they mentioned specific passages of the Oath. Leibbrand stood for, as he himself put it, an uncompromising "Hippocratic" standpoint, dismissing any experiments on humans that did not serve the needs of the subjects themselves as being unethical. Ivy, on the other hand, made a distinction "between the doctor as a therapist, the healer, and the doctor as a researcher". Different sections of the Hippocratic Oath should be applied to one or the other type, but Ivy did not specify which sections he meant.[4] Later on in the trial, the defendants also referred to the Hippocratic Oath. Karl Brandt, one of those responsible for Nazi "euthanasia", tried to justify the medical crimes as being a modern interpretation of the Hippocratic Oath.[5] The tribunal did not accept this interpretation of the Hippocratic Oath, though it did not try to disprove it either. As Alexander Mitscherlich, one of the attendants of the trials, put it, the Oath had proved ineffective as an ethical standard of modern medi̇cine.[6]

In 1947, with the aid of prosecution witnesses Andrew Ivy and Leo Alexander, the tribunal created and included in its decision a new ethical standard that was independent of the Hippocratic Oath and is now known as the Nuremberg Code, a ten-point statement delimiting permissible medical experimentation on human subjects.[7] The World Medical Association appeared to take no notice of this "breach with Hippocrates", when in 1948 it drew up a set of pledges serving as ethical guidelines for doctors throughout the world one year after the trial had ended. Confronted with accusations that members of their profession had backed the Third Reich, representatives of the German Medical Association also were keen on espousing the Hippocratic Oath as an argument for their own benefit.[8] The prosaic Nuremberg Code thus easily fell victim to the victorious myth of Hippocrates.

Hippocrates and *Hippocratic Corpus*

Although knowing the date when they were written is relatively trivial for most historical documents, not knowing when the Hippocratic Oath was written does lead to a number of problems. The Oath is to be seen in the context of the works associated with Hippocrates' name - the *Hippocratic Corpus*. In medieval manuscripts, the Oath takes up the first page of the

Corpus, a practice which often has been maintained in modern editions and translations.[9]

The approximately 60 writings (counting methods vary) contained in the *Hippocratic Corpus* cover all topics in medicine; they are not, as was realized as far back as antiquity, written all by one author named Hippocrates. Not only the breadth of topics, but also obvious contradictions and fundamental oppositions show that the work was done by various authors. In addition, there are the "differences in quality" of the writings that have been perceived in various ways throughout the ages. The *Corpus* originated over a period extending from the end of the 5th century B.C. until the late Hellenistic Age. Some texts may have been written in the post-Christian era. The body of writings was apparently first compiled under the author's name, Hippocrates, in Hellenistic Alexandria,[10] which is also the birthplace of Hippocratic exegesis. The latter used the literary form of commentaries on specific texts in the *Corpus* and was instrumental in creating the Hippocrates lexica. The earliest commentaries mentioned in the sources were probably written by Herophilus (approx. 330/320-260/250 B.C.); his pupil Baccheius of Tanagra (approx. 275-200 B.C.) created the first lexicon on the Hippocratic treatises.[11] The earliest existing commentary has been written by Apollonius of Citium (1st cent. B.C.). Commentaries were written then on the Hippocratic treatises partly in order to make them useful to contemporary medicine. This was still true of the last complete edition of Hippocrates by the French doctor and philologist, Émile Littré (1801-1881), published from 1839 to 1861.[12] Apart from the practical considerations, by espousing Hippocratic ideas doctors have been able to furnish themselves a quality seal for their own views, doing so ever since and far beyond the Hellenistic age. In an age of medicine which drew its authority from tradition, the adjective "Hippocratic" was especially attractive. In debates among various medical sects in antiquity, for instance between the "Herophileans" and the "Empiricists", one tried to prove that one's own ideas were "Hippocratic" while those of the others were "un-Hippocratic". In doing so, it was important to refer to the "real" Hippocrates - or at least to the author who was believed to be the real one.

The Greek doctor, Galen of Pergamon (approx. 129- 210 A.D.), contributed greatly to the image of Hippocrates and stylized himself as the purist "Hippocratic" physician. In doing so, in a sense he invented Hippocrates, and his interpretation rendition of the master from Cos has remained with us to this day.[13] For Galen, as well, it was obvious that not all of the writings in the *Hippocratic Corpus*, which had been edited again at the time of the Roman emperor Hadrian (117-138 A.D.), could possibly be written by one and the same author. For Galen, Hippocrates' fundamental doctrine was to be found in the treatise "On the Nature of Man" (De natura hominis). Ever since, Hippocrates has unquestionably been held as the father of the doctrine of the four humours, which was first touched upon in the aforementioned treatise.

The question involving the "authenticity" of single Hippocratic treatises is closely tied in with conjectures about the origins of the *Hippocratic Corpus*. The traditional view handed down to us from antiquity, which Galen also subscribed to, held that Hippocrates had founded a school on the island of Cos. The master himself was said to have written the best treatises of the *Corpus*. Among these high-quality texts are *Epidemics*, *Aphorisms*, *On the Sacred Disease* and *Prognosticon*, just to name a few. His pupils and successors were said to have draped garlands of "unauthentic" texts around this core of the *Corpus*. All texts were assumed to have been located on the island of Cos, where they constituted the "Library of the Doctors", From there, sometime during the early Hellenistic period, the omnibus of treatises was said to have found its way moved to the center of knowledge, the library of the newly founded city of Alexandria. There scholars allegedly catalogued and published the writings under the name of the *main* author, Hippocrates. The *Corpus* has thus been held to consist of some "genuine" texts by Hippocrates and some falsely attributed to him.

This widespread "traditional" theory, which has endured from antiquity to the present, is supported by several factors, some of which are inherent to the context of the treatises, others of which are extrinsic in nature. To begin with the inherent factors mentioned first, the treatises of "high quality" (*Epidemics I, III, Prognosticon* etc.) were written during Hippocrates' lifetime (around 400 B.C.). In the 20th century, the German classical philologist, Karl Deichgräber, was foremost in proving how these treatises are linked to each other and, in view of their historical background, when they were written.[14] Among the extrinsic arguments supporting the "traditional" theory, one states that the island of Cos was under the sphere of influence of the Ptolemaic kings of Egypt, who actively supported the doctors and scholars of Alexandria. Ptolemy II Philadelphus (reigned 283/82-246 B.C.) was born in the Ptolemaic winter quarters at Cos in 308 B.C. during a naval operation.[15] It is thus possible that the Ptolemaic kings, who in antiquity were notorious for their craving for books,[16] also transported the medical library from Cos to the capital. Galen, too, held this opinion, though none of the sources explicitly mentions the transfer of the Hippocratic books to Alexandria.[17]

Galen took his contemporaries' criticism of the authenticity of the Hippocratic writings seriously. This is obvious from the difficulties he had in justifying himself: Aristotle had attributed the treatise "On the Nature of Man", which Galen claimed was genuine "Hippocratic", to a certain Polybus (Aristotle, *Historia animalium* III 2; 512 b 12).[18] A later source, one of the so-called "Letters of Hippocrates" (which we will return to shortly) called this Polybus a son-in-law of Hippocrates,[19] while Aristotle did not mention any whatsoever connection between Polybus and Hippocrates. Thus, if we were to believe Aristotle, not even the programmatic treatise "On the Nature of Man" had been written by the master from Cos! Galen solved this serious problem by reasoning that the text mentioned probably consisted of several parts, an interpretation which can in fact be corrobo-rated by the text. Galen considered the first, more important section with its exposition of the doctrine of the humours to be "genuinely Hippo-cratic". He polemically disputed the fact that Polybus was supposed to have been the author of the text, as "some" (*enioi*) claimed.[20] The "genuinely Hippocratic" doctrine of the humours, Galen added, was the very doctrine that Plato had referred to in his *Phaidrus*[21] - a source which we will also return to. For Galen, this kind of "proof" seemed sufficient and he did not add further remarks.

Aristotle (*Historia animalium* III 2; 512 b 12) had certainly mentioned the Polybus in question as being the author of a treatise that is identical with at least some chapters of "On the Nature of Man", even if not the author of the entire treatise. This obvious contradiction - the platform of Hippocratic medicine as the work of a doctor about whom we have no in-formation other than his name, Polybus, - was intertwined with the legends involving Hippocrates, the so-called "Letters of Hippocrates" (in German: "Hippokrates-Roman"). Here, Polybus appears as the son-in-law and pupil of Hippocrates; he is thus directly associated with the master, his family and his school. The Hippocratic myth was thus able to combine the lore from other sources with the idealized portrait of the great doctor. Part of this idealized portrait of Hippocrates and his work was that only texts of "high quality" were considered "genuinely Hippocratic". Whenever this viewpoint was challenged, as in the debate about the authorship of "On the Nature of Man", the idealized portrait and the lore were reconciled by leg-endary details.

Attributing the principles of medicine of one's own age to an idealized forefather has been a matter of course for doctors since antiquity. But why was it at all possible to idealize Hippocrates' person and works to such an extent? What was the "historical" Hippocrates like?

The Historical Hippocrates and the "Letters Of Hippocrates"

In two dialogues, Plato mentions Hippocrates as a contemporary of Socra-tes (469-399 B.C.). In the fictitious setting of *Protagoras* (311 bc), datable to the years prior to 429 B.C., i.e. Socrates' conversation with Protagoras, Hippias, and Prodicus, Socrates mentions his contemporary "Hippocrates, the Coan, the *Asklepiades* [= physician]" who, like Protagoras, and other sophists of his time, for a fee trains young people to be doctors. For Plato, Hippocrates had the same rank in medicine as Polyclet or Pheidias in sculpture and Protagoras among the sophists (*Protagoras* 311c). In another Platonic dialogue, *Phaidrus* (270 a), one learns in passing that Hippocrates used a scientific method of seeing the body in the context of the "nature of the whole" (*tou holou physis*). It is open to question whether the nature of the whole body or the nature of the entire cosmos is meant. Plato's statements about Hippocrates' method, though seemingly parenthetical, were to play an important role in shaping the image future generations would have of the "Father of Medicine".

One generation later, Plato's pupil Aristotle (384-322 B.C.), mentioned that Hippocrates, although of diminutive stature, was outstanding as doctor (*Politics VII 4.* 1326 a 15f.). Aristotle thus adds nothing substantial to Plato's remarks. To Plato, Hippocrates was an outstanding doctor, who was the very epitome of medicine. Admittedly, the pre-Hellenistic reports about Hippocrates mention neither his medical theories nor any of his texts; the historical figure, Hippocrates, emerges a "name without works".[22] How is this statement to be reconciled with the fact that many texts, namely the *Hippocratic Corpus*, have been handed down under his name?[23]

In addition to the above-mentioned "traditional" theory, there is a "sceptical" theory that merits our attention. The former has been evolving since antiquity and still postulates that there is a core of "genuinely Hippocratic" treatises, consisting of the oldest and best works. Nonetheless, the "traditional" theory is also careful not to insist that Hippocrates is the author of certain works in this core, preferring instead to speak him as the probable author.

In contrast, the "skeptical" theory, originated at the end of the 19th century and making headway our century, argues in quite another way.[24] According to this theory, philologists in Alexandria had catalogued an anonymous collection of medical writings and selected as their author Hippocrates of Cos, the doctor whom the authorities of classical antiquity, Plato and Aristotle, had referred to as being the outstanding doctor of their time. Yet the Alexandrian philologists knew nothing about Hippocrates except for what Plato and Aristotle had mentioned. In any event, it was clear that Hippocrates was just as prominent among physicians as Pheidias and Polyclet were among sculptors.

The "skeptical" theory is based on the assumption that the historical Hippocrates has vanished behind the fictive author. It claims that, even in Alexandria, it was no longer possible to name the "genuine" treatises with any certainty, so the best were simply held to be "genuine", i.e. written by the master himself. The need to learn more about the author of these highly esteemed writings that were being used by medical practitioners was allegedly met in due time by legendary biographical texts. Such an idealized portrait of Hippocrates is to be found in a group of texts of the *Hippocratic Corpus* known as the "Letters of Hippocrates".[25] Within the *Corpus*, Hippocrates only in these texts appears as an active figure (in no other Hippocratic text Hippocrates is mentioned by name): he proves to be a Greek patriot who refuses to help the Persian barbarians, not even for a high sum. He becomes prophylactically active against a plague that is threatening Greece, and is highly honored by the Athenians.

The general opinion among researchers is that these "Letters", creating in all a novel (therefore the German term "Hippokrates-Roman"), were written at a later date, at a time when the *Hippocratic Corpus* had long been in existence. The "skeptical" theory thus emphasizes that the image obtained through the "Letters" does not suffice to confirm the authenticity of the writings in the *Corpus*; instead, the "Letters" show the yearning for biographic details about the life of the alleged "Father of Medicine" whose writings were already being put to good use. Hippocrates appears in the "Letters" as the kind of figure needed to explain the heterogeneous character of the *Hippocratic Corpus*: a long-lived, widely traveled physician cloaked in the confines of mystery. After Plato and Aristotle had praised him merely as an important, if not the most important doctor, according to the "sceptical" theory, the need for biographical details about his character was filled by the "Letters" and the *Vitae* of Hippocrates that exist in various versions.

Such a sceptical view, one which in particular the classical philologist, Ludwig Edelstein (1902-1965), professed in the 20th century, since the thirties, leaves little untouched of Hippocrates except his name: *no* work remains that has been attributed to him in the textual tradition since antiquity. Any attributing of works to Hippocrates referred to arguments of "quality": a treatise should be "genuine" because its quality fits with the rank of the "Father of Medicine". Against this view, Edelstein, without disputing the existence of the historical figure, claimed that Hippocrates has to be regarded as "a name without any tangible historical reality".[26]

Against Edelstein's "iconoclastic" theory, those adherent to the "traditional" theory collected some evidence. The "traditional" theory is still supported by the fact that the best texts (*Epidemics I, III, Prognosticon* etc.) originated in Hippocrates' lifetime. Why should they not have been written by the master himself? No strict evidence really supports this view, and until 100 years ago nothing spoke against it. But in 1893, the text of the so-called *Anonymus Londinensis* was found on a papyrus in the British Museum. This text is a fragment of an excerpt, datable to late antiquity (1st/2nd century A.D.); the excerpt refers to a doxographic text, a brief outline of medical history in which the teachings of 20 famous Greek doctors (among them Plato's *Timaius*, which was accepted as a medical authority during antiquity) are explained. Apparently, the *Anonymus Londinensis* is the excerpt of a work written by one of Aristotle's pupils, namely Menon, entitled *Iatrika* ("Medicine") of his pupil Menon (2nd half of the 4th century B.C.).[27]

Although Hippocrates is mentioned in the *Anonymus Londinensis*, he is not acclaimed as the "Father of Medicine", but rather as one doctor among many. Surprisingly, a medical doctrine is attributed to this Hippocrates that is not to be found in the knowledgeable "genuine" writings of the *Corpus*, i.e. those treatises that the "traditional" theory holds to be "genuine". Instead, the doctrine which is attributed to Hippocrates by the *Anonymus Londinensis*, resembles a doctrine found in a treatise "On Breaths" (*De flatibus*). This treatise for the "traditional" theory always belonged to the "spurious" text of the *Hippocratic Corpus*, a text denounced as "sophistic" by classical philologists.

According to the doctrine of "On Breaths", air trapped in the body is the cause of all illness. Now, this would be the doctrine of the "historical" Hippocrates (and not e.g. the doctrine of the four humours). The inconsistency was apparent even to the anonymous author of late antiquity who wrote the excerpt of Menon's text. But he did not stop at merely reproducing Menon's version of the teachings of Hippocrates; he also argued that Menon (the text mentions Aristotle, Menon's teacher) was wrong. The "genuine" Hippocratic doctrine about illness should be different, namely the theory of the four humours. The anonymous epitomizer explicitly makes reference to the text "On the Nature of Man". This not surprising since in the 1st/2nd century A.D., when the epitomizer was working on Menon's text, the theory of the four humours was regarded as the Hippocratic doctrine per se. The *Anonymus Londinensis* is important as a report of Menon's opinion, which takes us back some two generations after the death of the historical Hippocrates. The fact that the *Anonymus Londinensis* himself called Menon's view erroneous, in this case argues for the credibility of Menon. Menon had written his account of Hippocrates' doctrine independant of the later image of the "Father of Medicine".

When the *Anonymus Londinensis* in late antiquity made his excerpts from Menon, the Hippocratic myth was already so well established that he was more prone to doubt the source than revise his view of medical history. A similiar thing happened when the *Anonymus*/Menon was rediscovered at the end of the 19th century.[28] For the first editor of the *Anonymus Londinensis*, the philologist Hermann Diels, "On Breaths" was "a frightening example of the rampant iatrosophistics around the turn of the fifth and fourth centuries".[29] He saw it as a "great error" of Menon's to have thought the treatise "On Breaths" held in such low esteem by modern researchers of the *Hippocratic Corpus* to be "genuine".

Menon's text is so important for the "Hippocratic question" because it decisively complements Plato's pre-Hellenistic report; Menon's work is the source closest to the time of Hippocrates to mention his doctrine (Plato, as we have to remember, had not mentioned Hippocrates' doctrine but his scientific method, see above). Menon wrote his *Iatrika* before the *Hippocratic Corpus* was compiled in Alexandria. His report on the historical Hippocrates as the author of a doctrine that is most apt to be found in "On Breaths" thus merits more credibility than the idealized Hippocratic tradition of Hellenism. In Menon's account, as it is shown by the *Anonymus Londinensis*, the historical Hippocrates is more of a medical sophist than the "Father of Medicine". The apparent strength of the "traditional" theory that postulates Hippocrates as the "Father of Medicine" and the author of the best writings in the *Corpus* is, in reality, its weakness. Largely under the influence of Plato's image of Hippocrates, scholars since antiquity haved believed to know what "Hippocratic" means: the best and most original texts and ideas in the *Hippocratic Corpus*, which address doctors of all epochs. This idealized image of Hippocrates, however, has always been the projection of a later Hippocratic myth back into the classical age, and thus also an idealization of later medical reality.

Hippocratic Oath and *Hippocratic Corpus*

The attempts at resolving the "Hippocratic question" [Are there "genuine" works of Hippocrates within the Corpus?] that have been briefly described here also have relevance for the Hippocratic Oath. The authorship and date of this text, as with all texts in the *Hippocratic Corpus*, is unclear.[30] Unlike other Hippocratic texts (e.g. *Epidemics I, III*) that can be clearly traced back to the time around 400 B.C. and thus to Hippocrates' lifetime, establishing the date of the Oath is very difficult. It seems to have been unknown in Hippocrates' day and for a long time afterwards. Yet in (ancient) editions of the *Hippocratic Corpus* the Oath has been placed on the first page, as can be viewed in the Byzantine manuscripts.[31] By virtue of being accorded such a prominent position, the Oath became (and still is being regarded as) the essense of the *Hippocratic Corpus*, the "the actual legacy of Hippocrates, the credo of all of his doctrines and the quality seal of his medical teachings", in terms of "paratextuality".[32] To this day, the Oath is the quintessential Hippocratic text, the only one to be quoted when one wants to give a brief impression of Hippocrates.[33]

It is commonly accepted that the Oath has not been formulated by the historical Hippocrates, this is accepted even by supporters of the "traditional" theory who view Hippocrates as the author of the best writings in the *Corpus*.[34] Nevertheless, the Oath, even if not considered to be a work of the master from Cos, is deemed "Hippocratic" since it meets the quality criteria attributed to the "Hippocratic school". W.H.S. Jones, editor of Hippocratic texts, among them the Hippocratic Oath and its variants, admitted in 1923 that the Oath does not always correspond to other texts in the *Corpus* but then he continued:

> So some [Greek] physicians did not feel bound by all the clauses, and some may not have felt bound by any. We may suppose, however, that no respectable physician would act contrary to most of the Oath, even if he were ignorant of its existence.[35]

The classical philologist, Hans Diller (1905-1977), one of the most influential research scholars of the *Hippocratic Corpus* and for the most part a supporter of the "traditional" theory, emphasized that "the greatest ability of the Greek classical age, could be seen at work in this document, namely to draw appropiate conclusions from a problem".[36]

Karl Deichgräber, whose research on Hippocratic medicine has been mentioned above, was a "conservative" opponent of his contemporary "iconoclast" Ludwig Edelstein. Deichgräber, too, did not believe that the historical Hippocrates had written the Oath.[37] But he did assume that the "so beautiful and authoritative document" was written around 400 B.C. (i.e. in Hippocrates' lifetime). Like Diller, Deichgräber maintained that the Oath "survived due to its greatness, in other words thanks to its relative distance to reality".[38] The Oath appears thus to be "genuinely Hippocratic" in a higher sense of the term.[39] If Hippocrates did not compose it himself, then the Oath at the very least is held to reflect Hippocratic ideas as they are known to us in the earliest and best texts of the *Corpus*.

So when was the Oath actually written, and where is it cited in antiquity?[40] One would expect such a key text of Hippocratic thought to be mentioned frequently in antiquity. This is not the case. Although the Oath does correspond with - or at least does not contradict - the ethical rules inherent to the *Hippocratic Corpus*, not a single text in the Corpus refers to it. This is also true for the so-called "deontological" texts of the *Corpus* that deal with ethical aspects of medical praxis, such as "On the Art", "The Law", "On Ancient Medicine", "On the Doctor", as well as the later texts "Decorum", and "Guidelines".[41] These texts, written by various "Hippocratic" authors (and hence anonymous), all of which most likely originated in the 4th century B.C., except for the last two (1st/2nd century A.D.), deal with basic ethical problems in medicine: the doctor's personal conduct, the distinction between "true" and "false" doctors, the behavior of doctors toward patients, including the question of the fee. In all these deontological texts, there are no direct parallels to the Hippocratic Oath. It seems as if this text was not known to the followers and collegues of Hippocrates or in Greek antiquity in general. There is, in addition, no direct tradition of the text going back to Hippocrates' time. Indeed, the Oath is rarely cited or mentioned in literature from later antiquity, too.

A *terminus ante quem* is certain: the Oath was written *before* the 1st century A.D. since it was first mentioned at this time by Erotianus, who counted it among the "genuinely Hippocratic" writings.[42] Additonally the Oath is mentioned by Scribonius Largus, the personal physician of the Roman emperor Claudius (41-54 A.D.).[43] Soranus of Ephesus, who was active in Rome at the end of the 1st century A.D., paraphrases a passage from the Hippocratic Oath in his gynecological writings: Hippocrates says, "I will not give an abortivum to anyone".[44] Soranus' Greek wording admittedly differs from the Greek text of the Oath in this passage. The so-called "ban on abortion" of the Hippocratic Oath is difficult to grasp in terms of its literal meaning. It was later, in the European tradition beginning from Christian middle ages, understood as a *general* ban on abortion, but we cannot be certain whether the text of the Oath originally intended a *partial* ban, i.e. a special form of application by pessary.[45]

An inscription encarved at the beginning of the 3rd century A.D. in the Asclepieum at Athens contains a poem by the stoic philosopher Sarapion (approx. 100 A.D.) in which an "Oath" is mentioned under the title "Duties of the Physician"; presumably, the Hippocratic Oath is meant.[46] In Galen's extant Greek writings (2nd century A.D.), which often reflect the idealized portrait of Hippocrates, oddly enough no reference is made to the Hippocratic Oath (nor to any of the other deontological texts).[47] None of the writers of antiquity who have dealt with Galen's writings mentioned him having written anything about the Oath. However, in medieval Arabic texts, a commentary on the Hippocratic Oath is attributed to Galen. Hunain Ibn Ishaq (808-873), an Arab Christian physician and philologist active in Bagdad, was the first to mention this commentary, which he translated from Greek into Syrian.[48] The text has survived in fragments in the form of quotations by later Arab writers. And it is interesting that the quite detailed fragments do not focus on the ethical rules of the Oath, but rather on questions of the (mythical) origin of medicine, Asclepius and his iconography.[49] Even if this commentary on the Oath is to be attributed to Galen, it contains medico-historical, not ethical discussions - at least in the parts that have survived.

In late Christian antiquity, the Hippocratic Oath is mentioned sporadically. Saint Jerome (approx. 340- 420 A.D.), author of the Vulgate, mentions in a letter at the end of the 4th century the Oath that Hippocrates had beginning students swear to. It is, however, not clear whether Jerome is talking about the training of doctors in his lifetime. His Greek contemporary Saint Gregory of Nyssa (approx. 328-390 A.D.) praises his brother, the doctor Caesarius, who, perhaps due to the Christian ban on oaths, did not swear the Hippocratic Oath.[50]

Back to Hippocrates

The Hippocratic Oath only attained its influence in Christian (and Islamic) times. Text variations in the manuscripts show that the Hippocratic Oath was not only handed down, but also adapted in the Middle Ages. There are e.g. Byzantine manuscripts of the Oath, beginning with invocations altered to suit the Christian audience (similiar phenomena can be seen in an Islamic context). Two Greek manuscripts (Vatican, *Urbinas graec.* 64 and Milan, *Ambrosianus* B 113 sup.) present the text of the Oath with its Christian modifications and written in the form of a cross to show graphically that Hippocratic and Christian ethics were congruent. In Latin translations of the Oath, there were characteristic changes, e.g. concerning the so-called "ban on abortion", which was definitively understood by Christians as a general ban. Renaissance medicine took a growing interest in the text of the Oath, which was primarily read in Latin and adopted for new purposes.[51] The relevant passage of the "ban on abortion" was "unambiguously" translated into Latin with the various means of abortion named. In early modern times, the Oath also served professional, academically trained doctors as a means of separating themselves from non-academic healers of all kinds.

Sections of the Oath are to be found in graduation oaths and faculty statues of medical schools from the past few centuries. Here, the Hippocratic Oath, or sections of it, were sworn for the first time in history

(Wittenberg 1508, Basel 1570).[52] The complete text of the Hippocratic Oath was first recited by medical school graduates in the (post-revolutionary) year 1804 at Montpellier.[53] Other universities, especially in the United States, followed the example and introduced a "Hippocratic" oath for their graduates. In the second half of the 19th century, the interest in Hippocrates diminished among the doctors, who were now oriented towards the natural sciences. After the initial optimism of progress, fostered by new technology and possibilities of development, was disappointed in the early 20th century, the ideal of Hippocrates reappeared on the horizon. In the notorious "crisis of medicine" after the First World War, the adjective "Hippocratic" became attractive and various branches of medicine were eager to label their activities with it. In 1928, the journal "Hippokrates" was first published by the publishing house at Stuttgart, bearing the same name as the journal.[54] This fashionable "Hippocratism" united "biological", "holistic", and "natural" attempts by such diverging characters as Georg Honigmann, Erwin Liek and Henry E. Sigerist.[55] Since 1931, the medical dissertation (!) of the French doctor Gaston Baissette, entitled "Hippocrate", became popular in the whole of Europe. This book presumably covered the life and work of the "real" Hippocrates, but in fact it was a kitschy doctor's novel.[56] The label "Hippocratic" had no specific meaning for these doctors proclaiming a new "Hippocratism"; for them "hippocratic" meant finally something good and genuine, in other words exactly what apparently seemed characterize their own concept of medicine. Dissatisfied with the present these outsiders looked into the past to find some authority for their (often modest) new approaches. This "Hippocratic" direction in medicine proved, however, very quickly to lack content.

The only thing remaining of Hippocrates' myth in German medicine after 1933 was the Oath. Franz Büchner (1895-1991), pathologist at Freiburg, used it as an argument against the killing of the ill and disabled ("Nazi euthanasia") when he held an open lecture on 18 November 1941 at the University of Freiburg entitled "The Oath of Hippocrates".[57] As courageous as Büchner's open resistance to the regime was, his argument was anachronistic: it was not the Hippocratic Oath which outlawed the killing of mentally ill in Germany, but the the *Reichsstrafgesetzbuch* (penal code of the Reich). Non-medical opponents to the "euthanasia", e.g. Clemens August Graf von Galen, cardinal at Münster, referred in public (August 1941) to the penal code to oppose the "euthanasia".[58]

The Hippocratic Oath was a problematic argument against the ethical crimes of the Nazi. The Oath could even be used, one would say *mis*used, to justify the atrocities. This was the case, as we have seen, in the Nuremberg trials when Karl Barndt claimed that the Nazi "euthanasia" had been an actual adaptation of Hippocratic ethics.

Considering the problematic meaning of the word "Hippocratic" for modern medicine, it is all the more surprising that the World Medical Association in 1948 referred to the Hippocratic tradition in content and form.

The myth of Hippocrates has ever been substantial for shaping the (self-) image of physicians. The (usually modernized) "Hippocratic" Oaths sworn at many American universities today belong in this category. The "return" back to Hippocrates as a point of orientation comes at a time when bioethics has obscured the traditional forms of "medical ethics" and the absolute points of orientation are lost in a pluralism of values.[59]

The Invention of Hippocrates

The fact that the Hippocratic Oath, presumed to be the key document of medical ethics in antiquity, was unknown to Greek physicians of the classical age and cited only rarely in later antiquity, suggests that the Oath was less important and influential than is assumed today. And yet, this "sceptical" conclusion does not harmonize with an idealized portrait of Hippocrates. How could we accept that the Hippocratic Oath, re-shaped in the Declaration of Geneva, should rule modern medicine, if it did not govern ancient Hippocratic medicine? The aforementioned "sceptic," Ludwig Edelstein, in 1943 suggested a theory, fundamentally opposed to the "traditional" view.[60]

Table 1 Hippocratic Oath, Translation by Ludwig Edelstein, 1943

I swear by Apollo Physician and Asclepius and Hygieia and Panaceia and all the gods and goddesses, making them my witnesses, that I will fulfil according to my ability and judgement this oath and this covenant.

To hold him who has taught me this art as equal to my parents and to live my life in partnership with him, and if he is in need of money to give him a share of mine, and to regard his offspring as equal to my brothers in male lineage and to teach them this art - if they desire to learn it - without fee and covenant; to give a share of precepts and oral instruction and all the other learning to my sons and to the sons of him who has instructed me and to pupils who have signed the covenant and have taken the oath according to the medical law, but to no one else.

I will apply dietetic measures for the benefit of the sick according to my ability and judgement; I will keep them from harm and injustice.

I will never give a deadly drug to anybody if asked for it, nor will I make a suggestion to this effect. Similarly I will not give to a woman an abortive remedy. In purity and holiness I will guard my life and my art.

I will not use the knife, not even on sufferers from stone, but will withdraw in favor of such men as are engaged in this work.

Whatever houses I may visit, I will come for the benefit of the sick, remaining free of all intentional injustice, of all mischief and in particular of sexual relations with both female and male persons, be they free or slaves.

What I may see or hear in the course of the treatment or even outside of the treatment in regard to the life of men, which on no account one must spread abroad, I will keep to myself holding such things shameful to be spoken about.

If I fulfil this oath and do not violate it, may it be granted to me to enjoy life and art, being honored with fame among all men for all time to come; if I transgress it and swear falsely, may the opposite of all this be my lot.

Note: Guided by his theory that the Oath should reflect Pythagorean philosophy, Edelstein translated, i.e. interpreted, the Greek text in terms of an absolute prohibition of surgery and of abortion.

Edelstein analyzed some - even today - puzzling passages of the text, such as the so-called "ban on surgery" and concluded that the Oath had been formulated in the 4ᵗʰ century B.C. as an esoteric oath of a small *Pythagorean* group of doctors. According to Edelstein, it could be helpful for scholars of Hippocratic medicine to understand the Hippocratic Oath in its context, by realizing "that the Hippocratic Oath is a Pythagorean manifesto and not the expression of an absolute standard of medical conduct".[61]

At the beginning of the 1930s Edelstein had solved the problem of the "genuine" works of Hippocrates by arguing that no "genuine" works can be identified at all. Now, in 1943, he tore down another pillar of Hippocrates' idealized image. According to Edelstein, the Hippocratic Oath was not a document expressing timeless values for doctors of all epochs, but a enigmatic text, specific for a certain time and bound to a certain esoteric philosophy - Pythagoreism. Admittedly, a secret Pythagorean doctor's oath does not go well with an idealized, timeless image. Looking back, Edelstein remarked with some bitter humor that already with his initial works on the "genuine" works of Hippocrates he "shaved off Hippocrates' beard".[62] His scepticism did not make him any friends among his German colleagues, as had become clear. Shortly after his first publications which created a lot of dispute, although on a scientific level, Edelstein as a jew was forced to emigrate and took with him his "sceptical" theory about Hippocrates. His views, transplanted to the USA, were lost for German medical history. Edelstein published his translation and commentary of the Hippocratic Oath in English in 1943; it was only taken note of 20 years later in Germany and, at any rate, was rejected. Today, Edelstein's view is nearly accepted as the norm in American publications, while it is still considered an exotic in Germany.[63]

It should be emphasized that Edelstein's theory of the Pythagorean character of the Oath is only a hypothesis that on the one hand plausibly solves many problems - e.g. origin, date, and dissemination of the Oath; on the other hand, the Pythagorean character remains highly speculative. Edelstein's theory therefore is now in a defensive position,[64] and new translations and commentaries on the Hippocratic Oath have definitely turned away from assuming Pythagorean influence. The Oath is now being interpreted in the historical context of the *Hippocratic Corpus* (see e.g. von Stadens translation in Table 2).

Table 2 Hippocratic Oath, Translation by Heinrich von Staden, 1996

I swear by Apollo the Physician and by Asclepius and by Health and Panacea and by all the gods as well as goddesses, making them judges [witnesses], to bring the following oath and written covenant to fulfillment, in accordance with my power and my judgement; to regard him who has taught me this techne as equal to my parents, and to share, in partnership, my livelihood with him and to give him a share when he is in need of necessities, and to judge the offspring [coming] from him equal to [my] male siblings, and to teach them this techne, should they desire to learn [it], without fee and written covenant, and to give a share both of rules and of lectures, and of all the rest of learning, to my sons and to the [sons] of him who has taught me and to the pupils who have both made a written contract and sworn by a medical convention but by no other.

And I will use regiments for the benefit of the ill in accordance with my ability and my judgement, but from [what is] to their harm or injustice I will keep [them].

And I will not give a drug that is deadly to anyone if asked [for it], nor will I suggest the way to such a counsel. And likewise I will not give a woman a destructive pessary.

And in a pure and holy way I will guard my life and my techne.

I will not cut, and certainly not those suffering from stone, but I will cede [this] to men [who are] practitioners of this activity.

And as many houses as I may enter, I will go for the benefit of the ill, while being far from all voluntary and destructive injustice, especially from sexual acts both upon women's bodies and upon men's, both of the free and of the slaves.

And about whatever I may see or hear in treatment, or even without treatment, in the life of human beings - things that should not ever be blurted out outside - I will remain silent, holding such things to be unutterable [sacred, not to be divulged].

If I render this oath fulfilled, and if I do not blur and confound it [making it to no effect], may it be [granted] to me to enjoy the benefits both of life and of techne, being held in good repute among all human beings for time eternal. If, however, I transgress and perjure myself, the opposite of these.

Note: According to von Staden, the Oath is not an esoteric document alien to the other Hippocratic tracts; thus, von Staden, without suggesting a new dating of the Oath, interpretes it in the context of the Hippocratic Corpus.

Still convincing in Edelstein's theory is, however, his conviction that he does not accept the timelessness of medical ethics. Edelstein demands that the Hippocratic Oath, instead of being the fundamental document of medical ethics, has to be seen as a myth and a backward projection into history of contemporary desires. Thus it is justified to speak, in terms of the history of interpretations of the Hippocratic Oath, of a "post-Edelstein" era.[65]

Edelstein's view challenges us to understand and analyze the long history of the Oath and its influence on medical ethics, from the Middle Ages to modern times, as the history of the reception of an ambiguous text. Hippocrates and the surviving treatises bearing his name thus become the object of historical study. Demands to "go back to Hippocrates", as are commonly heard among doctors, turn out to be instrumentalized historical myths.

Notes

1   Text in the *Encyclopedia of Bioethics*, Vol V, p. 2646f.; see references for the abbreviations used in the notes.

2   Mitscherlich/Mielke: *Medizin ohne Menschlichkeit*; Annas/Grodin: *The Nazi Doctors and the Nuremberg Code.*

3   Annas/Grodin: *The Nazi Doctors and the Nuremberg Code*, p. 87; cf. Leven: *Der Hippokratische Eid im 20. Jahrhundert.*

4   Mitscherlich/Mielke: *Medizin ohne Menschlichkeit* 1960, p. 47 (= ed. 1995, p. 63).

5   Leven: *Hippokrates im 20. Jahrhundert*, p. 78.

6   Mitscherlich/Mielke, 1960, p. 47f. (= ed. 1995, p. 63f).

7   Annas/Grodin: *The Nazi Doctors and the Nuremberg Code*, pp. 121-144.

8   Leven: *Hippokrates im 20. Jahrhundert*, p. 84.

9   Rütten: *Hippokrates im Gespräch*, p. 51f.

10   Smith: *The Hippocratic Tradition*, p. 199.

11   Von Staden: *Herophilus* p. 427f.

12   Littré, É. (ed.): *Œuvres complètes d'Hippocrate*. Traduction nouvelle avec le texte Grec en regard,10 Vols, Paris 1839-1861 (repr. Amsterdam 1973-1982).

13   Smith: *The Hippocratic Tradition*, p. 175; Lloyd: *Galen on Hellenistics and Hippocrateans*, p 416.

14   Deichgräber: *Die Epidemien und das Corpus Hippocraticum.*

15   Hölbl: *Geschichte des Ptolemäerreiches*, p. 20, p. 26.

16   Galen: In *Hipp. Epid. III* comment II 4 (ed. E. Wenkebach, CMG V, 10. 2. 1), Leipzig, Berlin 1936, p. 79, lines 8-15).; cf. Blank, H.: *Das Buch in der Antike*, München 1992, p. 139.

17   Nutton: *Healers in the Medical Market Place*, p. 31; Smith: *The Hippocratic Tradition*, p. 201, adds: "That modern scholarly myth can be ignored because it would be in the sources if it had any basis at all".

18   Grensemann: *Polybos*, p. 57.

19   *Presbeutikos* (ed. Littré, Vol. IX, p. 420, 2 = ed./transl. Smith, W.D.: *Hippocrates. Pseudepigraphic Writings* (=Studies in Ancient Medicine, 2), Leiden, New York 1990, p. 118.

20   Galen: In *Hipp. Nat. Hom. comment., Prooemium* (ed. J. Mewaldt, CMG V 9, 1), Leipzig, Berlin 1914, p. 7-11); cf. Jouanna, J. (ed./transl.): *Hippocrate. La nature de l'homme* (CMG I 1, 3), Berlin 1975, Introduction, p. 19-22, 55-59.

21 Galen: In *Hipp. Nat. Hom.* comment., Prooemium (ed. J. Mewaldt, CMG V 9, 1), Leipzig Berlin 1914, p. 8, line 30f.

22 Edelstein, RE-*Hippokrates*, col. 1328.

23 Jouanna: *Hippocrate*, p 85, gives the amusingly appropriate heading "Des écrits en quête d'auteur" to chapter IV of his book.

24 Smith: *The Hippocratic Tradition*, pp. 31-44.

25 Hippocrates. *Pseudepigraphic Writings* (ed./transl. Smith); Pinault: *Hippocratic Lives and Legends*.

26 Edelstein, RE-*Hippocrates*, col. 1328; cp. Smith: *The Hippocratic Tradition*, p. 43.

27 Mentioned in the index of Aristotle's writings by Diogenes Laertius, V 25, cp. Aristotle: *Problemata Physica*. Translated and annotated by H. Flashar (= Aristoteles. Werke in deutscher Übersetzung, Bd. 19), Berlin 4th ed., 1991, p. 318; Text: Diels, H. (ed.): *Anonymi Londinensis ex Aristotelis Iatricis Menoniis et aliis medicis ecologae* (= Supplementum Aristotelicum, Vol. III 1), Berlin 1893, here pp. 8-12 (= cols. V 35-VII 40); reprinted in Gigon, O. (ed.): *Aristotelis opera*, Vol. III, Berlin, New York 1987, pp. 511-521, here p. 513.

28 Smith: *The Hippocratic Tradition*, p. 37.

29 Diels: *Ueber die Excerpte von Menons Iatrika*, p. 424.

30 Rütten: *Die Herausbildung der ärztlichen Ethik*, pp. 57-66.

31 Rütten: *Hippocrates im Gespräch*, p. 51.

32 Rütten: *Hippocrates im Gespräch*, p. 52.

33 For a recent example cf. Kytzler: Reclams *Lexikon der griechischen und römischen Autoren*, pp. 158-160; Rütten: *Hippokrates im Gespräch*, p. 53, comments on this circular logic (transl.): "Hippocrates explains the Oath, and the Oath explains Hippocrates".

34 One exception is Lichtenthaeler: *Der Eid des Hippokrates*, who claims to have proved that Hippocrates is not only the author of the best writings of the *Corpus*, but also, "with cumulating evidence", the author of the Oath (p. 323).

35 Jones, W.H.S. (ed./transl.): *Hippocrates*. Vol. I, Cambridge/Mass., London 1923, p. 296.

36 Diller, H. (ed.): *Hippokrates*. Schriften, p. 7.

37 Deichgräber: *Der hippokratische Eid*, p. 13, p. 23.

38 Deichgräber: *Der hippokratische Eid*, p. 30.

39 See also Flashar: *Griechische Welt*, p. 355 (translated): "Whether the famous Oath is really written by Hippocrates (born 460 B.C.) or not is uncertain. But it does reflect the ethos of the schol at Kos impressively".

40 Rütten: *Receptions of the Hippocratic Oath*, p. 467.

41 Edelstein: *The Professional Ethics of the Greek Physician*; Gourevitch: *Le triangle hippocratique*, pp. 251-288; Nutton: *Beyond the Hippocratic Oath*; von Staden: *Personal and Professional Conduct in the Hippocratic Oath?*, pp. 404-437.

42 *Erotiani vocum Hippocraticarum collectio cum fragmentis*, E. Nachmanson (ed.) (= Collectio Scriptorum Veterum Upsaliensis), Göteborg 1918, p. 9, p. 19.

43 *Scribonius Largus: Compositiones*, Prooimion, G. Helmreich (ed.), Leipzig 1887, p. 2; cp. Temkin: *Hippocrates in a World of Pagans and Christians*, p. 21; it is unclear whether the earliest direct mention of a "Hippocratic Oath" attributed to Cato the Elder (234-149 B.C.) by Plutarch (Life of Cato the Elder, chap. 23, 3) refers to this Oath.

44 *Sorani Gynaeciorum libri* IV (ed. J. Ilberg, CMG, IV), Leipzig, Berlin 1927, here I 19, 60, 2 (p. 45, 9f.).

45 von Staden: *Personal and Professional Conduct in the Hippocratic Oath?*, p. 407, translates this passage: "I will not give a woman a destructive pessary"; Lichtenthaeler: *Der Eid des Hippokrates*, translates: "Ich werde keiner Frau ein keimvernichtendes Vaginalzäpfchen verabreichen"; on the "ban on abortion" in the Oath and its difficult meaning cp. Rütten: Receptions of the Hippocratic Oath; and Rütten: *Medizinethische Themen in den deontologischen Schriften*, pp. 91-98.

46 Oliver: *An Ancient Poem of the Duties of a Physician*, p. 315-323; Gourevitch: *Le triangle Hippocratique*, pp. 278-280; Temkin: *Hippocrates in a World of Pagans and Christians*, p. 72.

47 Nutton: *Beyond the Hippocratic Oath*, pp. 19-21; Galen set forth his ideal of the good doctor in a commentary on a passage in the Hippocratic treatise *Epidemics* (VI 4,7), cp. Deichgräber: Medicus gratiosus.

48 Rosenthal: *An Ancient Commentary on the Hippocratic Oath*, p. 53f.

49 Rosenthal: *An Ancient Commentary on the Hippocratic Oath*, pp. 54-81.

50 Hieronymus: *Epistula* 52, 15 (Select Letters of St. Jerome, ed. with an English Translation by F.A. Wright, Cambridge/Mass., London 1933, p. 224); Gregorius of Nazianzus, Oratio VII, Funebra in laudem Caesarii fratris, ed. J.P. Migne, Patrologia Graeca, Vol. 35, col. 767 A; cf. Temkin: *Hippocrates in a World of Pagans and Christians*, p. 182.

51 Rütten: *Die Herausbildung der ärztlichen Ethik*, p. 65; Rütten: *Receptions of the Hippocratic Oath*, p. 469f.; Nutton: *Beyond the Hippocratic Oath*.

52 Nutton: *What's in an Oath?*, p. 521.

53 Nutton: *What's in an Oath?*, p. 522.

54 On the "crisis of medicine" in the 1920s and on Georg Honigmann, the founding editor of the journal *Hippokrates* cf. Wiesing: *Die Persönlichkeit des Arztes*, pp. 185-188; pp. 194-199; the journal *Hippokrates* was edited until 1978.

55 Bothe: *Neue deutsche Heilkunde*.

56 Wiesing: *Die Persönlichkeit des Arztes*, p. 203; Liek and Sigerist went separate ways at the very latest on this issue.

57 Büchner: *Der Eid des Hippokrates*. Wortlaut, pp. 131-151; cf. Leven: *Hippokrates im 20. Jahrhundert*, pp. 65-74.

58 Leven: *Der Hippokratische Eid im 20. Jahrhundert*, p. 123.

59 Nutton: *Beyond the Hippocratic Oath*; Nutton: *What's in an Oath*, p. 522.

60 Edelstein: *The Hippocratic Oath*.

61 Edelstein: *The Hippocratic Oath*, reprint in: Edelstein: *Ancient Medicine*, p. 63.

62 Temkin: Introduction to Edelstein: *Ancient Medicine*, p. vii.

63 For instance, Edelstein's translation of the Hippocratic Oath is the only one cited in the *Encyclopedia of Bioethics* (Vol. V, p. 2632), without mentioning his name, as if Edelstein's translation were the only possible or "correct" one.

64 Flashar: *Ethik und Medizin – Moderne Probleme und alte Wurzeln*, p. 3; Rütten: *Medizinethische Themen in den deontologischen Schriften*, p. 69.

65 Rütten: *Medizinethische Themen in den deontologischen Schriften*, p. 68, has coined the expression "nachedelsteinsche Ära".

References

Annas, G.J., Grodin, M.A. (1992), *The Nazi Doctors and the Nuremberg Code. Human Rights in Human Experimentation.* New York, Oxford University Press.

Bachmann, M. (1952), *Die Nachwirkungen des hippokratischen Eides. Ein Beitrag zur Geschichte der ärztlichen Ethik,* Med. Diss. Mainz, Würzburg.

Baissette, G. (1931), *Hippocrate.* Paris [German transl.: *Leben und Lehre des Hippokrates.* Stuttgart 1932].

Bothe, D. (1991), *Neue Deutsche Heilkunde 1933-1945. Dargestellt anhand der Zeitschrift "Hippokrates" und der Entwicklung der volksheilkundlichen Laienbewegung* (= Abhandlungen zur Geschichte der Medizin und der Naturwissenschaften, 62). Husum.

Büchner, F. (1985), *Der Eid des Hippokrates.* Wortlaut des am 18. November 1941 in der Aula der Universität Freiburg gehaltenen öffentlichen Vortrages, in: Büchner, F., *Der Mensch in der Sicht moderner Medizin.* Freiburg, Basel, Wien, pp. 131-151.

Deichgräber, K. (1933), '*Die Epidemien und das Corpus Hippocraticum. Voruntersuchungen zu einer Geschichte der Koischen Ärzteschule*'. Abhandlungen der Preußischen Akademie der Wissenschaften, *Phil.-Hist. Klasse* Nr. 3, Berlin (Augmented repr. Berlin, New York 1971).

Deichgräber, K. (1970), *Medicus gratiosus. Untersuchungen zu einem griechischen Arztbild.* Mit dem Anhang "Testamentum Hippocratis" und Rhazes' "De indulgentia medici," Abhandlungen der Akademie der Wissenschaften und der Literatur, Mainz, Geistes- u. sozial- wissenschaftliche Klasse, Nr. 3.

Deichgräber, K. (1955), *Der Hippokratische Eid,* Stuttgart.

Diels, H. (1893), *Ueber die Excerpte von Menons Iatrika in dem Londoner Papyrus 137. Hermes* 28, pp. 407-434.

Diller, H. (ed.) (1962), *Hippokrates. Schriften. Die Anfänge der abendländischen Medizin.* Reinbek bei Hamburg, reprinted with bibliographical supplement by K.-H. Leven, Stuttgart 1994.

Edelstein, L. (1956), 'The Professional Ethics of the Greek Physician', *Bulletin of the History of Medicine* 30, pp. 391-419, reprinted in: Edelstein, L.: *Ancient Medicine,* pp. 319-348.

Edelstein, L. (1931), *Peri aeron und die Sammlung der hippokratischen Schriften* (= Problemata, 4), Berlin.

Edelstein, L. (1935), 'Hippokrates' in: Pauly's *Realencyclopädie der classischen Altertumswissenschaft,* Supplement VI, Stuttgart, cols. 1290- 1345.

Edelstein, L. (1967), *Ancient Medicine.* Selected Papers of Ludwig Edelstein, edited by O. and C.L. Temkin. Baltimore.

Edelstein, L. (1939), 'The Genuine Works of Hippocrates', *Bulletin of the History of Medicine* 7, pp. 236-248; reprinted in Edelstein, L.: Ancient Medicine. Selected Papers, pp. 133-144.

Edelstein, L. (1943), 'The Hippocratic Oath. Text, Translation and Interpretation', *Supplements to the Bulletin of the History of Medicine,* No. 1, Baltimore [German translation ed. by H. Diller, Zürich, Stuttgart 1969].

Encyclopedia of Bioethics. Revised Edition, ed. by W.T. Reich (1995), Vol. 1-5, New York, London.

Flashar, H. (ed.) (1997), *Griechische Welt,* Frankfurt/M.

Flashar, H. (1997), 'Ethik und Medizin - Moderne Probleme und alte Wurzeln' in: *Médicine et morale dans l'Antiquité, Entretiens sur l'Antiquité Classique,* 43, Fondations Hardt, Geneva, pp. 1-29.

Gourevitch, D. (1984), *Le triangle hippocratique dans le monde gréco-romain - le malade, sa maladie et son médecin.* Paris, Rom.

Grensemann, H. (1968), *Der Arzt Polybos als Verfasser hippokratischer Schriften,* Abh. Akad. Wiss. Lit. Mainz, geistes- u. sozialwiss. Kl., Jg. 1968, Nr. 2.

Hölbl, G. (1994), *Geschichte des Ptolemäerreiches,* Darmstadt.

Jones, W.H.S. (1924), *The Doctor's Oath. An Essay in the History of Medicine,* Cambridge.

Jouanna, J. (1992), *Hippocrate,* Paris.

Kollesch, J., Harig, G. (1978), 'Der hippokratische Eid. Zur Entstehung der antiken medizinischen Deontologie', *Philologus* 122, pp. 157- 176.

Kollesch, J., Nickel, D. (Eds.) (1994), *Antike Heilkunst,* Stuttgart.

Kudlien, F. (1978), 'Zwei Interpretationen zum Hippokratischen Eid', *Gesnerus* 35, pp. 253-263.

Kytzler, B. (1997), *Reclams Lexikon der griechischen und römischen Autoren,* Stuttgart.

Leven, K.-H. (1994), *Hippokrates im 20. Jahrhundert: Ärztliches Selbstbild, Idealbild und Zerrbild* in: Leven, K.-H./Prüll, C.-R. (Hg): *Selbstbilder des Arztes im 20. Jahrhundert. Medizinhistorische und medizinethische Aspekte* (= Freiburger Forschungen zur Medizingeschichte, N.F., 16), Freiburg, pp. 39-96.

Leven, K.-H. (1997), *Der Hippokratische Eid im 20. Jahrhundert* in: Toellner, R., Wiesing, U. (Eds.): *Geschichte und Ethik in der Medizin. Von den Schwierigkeiten einer Kooperation* (= Jahrbuch Medizinethik, 10), Stuttgart, Jena, pp. 111-129.

Lichtenthaeler, Ch. (1984), *Der Eid des Hippokrates. Ursprung und Bedeutung* (=XII. hippokratische Studie), Köln.

Lloyd, G.E.R. (1975), 'The Hippocratic Question', *Classical Quarterly n.s.* 25 , pp. 171-192; reprinted with an "Introduction" (1991) in: Lloyd, G.E.R.: 'Methods and Problems in Greek Science'. *Selected Papers,* Cambridge 1991, pp. 194-223.

Lloyd, G.E.R. (1991), *Galen on Hellenistics and Hippocrateans. Contemporary Battles and Past Authorities* in: Lloyd, G.E.R.: *Methods and Problems in Greek Science. Selected Papers,* Cambridge, pp. 398-416.

Mitscherlich, A., Mielke, F. (1960), *Medizin ohne Menschlichkeit.* Dokumente des Nürnberger Ärzteprozesses, Frankfurt/M., revised edition 1995.

Nutton, V. (1992), 'Healers in the Medical Market Place. Towards a Social History of Graeco-Roman Medicine' in: Wear, A. (ed.): *Medicine in Society. Historical Essays,* Cambridge, New York, pp. 15-58.

Nutton, V. (1993), 'Beyond the Hippocratic Oath' in: A. Wear and J. Geyer- Kordesch/R. French (Eds.): *Doctors and Ethics. The Earlier Historical Setting of Professional Ethics, Clio Medica* 24, pp. 10-37.

Nutton, V. (1995), 'What's in an Oath?' College Lecture, *Journal of the Royal College of Physicians of London* 29, pp. 518-524.

Oliver, J.H. (1939), 'An Ancient Poem of the Duties of a Physician', *Bulletin of the History of Medicine* 7, pp. 315-323.

Pinault, J.R. (1992), *Hippocratic Lives and Legends,* Leiden, New York.

Rosenthal, F. (1956), 'An Ancient Commentary on the Hippocratic Oath'. *Bulletin of the History of Medicine* 30, pp. 52-87.

Rütten, Th. (1993), *Hippokrates im Gespräch.* Katalog der Ausstellung des Instituts für Theorie und Geschichte der Medizin und der Universitäts- und Landesbibliothek Münster, 10. Dez. 1993 - 8. Jan. 1994 (= Schriften der Universitäts- und Landesbibliothek Münster, 9), Münster.

Rütten, Th. (1996), 'Die Herausbildung der ärztlichen Ethik. Der Eid des Hippokrates' in: Schott, H. (ed.): *Meilensteine der Medizin,* Dortmund, pp. 57-66.

Rütten, Th. (1996), 'Receptions of the Hippocratic Oath in the Renaissance. The Prohibition of Abortion as a Case Study in Reception', *Journal of the History of Medicine* 51, pp. 456-483.

Rütten, Th. (1997), 'Medizinethische Themen in den deontologischen Schriften des Corpus Hippocraticum' in: *Médicine et morale dans l'Antiquité, Entretiens sur l'Antiquité Classique*, 43, Fondations Hardt, Genf, pp. 65-120.

Smith, W. D. (1979), *The Hippocratic Tradition*, Ithaca, London.

Staden, H. von (1989), *Herophilus. The Art of Medicine in Early Alexandria*. Edition, Translation and Essays, Cambridge.

Staden, H. von (1996), 'In a pure and holy way. Personal and Professional Conduct in the Hippocratic Oath?' *Journal of the History of Medicine* 51, pp. 404-437.

Temkin, O. (1991), *Hippocrates in a World of Pagans and Christians*, Baltimore, London.

Triebel-Schubert, Ch. (1985), 'Bemerkungen zum Hippokratischen Eid', *Medizinhistorisches Journal* 20, pp. 253-260.

Veatch, R.M. (1995), 'Medical Codes and Oaths. I. History. II. Ethical Analysis' in: *Encyclopedia of Bioethics*. Revised Edition, ed. by W.T. Reich, Vol. 3, New York, London, pp. 1419-1427; 1427-1435.

Wiesing, U. (1996), 'Die Persönlichkeit des Arztes und das geschichtliche Selbstverständnis der Medizin. Zur Medizintheorie von Ernst Schweninger, Georg Honigmann und Erwin Liek'. *Medizinhistorisches Journal* 31, pp. 181-208.

2 Medical Science and Ethics before 1947

Anne-Marie Moulin

To characterize the medical profession at the crossroad of science, myths and medicine, before the Nuremberg Trials and the writing of the Nuremberg Code, is to become aware that progress of knowledge and sense of responsibility in the profession developed inequally during the course of history.

This does not mean that modern medical ethics is a complete innovation. The recently praised "increase in the popularity of ethics"[1] corresponds in fact more to a rediscovery than to an invention.[2] Michel Serres rightly grew angry at the neologism "bioethics": "Sometimes, novelties only originate from what we have forgotten. We are importing at great cost of translations an ethics fragmented in plastic pieces whereas our European tradition had carved the same one in granite and gold over more than two millennia".[3]

Medical practice since Antiquity has never been devoid of ethical concern. In the Middle-Ages,[4] a period often taxed with obscurantism, the corporate body of doctors carried on some supervision of practices and relied on consensus for the appreciation of what course of action was to be taken in response to which diagnosis. Municipalities gave an unequal but real support to those attempts at making the profession more sound, as in London,[5] for instance, where a sort of medical insurance intervened in cases of medical negligence or mistake. The official hierarchy of scientists entailed the obligation of consultation on serious cases and deontology was based on the adage *primum non nocere* and on respect for the patient.

The optical illusion caused by the so-called emergence of medical ethics after Nuremberg is explained by the fact that the sense of responsibility in the profession and the exercise of medical power started slowly but surely to break from one another from the last century onward. Thus, to restrict the history of medicine in the last hundred years comes down to misjudging the ancientness of a moral reflection and questioning which nevertheless greatly contributed to the shaping of today's medical identity and of its self-image.[6] The physicians who emphasize today the crisis in the trade may not be aware of the exceptional character of the last 100 years for their corporation.

The long century which began in the 1870s was marked by a paradox. In France as in most European countries, the medical profession underwent an unprecedented numerical development: limited to a few hundred of practitioners at the time of the Revolution, it numbered twenty thousand practitioners in 1890, to which 2500 health officers must be added. This development took place hand in hand with an increased visibility on the political scene. Under the Third Republic, the Chamber of Deputies was peopled with men of higher rank, among which doctors held an important place.[7] The alliance with laboratories sealed a firm belief in the ongoing development of medical knowledge.[8] Especially in France, pasteurism provided medicine with an official revolution often compared to the drastic changes in Galilean and Newtonian physics.

At the same time, what would later be called the medicalization of society was beginning to develop.[9] The intervention of doctors expanded to numerous areas. Schools[10] and factories received their mark, as shows the law on medical assistance passed in 1893. In courts, forensic scientists were called in to determine the cause of death, to measure the defendants' responsibility, to evaluate the psychological condition of the accused and to testify to extenuating circumstances. In his characterization of *fin de siècle* medicine, the historian of medicine Jacques Léonard used the striking phrase "medicine between power and knowledge",[11] and the end of the 19th century registered the *de facto* rise of the former as well as of the latter.

The paradox here is that the doctor, by his participation in the making of the laws and in a way his absorption in them and by his more and more frequent contact with magistrates as an expert, seemed at the same time to have taken refuge in an area shut off by the law where his responsibility could be judged only by his peers, and, in some way, only by himself.

The reason for this is partly to be looked for in the fact that medicine changed its status and became experimental with Claude Bernard. Yet, if this addition marked the coming, first a modest one as we know, of research laboratories, it also meant that clinical medicine acquired a heuristic significance to a point unknown before. The pasteurian Emile Sergent used in this respect the phrase "spontaneous experimentation".[12] On the one hand, general physiology, the science of the laws of the living that now instructed medical actions, established a continuity between clinical matters and laboratory experiences: the disease is nothing but a borderline case. On the other hand, for the generation listening to Claude Bernard, the pharmacological analysis of a particular poison which can turn to a remedy[13] must be made on the living in order to determine the modalities of application, which strengthened even more the continuity between laboratories and doctors' offices, between animal models and human guinea-pigs.[14] The opening of medicine to experimental procedures appeared as a condition for the lightning progress expected in France as in Germany after the works of Bernard and Du Bois-Reymond, Pasteur, Ehrlich and Koch, to name a few names only.

On the grounds of progress, real or anticipated, the doctor of the 19th century was not bound anymore to limit himself to a sort of recognized know-how. He liberated himself from the community framework of his profession and from prescribed actions. With his therapeutic audacities, he was now on the way to becoming a researcher. As Canguilhem says, the doctor "experiments, that is to say treats only in fear".[15] In other words, the ideal of experimental medicine in all the senses of the term became fact at the end of the 19th century, with the requirement to explore unbeaten tracks. What is today called "therapeutic contingency" was integrated into practical medicine. As Charles Nicolle said about the men of his generation in 1933, "any physician can claim a part in the discoveries by the chosen ones of his science. Does he not often participate with them by the tests he involves himself with?"[16]

This experimental change in general medicine makes even more striking a certain gap between medicine and law.

Medicine and Law

Two mental universes, different, but called to meet up with one another in many respects, confront each other here: law and medicine. In the 19th century, the body of medical law, especially in matters of legal responsibility, was still to be developed. In the Napoleonic Civil Code, there was neither reference to physicians nor to the human body, which was mentioned only in Articles 319 and 320 on involuntary injury under criminal law.[17] For this reason, one must follow the development of ideas more on the side of jurisprudence than that of legislation. For most doctors, so Dr. Double in his important report on the profession to the Academy of Medicine in 1829, this gap in the law did not reflect the legislators' negligence, but rather confirmed the "natural" irresponsibility of medicine, a conjectural art *par excellence*, with the practitioners' semi-competence being opposed to the complete incompetence of the non-practitioners, whether they be patients or magistrates.[18]

Here, the argument put forward is double. On the one hand, practitioners were supposed to be answerable only to themselves for their actions. On the other hand, the results of their professional actions could be really appreciated only by competent persons, that is to say by professional peers. Therefore, the Articles 1382 and 1383 in the Civil Code, which obliged any citizen to redress wrongs he or she had caused, would be applicable only after advice of a medical jury. Paradoxically, but only seemingly so, the extension of knowledge, or, to put it another way, of progress, reinforced the doctors' skepticism and their conviction that prevailing common rules for evaluating human behavior were not applicable. The "leitmotiv" of the medical defense was that the medical arts forbid any final rational judgement in the absence of empirical regularities which allow for the wording of a law. Education was considered as being there for providing training and broad knowledge, but not practical rules of behavior and decision-making.

Let us recall here that medical education under the *Ancien Régime* was extremely heterogeneous. Colleges provided introductory knowledge before the access to the Medical Faculties did. Parallel education was also given at the *Muséum d'Histoire Naturelle* and *Jardin du Roi*. The State had made repeated but unsuccessful attempts at reducing this diversity and at unifying testing procedures. The king had created the Royal Academy of Surgery in 1731 and the Royal Society of Medicine in 1776, responsible for the large scale epidemiological surveys so well-known to historians.[19] These institutions aimed at producing, coordinating and sanctioning medical knowledge without any distinction being made between practice and research as we understand it today. The area of public health had made its official appearance with the topics of epidemics, of supervision of thermal springs which had played such an important role since antiquity in pre-revolutionary France, of assistance to the needy poor and finally of control of "secret remedies".[20] On the other hand, the Royal Society showed no concern for the question of the therapists' responsibility.

At the time of the Revolution, the medical trade escaped for a short time any form of control until the Imperial takeover. Three Medical Faculties were then founded in 1803 and integrated into the University of Napoleon I in 1808. The control of the evolultion of knowledge and of medical practice rested in the first place with the Faculty and Academy of Sciences. The diploma in medicine entitled the holder to practice throughout all France. It represented a blank signature identifying a general competence more than a precise know-how (this vagueness still persisting today leads some officials to advocate a regular updating of knowledge marked by a reappraisal of diplomas). Against those advocating an early specialization, the general degree was maintained, and the old distinction between surgeons and physicians was not reestablished. This meant, at least in theory, that any practitioner could perform (and it is still true today any action of his trade and that only his conscience dictated to him to avoid performing operations he had not mastered, except in emergency cases, in which case Article 63 of the Civil Code on failure to come to the assistance of persons in danger applied.

The Restoration (1815-1830) wanted to mark the change. The King tactically separated the powers of the Faculty, filled with old revolutionaries who were in supreme control of medical practice, from those of an Academy directly dependent on royal authority for the nomination of its members and in charge of reflecting upon the development of knowledge. As in many other fields and beyond the break the French Revolution represented, the creation of the Academy of Medicine in 1820 by Louis XVIII marked a certain continuity in the state efforts to intervene in matters of public health.[21]

However, the Academy hardly functioned as a place for the articulation of medical truth. The genre the institution deployed was one of controversy.[22] Contradictory debates were the essence of the life of the Academy, a very lively one besides. Its constituent body seemed not to feel obliged to put an end to the divergences arising there. The isolated and individual character of therapeutic responsibility shone out in those discussions, comparable in advance to the researcher's freedom. Data accumulated in files without any consensus being elaborated. There were as many opinions as members of the Academy, as acknowledged by the surgeon Velpeau in 1853.

This controversial mood implicitly admitted the extremely volatile character of medical certainties, discouraging overall projects favored by the Ideologues at the beginning of the century. In medicine, there are indeed few great theoretical changes and so to say no scientific revolutions, contrary to the wishes of a Cabanis. The profession makes do with a mode of uncertain knowledge. Errors of yesterday are innovations of tomorrow. The variability of results discouraged efforts towards synthesis and left elbow room for practitioners guided only by the lights of their moral and intellectual consciousness:

> Practitioners are free in the cases addressed to them for treatment to accept or refuse the efforts made by those trying to enrich medical art with new procedures. They act at their own risks outside the intervention range of the Academy.[23]

Practitioners then considered themselves free to judge therapeutic innovations and to decide whether or not to use them,[24] as when, for instance, the use of anesthetics together with chloroform became quite a common practice.

The freedom to choose one's therapeutics and consequently to experiment personally with a treatment's efficiency was not only a response to the official uncertainty of the medical authorities, but also a celebrated medical value corresponding to the liberal ideas of the profession and its exaltation of the *honnête homme* in the classic cultural sense of the term. The emphasis put on the doctors' autonomy as a subject of moral values may correspond to what Robert Nye proposed calling an "honor code",[25] but can also be interpreted as a special case of the ideal of individual bourgeois freedom celebrated during the July Monarchy.

According to Georges Weisz, who studied in detail the Academy deliberations, a single debate stood out as an exception in which the venerable assembly spoke out unanimously, namely the question of syphilization.[26] It concerned the prophylactic inoculation with syphilis endorsed in France by Auzias-Turenne and a few German practitioners, but which was unanimously condemned. It is true that Auzias-Turenne had not merely set the example and tested the reality of his immunity by inoculating himself with syphilis, but he had also conceived a syphilis inoculation program for the whole population, or more precisely for the youth, based on the vaccinia model. Auzias-Turenne so followed the ways of a public health policy of prevention conducive to bodily restraint. The syphilization project went thus completely beyond the limits of common therapeutic experimentation and stood in the range of public health, calling as such for a concerted answer.

Freed from the yoke of the medieval guild and its conformism and sense of hierarchy, imbued with positivist thinking and a belief in the irresistible advance of knowledge, the doctors of the end of the 19th century stood so much alone in the face of the flow of knowledge that it seemingly depended only on them to perform practical experimentations. Consequently, the distance was narrow between clinical observation, therapeutic and even non-therapeutic experimentation which all seemed to go together. In his lectures on medical responsibility given in the evening of his career in the *Collège de France*, Nobel Prize recipient Charles Nicolle rightly noted "the faith in his own action" and the "faith in his own experience" characterizing what he called "the medical individualism" linked to the doctor's "full powers to act".[27] Although Nicolle belonged to the Pasteurian school, which he readily equated with a holy order, he gave those physicians acting independently the first role. Before World War I, and in order to judge the value of his home-made anti-gonococcal vaccine, Nicolle leaned on his network of doctor friends, as for instance, on Dr. Leredde, who also treated patients for venereal diseases.[28] As a therapist and researcher, the physician, in Nicolle's opinion, works in a grandiose and romantic solitude, freed from all obligations but that of work. The profession remains rebellious to statistics due to its inclination toward independence[29] and also on the basis of its daily familiarity with the complexity of therapeutic choices[30] and in the name of its experience with the biological singularity of the human being.

The idea according to which physicians could form a separate order free from ordinary laws was able to develop among a constituent body keeping some particularities of the *Ancien Régime* corporations, among which was the strong feeling of belonging to a community bound by an implicit code. Rather than an honor code, a remote reminiscence of the medieval aristocracy, I see in this the reflection of a sense of corporation developed and nourished by certain esoteric practices, such as that of dissection performed during medical studies at the Faculty,[31] which conferred an ethos of transgression in regard to the common taboos toward human life.[32] This sense of transgression could only be reinforced by ulterior practices during the career, familiarity with the patients' secrets, the permission to operate on living flesh and the leniency of the law which ordinarily punished the breach of corporal integrity as assault and battery. The surgical trade lay curled up under the cover of this legal protection and slowly evolved from the profession of the barber, who was almost an executioner and a butcher,[33] to the solemn figure in charge of the unveiling of nature which Paul Valéry presented in his famous address to surgeons in 1937.

These particularities explain why while hygiene spoke loudly in the Chamber of Deputies, physicians showed themselves so reluctant to directly support state action from the moment it interfered with their relations to the patients, and invoked medical secrecy when, for example, cases of infectious diseases had to be reported, despite the law which made this reporting compulsory in 1892.[34]

The Magistrates' Answer

The frontier between therapeutics and scientific experimentation was already difficult enough to draw considering the general observation that any treatment entails specific individual risks and can therefore teach us something. The physician experiments, that is to say treats as Canguilhem said. But non-therapeutic experimentation also tended to develop at the end of the last century. Often, doctors practiced on themselves and their nearest relatives and friends. They also operated occasionally on subjects already sick and in a way fallen under their power. For instance, they tested the transmission mode of a disease at a time when the notion of infectious disease overshadowed that of hereditary disease and the expectation of imminent breakthrough multiplied daring actions by ten.

In 1902, *Memoires*, written by a physician from Saint Petersburg and constituting a real indictment against lightly adopted medical innovations were published.[35] The chapter dealing with "experimentation in the living human being" reviewed numerous examples taken from a broad range of European medical publications. Many cited experiments were about the inoculation of venereal diseases. They were explained, if not justified, by the absence of any animal model and the social importance of syphilis and blennorrhagia. The author, Dr. Veressaief, drew up the tragic appraisal of progress by formulating the dilemma of the physician trapped between an appalling routine and the fearsome necessity to innovate.

Among all levels of society, magistrates were perhaps the least sensitive to the physicians' argumentation. Throughout the 19th century, they repeatedly and forcefully recalled that no citizen stands above the law, whatever his field of competence. In their eyes, common law sufficed to give a framework of reflection adaptable to the specificities of medical practice.

In 1859, an internist from Lyons experimented on the transmission of secondary syphilis to a scabious child and published the results of his observations.[36] Here, it is a matter of an experience determined, documented, controlled and finally published by a single person, in accordance with the ideal of the freelance profession. The child contracted syphilis and recovered later on. The incriminated physician pleaded his absence of ill intent and his wish to serve science. The tribunal in Lyons pronounced in 1859 an arrest stipulating the necessity of consent before any medical action. (Let us recall that in France, one will to have to wait until the 1988 law on experimentation in human beings without any direct benefit for the subject implied in the experiment to gain legal status.)

Physicians put forward the benefit for the collective and the rights of the science they serve. This recalls to mind the emphasis Pasteur put on "these holy places called laboratories". The magistrates retorted that the physician's right to pursue knowledge is not an absolute and that no one can put it forward for the justification of any kind research. Priority must be given to the benefit of the patients to whom the physicians were bound by the implicit contract resulting from the patients' call or request. The magistrates considered that, except for therapeutic intention, physicians fell under common law and could be answerable for the crime of intended battery caused by their Faustian hubris: they were personally responsible, although at different legal levels, for their therapeutics and research.

At the same time, the magistrates were perfectly aware of the stakes of the physicians' resistance to integrate under common law. Prosecutor Dupin said it in eloquent words in 1835:[37] the medical profession's way of thinking endangered society's foundations by creating a middle body standing in the way of power, which was the obsessive fear of lawyers of the Ancient as well as the New Regime. As early as the reign of Citizen King Louis-Philippe, Prosecutor Dupin clearly showed his fidelity to the idea of a nation composed of citizens not only equal in the face of the law, but also submitted to it.

During the whole century, magistrates declared their intention not to interfere with scientific controversies. Yet, they recalled that they needed to refer to an average norm of knowledge, yet open to changes in the course of time. The Court did not rule on scientific questions, but meant to pronounce the law based on the truth of the moment because the Court had to deduce from it the good practices opposable to the defendants. For instance, they accepted the concept of contagion for pragmatic reasons without pronouncing themselves on the details of its working. Interestingly, by their refusal to take sides in the struggle between those who believed in contagion and those rejecting it, the infectionist school (focus theory) and the contagionist, the Court anticipated the synthesis that would later occur between the ideas of both protagonists at the advent of bacteriology.[38]

With the hopes awakened by the development of microbiology, the plea for a certain irresponsibility of the physicians entailed the necessity to experiment frantically in order to clear the way for progress. This was an ode to wild freedom necessary for the experimenter venturing himself beyond the zone of certitude in which law can be established. Scientific logic was so strong that practitioners caught red handed while experimenting were truly surprised. The Hansen trial, which took place at the northernmost reaches of medical Europe was exemplary of the state of mind of the time.

The Hansen Trial

The name Gerhardt Armauer Hansen made Norwegian medicine known to the entire world. Indeed, Hansen proposed in 1873, at the beginnings of microbiology, that a bacterium made out under microscope in leprome extracts was the cause for a mysterious disease which had been taxing the clinicians' shrewdness for centuries: leprosy. Hansen strove for the acknowledgement of leprosy as an infectious disease (leprosy had rather been considered a hereditary disease), with all the changes it would imply for public health policy.

However, in order to fulfill the criteria requested by Henle for the definition of an infectious disease, perfectly known to Hansen, there was still a great deal of work to do. In spite of the repeated efforts of the Norwegian physician, there was no *in vitro* culture of the bacillus in question nor was it infectious for laboratory animals. In 1879, preyed upon by the wish to prove at any cost the infectious nature of leprosy, Hansen inoculated a leprome extract on the cornea of a female patient suffering from tuberculoid leprosy in the large Bergen hospital he was responsible for. The patient developed indeed a leprome on the cornea in the following weeks. But she had been strongly reluctant to be experimented upon, and the action gave rise to a general outcry in the hospital. With the help of a chaplain of the institution, the cause went to court.[39]

For his defense, Hansen argued he had merely transfered a basically curable disease since he had healed several lepers before by means of a surgical ablation of their corneous lepromes. The court accepted the charge of failure of consent and of therapeutic intention. The magistrate passed a true judgement of Solomon by distinguishing between two problems. First, the medical problem. In this respect, he pronounced Hansen's guilt for having omitted to obtain the patient's consent and having gone beyond her refusal. As a result, Hansen was bereft of his position at the hospital. Then, the problem related to science, to whose advance he had contributed. For this reason, he was maintained in his position of general inspector for leprosy in the entire Norwegian Kingdom. Hansen would later chair the great international leprosy congress in 1909. In this way, the divergence between man's and science's rights - two orders able to contradict one another - was officially acknowledged.

Liberal Practice and the 1927 Code of Deontology

Thus, a set of rules was progressively constituted in jurisprudence. These rules referred to the doctrine of a *sui generis* contract signed between the physician and the patient. This contract was consensual and signed against valuable consideration (that is to say involving the payment of fees). It was also *intuitu personae*, that is to say signed from person to person. It depended on the confidence placed by the patient in the doctor, but while it entailed on both sides rights and duties like any contract, it confirmed the radical asymmetry of the roles. The limited character of the actual results opposed to the expected ends restricted the doctor-patient contract to an *obligation of means* and not of results, which did not go as far as certain earlier practices, in particular practices in the Middle Ages which specifically mentioned recovery as a condition for fee payment. Practitioners in the past could be condemned for not having cured or for having aggravated a disease through a risky treatment without seeking the elder's advice, and they had to repay their fees as well as a fine. It is an irony of history that the restrictive doctrine of obligation of means was strengthened at the height of the Pasteurian era, contemporary with the advance of surgery thanks to the combination of asepsis and anesthesia and the rapid development of modern chemotherapy stemming from the dyestuffs industry before World War I. It partly shielded physicians from the authority of law and underlined the exceptional character of medical practice.

The physician and writer Georges Duhamel would speak later of a "colloque singulier". The asymmetrical character of the contract was officially balanced out by the moral commitment and the assessment of the ethical values specific to the trade. Louis Portes, President of the *Conseil de l'Ordre* in 1943, would express it later in his famous phrase of "confidence encountering conscience".[40] The autonomy of the medical sphere was therefore based as much on the esoteric and initiatory nature of the science defining it as on the affirmation of the moral values and authority of the profession.

The doctrine of the interpersonal contract developed in the special context of liberal medicine, whose Charter was written in France in 1927 by the medical syndicates. It corresponded to a type of social organization of medicine characterizing most European countries at that time. The code of deontology embodied in this charter affirmed a certain number of principles, all putting the emphasis on the freedom of the contracting parties: freedom for the patient to choose his doctor (Article 6), freedom of prescription for the doctor (Article 8), and medical secrecy as a guarantee for the intimacy of the relationship (Article 4).[41]

Written a few years before the Popular Front (the government of the Left Union which ruled during the whole year of 1936 and marked in France an intensified reflection on public health questions and initiated a project for re-organizing medicine), this charter mirrored a philosophy of law more Hegelian than Marxist. It made no distinction between the two types of free-dom: that of a learned person enjoying the command of his knowledge and that of a human being whose balance and reason can be disrupted by suffer-ing. Finally, it arbitrarily isolated this interindividual contract from the social context affecting it and from the intervention of the state, which was not only the warrant for individual agreements but also intervened more and more in the sphere of public health viewed as the sum of the health of the collective of individuals.

The recurrent demands for the creation of a modern medical guild, a *Conseil de l'Ordre du Médecin*, during the last hundred years obviously took on quite different forms in the course of time. In the last century, it showed the profession's aspirations for a corporatist autonomy on the model of attorneys who had had their association since 1803, as well as its concern to protect it-self from the law. At the turn of the century, the claim aimed at distinguish-ing between the concern for the profession's honor and integrity and the de-fense of its material interests which syndicates started to take care of. After World War I, it meant then a search for a guarantee against the state's en-croachments, or it showed on the contrary an intention of establishing an authority controlling the profession and responsible for the citizens' health, an indispensable partner for the signing of collective agreements towards a social medicine outlined during the Popular Front period.

After the defeat of several older plans which had been logged down in parliamentary procedures since 1923, the *Ordre des Médecins* was hastily created on October 7, 1940 by the Government of Marshal Pétain after the dissolution of the medical syndicates because of the new situation created by the armistice and the occupation of France by the German troops. For some people, the purpose was to constitute immediately a body representative of all doctors against the occupying forces' interference.

The *Ordre* was immediately assigned the writing of a Code of Deontol-ogy (1942). As a matter of fact, its activity was mostly limited at the begin-ning to prosaic tasks such as the tentative control of gas or drug shortages, the issuing of travel permits (*Ausweise*) to practitioners, etc.

The *Ordre* was reorganized September 10, 1942 through a law creating the National Council, disciplinary regional councils and substituting elected counsellors for counsellors appointed by the state. The defense of medical secrecy turned out to be crucial at the beginning of 1944 when, as the members of the Resistance harassed the occupation troops, the German authorities published in the press of the Northern Occupation Zone a notice obliging any person having treated persons wounded by firearms or explosives to reveal the latter's name and address to the German administration. Dr. Louis Portes, President of the National Council and supported by Dr. Grasset, Minister of Health, officially pointed out to the German authorities that French law and tradition were absolutely contrary to the violation of medical secrecy. The German repression continued to be exerted, but in a letter addressed July 4, 1944 to the Head of Government Pierre Laval, General von Neubronn declared that he declined to ask for the promulgation of a law on the violation of medical secrecy.[42]

Dissolved in 1945, the Association was recreated that same year at the *Libération*. It is interesting to note that in 1943, in liberated Algeria, the idea of a competing *Ordre* had been committed to paper. The rebirth of the *Ordre* in 1945 was a sign for a general need expressed under highly different regimes and reconciled various acceptations: this Association still exists to˙ day.[43] Yet, the revision of the Code of Deontology in 1945 did not mark a clear break with either the code of 1927 or 1942.

From this point of view of manifest historical continuity, one is entitled to ask if the year 1947, despite the echoes of the Nuremberg Medical Trial, truly marked a milestone in the history of European and French medicine and was the starting point of a radical calling into question of recent history. After 1947 for Louis Portes, President of the *Ordre*, as for many of his colleagues, traditional liberal medicine appeared as a shield against totalitarianism. At the same time, in the United States the powerful Association of American Physicians protested against the premises of a right to health[44] laid down by the *World Health Organization (WHO)* as an infringement on their prerogatives.[45] It was once again on the doctors' conscience that most practitioners meant to base the judgement of responsibilities. Neither the State, suspected of totalitarism after the monstrous deviation of Nazism, nor the sick laypeople were really asked to take part in the debate on therapeutic and experimental responsibility which remained the specialists' affair.

It has been repeated time and again that the Nazi cruelties did not stem from the doctors' scientific hubris, but from a scandalous ignorance of the various ethical provisions which had acted as brakes and safeguards in the past and that even in Germany, doctors disposed of all the texts which should have fundamentally restrained their activity and told them their duty. For example, during the BCG trial in Lübeck, indicted doctors had been severely blamed by judges for ignoring elementary rules of conduct sketched by law, such as obtaining the patient's consent.[46] Nevertheless, another reading can allow us to see in Nazi violence the monstrous leading astray of a medical pretension to place itself above the law. For this reason, the Nuremberg Code is not so much an act of theoretical novelty as a historical knot of international ethical reflection. At the Nuremberg Trials, all countries were summoned to appear.[47]

Today, in the face of science's rights, certainly hypertrophied at the end of the 19th century primarily because of the hopes aroused by science and the positivist credo, a consciousness for the patients' own rights has awakened: on the one hand, the right to health, supposing a patients' submission to all kinds of potentially dangerous inquisitory procedures and, on the other hand, a social urge to limit medical omnipotence, such as the obligation to obtain informed consent, in spite of all the difficulties raised by its appreciation. In France, the law has for a long time absolutely linked medical actions to a curative intent, rejecting non-therapeutic experimentation as illegal until the law of 1988 was passed. Modern ethicists are now defending what they call the patient's autonomy, reaching far beyond the simple right to choose one's practitioner. We are dealing here with an attempt to reestablish a parity in the contract doctrine, the claim of a true partnership in the therapeutical choices and the practice of research in the spirit of the common good.[48]

To recall the Hippocratic oath marks today in an almost mythical way the need to take up again a past tremendously rich in lessons. The Hippocratic oath is not contemporary with Hippocrates, and one does not even know from which time onward it played an effective part in the practice of the profession, but it became, during the course of history, emblematic for traditional ethical concerns and was at the same time a sign for the old wish to secure the autonomy of the profession based on its singular vocation.

1947 became retrospectively a milestone in the history of European medical deontology,[49] at a time when the profession drew the ethical lesson at the crossroad of its powers and its knowledge and reformulated its responsibilities in therapeutics and/or in experimentation. Georges Canguilhem[50] stamped at that time the debate by pursuing two historical logics to their end, which in his eyes, did not oppose but marked the two poles of a strong dialectic.[51] According to him, any medical action is an experimentation and supposes the conscience clause: A doctor is called to answer before "the court of his conscience". But any doctor is also called to answer "before a court of law".[52] Interestingly, Canguilhem cast in the same mould the Bernardian affirmation of the experimental nature of medicine and the democratic concern to submit physicians to common law. He marked at the same time the historical continuity in the process of knowledge construction and the break in the optimism of the last century, the mistrust in front of a certain medical irresponsibility.[53] The legislative unrest of the last years in France, following the trial on blood transfusion[54] which led to the 1988 law on non-therapeutic experimentation, can be considered as a remote consequence of the Nuremberg Trials and the Nuremberg Code. This legislation reformulated at the same time the rights and duties of the profession, consecrating the alliance of the Hippocratic oath with modern science.

Notes

1   Huriet C. (1995), *L'exercice médical dans la société: hier, aujourd'hui, demain*, Masson, Paris, p 59.

2   Moulin A. M. (1989), 'Medical Ethics in France', *Theoretical Medicine*, 9, 271-285.

3   Serres M. (1986), Foreword to *L'oeuf transparent*, Flammarion, Paris.

4   Pelner Cosman M. (1996), 'Medieval medical malpractice, the dicta and the dockets', *Bulletin of the New York Academy of Medicine*, pp 22-47.

5   Rawcliffe C. (1981), 'Medicine and medical practice in later medieval London', *Guidhall Studies in London History*, 5, pp 13-25.

6   Herzlich C. (1981), Représentations de la médecine et mémoire des médecins français, *L'exercice médical dans la société...*, pp 105-114.

7   Ellis J. (1990), *The Physician-Legislators of France, Medicine and Politics in the Early French Third Republic, 1870-1914*, Cambridge University Press, Cambridge.

8   Cunningham A., Williams P. eds. (1992), *The Laboratory Revolution in Medicine*, Cambridge University Press; Moulin A. M., Bacteriological Research and Medical Practice in and out the Pasteurian School, *Medical French Culture in the XIXth and XXth centuries*, in: Laberge A. and Feingold M. eds. (1994), Oxford University Press, Oxford, pp 327-349.

9   Moulin A.M. (1985), 'La biologie s'en mêle', *L'Histoire*, 76, pp 100-103.

10   Rosenberg C. (1995), 'Catechism of health : the body in the prebellum classroom', *Bulletin of the History of Medicine*, 69, pp 175-197.

11   Léonard J. (1981), *La médecine entre les pouvoirs et les savoirs. Histoire intellectuelle et politique de la médecine française au 19e siècle*, Aubier, Paris; Faure O. (1993), *Les Français et leur médecine au XIXe siècle*, Berlin, Paris.

12   Quoted by Nicolle C. (1936), *Responsabilités de la médecine*, Alcan Paris, p 11.

13   Beaune J.-C. ed. (1993), *La Philosophie du remède*, Champ Vallon, Seyssel.

14   Bynum W. (1993), "C'est un malade". Animal models and concepts of human disease', *Journal of the History of Medicine and the Allied Sciences*, 45, pp 401-415.

15   Canguilhem G. (1989), 'Thérapeutique, expérimentation, responsabilité (1959)', *Etudes d'histoire et de philosophie des sciences*, Vrin, Paris, p 389.

16   Nicolle C. (1936), *Responsabilités de la médecine*, p 9.

17   Baud J.-P. (1993), *L'affaire de la main volée. Histoire juridique du corps*, Seuil, Paris.

18   Weisz G. (1995), *The Medical Mandarins, The French Academy of Medicine in the nineteenth and early twentieth centuries*, Oxford University Press, Oxford, pp 21-25.
     Hermitte M.-A. (1996), *Le sang et le droit*, Seuil, Paris, p 52.

19   Peter J.-P. ed. (1972), *Médecins, climat et épidémies à la fin du XVIIIe siècle*, Mouton, Paris.

20   Ramsay W. (1988), *Professional and popular medicine in France, 1770-1830, The social world of medical practice*, Cambridge University Press, Cambridge.

21   Gelfand T. (1900), *Professionalizing modern medicine. Paris surgeons and medical science and institutions in the 18th century*, Westport, Conn.

22   Weisz G. (1995), *The Medical Mandarins*, pp 60-86.

23   Dr Gibert, *Bulletin de l'Académie impériale de Médecine* (1853) 19, p 973, quoted by Weisz G. (1995), *The Medical Mandarins*, p 75. Cf. the report on experiments on transmission of syphilis by the same author, *Bulletin de l'Académie impériale de Médecine* (1858), 24, pp 888-890.

24   Vogel M.J. ed. (1979), *The Therapeutic Revolution*, Pennsylvania University Press, Philadelphia; Warner J. W. (1986), *The Therapeutic Perspective. Medical Practice. Knowledge and Identity in America, 1820-1855*, Harvard University Press, Cambridge.

25   Nye R. (1995), 'Honor code and medical ethics in modern France', *Bulletin of the History of Medicine*, 69, pp 91-111.

26   Moulin A.M. (1991), *Le dernier langage de la médecine, Histoire de l'immunologie de Pasteur au Sida*, Presses universitaires de France, Paris, p 387 et sqq.

27   Nicolle C. (1936), *Responsabilités de la médecine*, p 9.

28   Correspondance Leredde-Nicolle, Fonds Nicolle, Archives départementales de Rouen. Pelis K. (1995), *Pasteur's imperial missionary*, Johns Hopkins University, Baltimore.

29   Matthews J.R. (1995), *Quantification and the Quest for Medical Certainty*, Princeton University Press, Princeton.

30   Tröhler U., 'To operate or not to operate ? Scientific and extraneous factors in therapeutical controversies within the Swiss Society of Surgery, 1913-1988', in: Bynum W.F. and Nutton V. eds. (1991), *Essays in the History of Therapeutics*, Rodopi, Amsterdam, p 89-113.

31   Richardson R. (1988), *Dissection, Death and the Destitute*, Routledge, London.

32   Moulin A. M. (1995), 'La crise éthique de la transplantation d'organes. A la recherche de la "compatibilité" culturelle', *Diogène*, 172, pp 76-96.

33   Pouchelle M.-C. (1983), *Corps et chirurgie à l'apogée du Moyen-Age*, Flammarion, Paris.

       Drouard A. (1995), 'Aux sources de l'eugénisme français', *La Recherche*, 26, pp 648-654.

34   Zylbermann P. (1994), *L'Hygiène dans la République*, thesis, Paris VI.

35   Dr Veressaieff (1902), *Mémoires d'un médecin*, Perrin, Paris.

36   *Gazette hebdomadaire de médecine et de chirurgie* (1859) 15.

37   For a stimulating account on the relationships between law and medicine, cf. Hermitte M. A. (1996), *Le sang et le droit*, Seuil, Paris, pp 47-63.

38   Delaporte F. (1990), *Le savoir de la maladie*, Presses universitaires de France, Paris.

39   Blom K. (1973), 'A Hansen and human leprosy transmission. Medical ethics and legal rights', *International Journal of Leprosy*, 41, pp. 199-207.

40   Portes L. (1954), *A la recherche d'une éthique médicale*, Presses universitaires de France, Paris.

41   Villey R. (1986), *Histoire du secret médical*, Seghers, Paris.

42   A "personal" anecdote related to this question can be related here. In 1944, a French surgeon, Dr. J. A. Barrier, a friend of my family, was summoned before a German officer in Clermont-Ferrand to answer for medical aid he had given to a wounded man from the *maquis*. He acknowledged the deed, but refused to reveal the name and address of the

wounded man. The officer, considering the moral and juridical imperatives invoked above, released him again.

43 Peter J.-P. (1975), 'Le grand rêve de l'ordre médical, en 1770 et aujourd'hui', *Autrement*, 4.

44 Moulin A. M. (1993), 'AIDS and the History of the Right to Health', *AIDS, Health and Human Rights*, Fondation Marcel Mérieux, Les Pensières, pp 67-73

45 Kickbusch I. (1996), 'Cinquante ans d'évolution des concepts de santé à l'OMS', *Prévenir*, 30, pp. 43-54

46 Menut L. (forthcoming), 'BCG Trial in Lübeck (1930-33)', in: Moulin A. M. ed., The Adventure of Vaccination.

47 The historian Paul Weindling raised the question of the dehumanizing consequences of coercive public health policies and of a certain sliding from mass treatment toward an isolation of social groups at risk, with the consequences we know of. P Weindling (1993), 'Typhus and the Holocaust', *Medicine and change, Historical and sociological studies of medical innovation*, I Lôwy ed., Ed. INSERM, Paris.

48 Hoerni B. (1991), *L'autonomie en médecine. Nouvelles relations entre les personnes malades et les personnes soignantes*, Payot, Paris.

49 Ambroselli C. (1993), *L'éthique médicale*, PUF, Paris.

50 Canguilhem G. (1993), *Philosophe, historien des sciences*, Albin Michel, Paris.

51 Moulin A. M., 'La médecine moderne selon Georges Canguilhem'. Concepts en attente, *Georges Canguilhem...*, pp 121-134.

52 Canguilhem G. (1989), 'Thérapeutique, expérimentation, responsabilité (1959)', *Etudes d'histoire et de philosophie des sciences*.

53 Meyer P. (1993), *L'irresponsabilité médicale*, Grasset, Paris.

54 Moulin A. M. (1995), 'Reversible history: blood transfusion and the spread of AIDS in France', *AIDS and the public debate*; C. Hannaway, V. Harden and J. Parascandola eds, IOS Press, Amsterdam, pp 170-186.

3 Ethical Conduct and Ethical "Norms" up to 1947

Etienne Lepicard

> The tribunal before which the doctor of today has to appear - from a strictly professional point of view, that is to say in relation to his patients - is no longer the tribunal of his conscience, nor is it simply the highest court within the profession, but a civil court.
>
> — G. Canguilhem[1]

From the standpoint of ethics, modern physicians have always wanted to have to answer only to the court of his own conscience, and perhaps after that the court of experts from the community, but certainly not any court where the general public is involved. Is this position still possible after the Nuremberg trial of Nazi doctors in 1947? In the middle of the previous century, when Claude Bernard stated in his *Introduction à l'étude de la médecine expérimentale* the necessity of experimenting on living subjects, he added to this statement a vast ethical discussion on the (questionable) legitimacy of such procedures. On the other hand, in the experiments in vivo carried out at Auschwitz or in other camps, there were no ethical barriers. How did we go from the one position to the other? Is the "Nuremberg Code" of 1947 a simple call for the necessity of an open debate on the subject, such as Claude Bernard had called for, or are we dealing with something fundamentally different in light of the date of its composition: after these experiments in the camps? This essay will try to answer these basic questions. Much is at stake, since the implications concern the place the "Nuremberg Code" should occupy within contemporary ethical debates relating to medicine in particular and to health in general.

Claude Bernard wrote his *Introduction* when illness had forced him to take some time off. What he produced is a collection of considerations of his own experimental practice, starting with the notes he made in the laboratory. After a theoretical introduction on experimental reasoning, the author devotes the second section to experiments on the living. In the third paragraph of the second chapter of this section, we find his thoughts on the need to experiments on living subjects - that is, to carry out vivisections. He explains this need as follows:[2]

40

The laws of raw matter were not found without penetrating into bodies or inert machines; similarly, it is impossible to discover the laws and properties of living matter without opening up living organisms and probing their insides. It will thus be seen to be necessary, after we have been able to dissect the dead, to also dissect the living in order that we may discover the interior or hidden parts of the organism and see them functioning; these sort of operations are called vivisections, and without this mode of investigation no form of physiology or scientific medicine is possible: to learn how man and animals live, it is indispensable to see a great number of them die, because the mechanisms of life cannot be revealed and proved except through knowledge of the mechanisms of death.

Several formulations are important in this passage: the "seeing", seeing things functionning, seeing beings dying - not to mention the fact that a better understanding of the mechanisms of life requires the observation of many deaths. It goes without saying that the same pressing, macabre curiosity ran rampant at Auschwitz. After explaining the "need" to experiment on the living, Claude Bernard devotes two pages to legitimizing this need by listing the experiments carried out "throughout the ages" on those sentenced to death. Then he opens the discussion - one we could call a debate on ethics - in which he asks himself whether such practices would be morally defensible. He does this by asking four questions: do we have the right to carry out experiments and vivisections on human beings? Can we perform experiments or vivisections on criminals sentenced to death? Do we have the right to perform experiments or vivisections on animals? And finally, should we let ourselves be emotionally affected by the objections of gentlemen or of men outside the field of science?

We should keep two things in mind that the author himself states in response to the first of these questions. First, the connections he makes between the medical experimenter (le médecin expérimentateur) and what we nowadays call the experienced doctor (le médecin expérimenté). A good experimenter is one who above all has experience that goes beyond book and laboratory knowledge. There is thus no fundamental distinction between the role of the general practitioner and that of the researcher. Finally, he holds a clear-cut ethical position:[3]

It is our duty and our right to perform an experiment on man whenever it can save his life, cure him or gain him some personal benefit. The principle of medical and surgical morality, therefore, consists in never performing on man an experiment which might be harmful to him to any extent, even though the results might be highly advantageous to science, i.e. to the health of others. This does not mean that in always performing experiments and operations solely for the benefit of the subject undergoing them that science does not also profit from them at the same time.

Little room for interpretation is left here: there is only one person one is treating and carrying out experiments on. The same position is maintained as clearly when the subjects are criminals sentenced to death, although the common good plays a larger role in this case: "These kinds of experiments being especially important for science, and not being able to be performed on any other beings but human beings, they seem to me to be permissible as long as they do not involve any suffering or inconvenience for the subject undergoing the experiment".

In response, however, to the fourth question, Claude Bernard makes some remarks that could very well be associated with what happened at Auschwitz and jugded at Nuremberg. He reminds us, to begin with, that in science "it is the idea that gives the facts their value and their signification" before he goes on to state that the same could be said for all fields, also with respect to morals:[4]

> The physiologist is not a man of fashion (un homme du monde), but rather a scientist, a man who is absorbed by a scientific idea he is investigating: he no longer hears the cries of the animals, he does not see the blood dripping, he only sees his idea and does not perceive anything other than the organisms that are hiding the things he wants to discover. Similarly, the surgeon is not hindered by even the most moving cries and sobs because he only sees his idea and the goal of his operation. Along the same lines, the anatomist does not smell he is in a horrible ossuary; under the influence of a scientific idea, he pursues with delight a nerve within the stinking, pallid flesh that would be a source of disgust and horror for anyone else. According to this line of thinking, we should consider useless or absurd any discussion on vivisections. It is impossible that men who judge the facts with ideas as different as ours could ever agree; and just as it is impossible to satisfy everyone, the scientist should not worry himself overly about the opinion of other except those who also understand his field, and not draw any rules of conduct from anywhere but his own conscience.

We may note once again on the insistence on "seeing" - although this time the clear vision is reserved for the idea while the organism "hides". We note, too, the position of the surgeon: Claude Bernard uses surgeons from the very first question onwards to get his foot into the door, since they were already experimenting on the living as part of their day-to-day operations.[5]

Along with these two things, almost as a sort of echo, goes the retelling of an experiment in a camp as told by Simon Wiesenthal in his book, *Justice n'est pas vengeance*. The passage sheds much light on what Wiesenthal himself thought of the implications of what happened in the camps for medicine. It is important to keep both of these approaches: retelling and reflecting. In the following quotations from this history-narrative, the reader is asked to go beyond the obvious emotional content, as we are not concerned with this text as a social history but rather as cultural history - or, to be more exact, a history of values, one that tries to discover what is at work in all these fractions of history, to discover the meaning of events within the context of a certain number of common values. This kind of narrative history, it seems to me, is indispensable in achieving this end. What would ethical considerations be if every disturbing aspect had been obliterated? Perhaps it is one of the lessons to be learned from the Shoah: reason purely detached from emotions does not suffice to guarantee the ethical character of conduct. But to come back to Wiesenthal, he writes:[6]

> I believe there is a sort of relationship between the powerful desire to save the lives of men and the desire to hasten their death. This is one of the revelations from psychoanalysis, which has been remarkably interested in the surgeon: the surgeon must be capable of cutting open the flesh of a living being. The doctor must have a slight, barely perceptible sadistic drive to do this. ... the Third Reich allowed this impulse to reach terrible proportions, to destroy human life instead of serving it. Doctors who might have become excellent surgeons were reduced to merely dissecting living beings.

Wiesenthal then adds:

> While I was detained at Mauthausen, I heard people talking about a doctor who seemed to me to illustrate the problematic nature of this issue in exemplary fashion: when he had finished his duties as a camp doctor, Dr Aribert Heim began working as a field doctor on the front, where he saved many lives. But here is of what another camp prisoner in Mauthausen was witness when working as surgical nurse assigned to work with Dr Heim: a convoy of deported Jews had just arrived at the camp from Holland. The SS doctor examined all of them conscientiously on the central square of the camp, commanding them one after the other to open their mouths so he could check their teeth. He finally took two of them and asked them very politely if they wouldn't mind participating in a minor surgical operation that would be perfectly harmless. In exchange, they would be set free. The two who had been selected thought this was their chance and followed the doctor confidently all the way to the infirmary, where they undressed and one of them waited while the other lay down on the table. The doctor opened the thorax and the abdomen of the anesthetized man in order - as he put it - to be able to "study in vivo" the internal organs: "It's the first time I've ever seen the stomach of a living man at work". He then took his scalpel and, before the stunned eyes of his aid, dissected one organ after another, as if he were dissecting a cadaver. Once the heart had stopped beating, he had the corpse removed and called the second patient...

This passage, by its very cruelty, shows in my opinion how problematic the issue can be. To begin with, there is the basic ambivalent impulse that exists in everyone and that is more or less called for depending on the professional activity being carried out. At the same time, there is the curiosity of the mind stimulated by what one sees, something which is inherent in any scientific investigation and without which no scientific progress would be possible. And finally, other questions are raised, especially when we keep Claude Bernard's analysis in mind: how did we go from the problem of scientific progress in medicine and the hope that more knowledge will permit us to treat patients better to this "science of death", to borrow an expression from Benno Müller-Hill?[7] It should be kept in mind that Germany was the first country (in 1931) to give out regulations controlling experiments on humans. Beyond the inherent fragility of all legislation and beyond the written word, there is also the question of the extent to which such norms are part of common awareness. Historians are begining to examine the fact that doctors were the largest socio-professional group in the Nazi party.[8] The social function of the Hippocratic Oath must also be reanalyzed in such circumstances.[9] Why did these doctors not see a contradiction in killing for research's sake? Why the ethical debate we have seen present in Claude Bernard's reflection had been so missing in Auschwitz? Is Nazi ideology behind all this or is there something else in the development of modern medical thought that is equally at fault?

Actually, the conditions for the passage from the one to the other are "intellectually" known. In the first place, we have to mention the information given by German expert to the American Military Court that was dealing with the cases of some Nazi doctors.[10] Professor Leibbrand spoke of "biological thought" in describing the relation to the body that began with the advent of experimental medicine. I would like to mention two other here: first, the passage of the individual body to the social body as the object of care for physicians; and second, the so-called "non-humanity" or "sub-humanity" of the Jews, the Gypsies, and other people discriminated against such as the mentally ill and homosexuals. Nazi doctors were thus working, according to their own criteria, for the common good without committing homicide. This last point seems to be specific to the Nazi regime and to explain its uniqueness.

The idea on experiments on living human beings goes hand in hand with the somewhat troubling manner in which the discussion is covered by Celse (first century A.D.) in the Proemium of his *De Medicina*. Celse describes there the type of doctor who proposes a rational theory of medicine and, in raising the question of the treatment of internal illness, expresses the need of getting to know the ordering of the inner organs on cadavers. He further states that according to these practitioners, Hierophile and Erasistrate, used an even better way of getting at this knowledge by opening the bodies of still living criminals from the prisons of kings. A bit later he gives an ethical motivation to this practice: research for cures from which all the innocent people in all future ages will benefit.[11] I stated above that this approach of Celse's is somewhat troubling because these citations give a great historical depth to the questions posed here and already suggested by Claude Bernard. Experiments on living people are not a recent development, nor is the argument about the potential benefits for the common good, nor the "use" of those who have lost some of their rights. If society takes it upon itself in both cases to conduct experiments on prisoners, the difference is that Celse does not deny that a homicide has been committed. It is merely that the common good superimposes itself on the good of the condemned.

Such an interpretation of the historical process sheds light on dilemma between the representation of the Shoah as a unique phenomenon in history and an alternate view of it involving a coherent system. One way of overcoming the historical dilemma would be, in this particular case of links between medicine and the Nazi regime, to move "from Auschwitz to Nuremberg". Indeed, to a certain extent, everything that the name Auschwitz represents for the connection between medicine and the Nazi regime entered the public domain at Nuremberg. Admittedly only to a certain extent, for only the tip of the iceberg was ever made to answer for itself. A number of doctors involved - and not the lowest among them - were never called to the stand, not to mention everything that happened before 1939 and has still to be tried in a court of law. In this respect, the work of the historian will never replace that of justice. However, despite all that, it was the trials at Nuremberg that showed the world the extent of the horror of what we have come to know under the name of Auschwitz.

In this context, how are we to understand the fame of the "Nuremberg Code"? Indeed, if it is perfectly clear that Nazi doctors were criminals , it is also undeniable that these trials were a shock to the very people who were writing the law. This raises an even more radical question: why? Do we have, here, a criteria with which to judge the medical tradition in its entirety? In other words, what have the words "Nuremberg Code" come to mean? As with the term "Auschwitz", is there not more in the terms "Nuremberg Code" that what it historically attributed to it, and what connection has it kept to the historical event? We must keep in mind the great delay which has elapsed since the time of the trials themselves and the fame which is accorded to the "Nuremberg Code" nowadays.

I would like to propose several vantage points of this rather vast set of questions. I cannot hope to give any exhaustive answers but rather to touch upon some essential concepts that - let's hope - will turn out to be fruitful. These ideas came to me during some research carried out over some ten years involving a case study of Dr Alexis Carrel's, a French surgeon who won the Nobel Prize, in 1912, for his work on organ transplants and blood vessel sutures. He spent most of his professional years at the Rockefeller Institute for Medical Research in New York. The influence of Claude Bernard's work on Carrel as well as the attachment of the latter to the grand master of experimental methods are undeniable. For instance, during the 1920s Carrel repeatedly refused to have his department renamed otherwise than "Division of Experimental Surgery" although the work done there had little to do with the original title.

Undoubtedly, Carrel is more well-known for his 1935 book on a "medical reconstruction" of human beings, *Man, The Unknown*, which was quickly translated into German: *Der Mensch, Das Unbekannte Wesen*. This work became a best-seller at the time of its publication.[12] It was long considered a classic and several editions have been published since the end of World War II, including a pocket book version. The fact that, during the Nuremberg trials, Karl Brandt cited this work[13] was hardly taken note of. Brandt, among others, tried to show during the course of the trials that other countries than Germany had given their approval to the elimination of lives "that are not worth living". Nowadays, many voices can be heard denouncing such an ethics that supports the theses of that book. Thus, in France the medicine school at Lyon, which had been named after Alexis Carrel, was recently renamed. The fact that this book was such a best-seller over so many years thus raises questions about the "norms" that were proposed in it and the reciprocal interaction that exists between author and reader concerning the interiorisation of norms. His fall from grace in the past few years begs the question of the mode of production and reception of "norms" under the influence of historical events.

Without going into any details, let it suffice to say that Carrel thought science was a source of morality; our society degenerates, but science has given us - for the first time in history - the means of reconstructing human beings - or, more importantly, of reconstructing a moral human being. The form of expression of this scientific morality remains somewhat religious. Where does such a set of beliefs in science as source of morals come from? They are not made in a vacuum. It is possible by using methods from literary history to trace the development of the spirit that appeared also in the wake of Carrel's book. Signs of public awareness of Carrel-like's ideas can be found in the United States by 1925 in Sinclair Lewis' *Arrowsmith*,[14] the first non-science fiction novel that had a medical researcher as its protagonist. The credo of science for science's sake are spelled out in Lewis' novel in great detail. The protagonist, who winds up as a monk in the desert, comes to advocate the inhumane in the name of scientific progress, as Dooley points out.[15] It's the scene where Martin Arrowsmith struggles to conduct an experiment corresponding to scientific criteria during an epidemic that eventually takes his wife. It wasn't until the 60s - during the rediscovery of the work of Sinclair Lewis, the idol of the years before the war but forgotten in the meantime - that this "science despite humanity" was focussed on.

With this horizon of expectations in mind, one can see Carrel's book as the original answer, formulated by a scientist, to the crisis of civilization that struck the western world in 1929-30. Science, for a time, seemed to be called into question by this crisis, but not the medical world. Carrel's book could thus be viewed as the declaration of his own belief as a medical researcher in the "scientific method", taking account, however, of the expectations of the general public, which were clearly exhibited by the success of Arrowsmith but also revised by the crisis. Carrel, if he is the principle and final author of the book, also took part in a discussion group among a circle of his friends in which such public expectations were talked about. This circle was composed of people, representing some of the most influential spheres in American society: a lawyer specializing in international law; a preacher-philosopher; an engineer and former ambassador in America of the Russian Kerenzki government; a member of the "brain-trust" close to President Roosevelt, etc. This diversity rules out the possibility that Alexis Carrel was a sort of mad scientist who went wrong; a broader intellectual context is noticeable here.

But a book is not only the production of an author, mirror of his social group, it is also the product of the readers. It is also what it allows to come into being. As such, the success of Carrel's work - best-seller in 1936, translated into 13 languages in three years - turned out to be a breakthrough in Carrel's career. Having been pensioned off by the Rockefeller Institute in 1939, Carrel created a cross-disciplinary Foundation for scientific research in 1941 in France - the Fondation Française pour l'Étude des Problèmes Humains, which became after the end of the war the Institut National d'Études Démographiques (INED). Thus, the success of the 1935 book re-created the author, not only in the public eye but also in politics. This resonance led to the creation of such an important institution. What was the nature of this resonance? This question is far too vast to answer even in summary fashion. However, it seems undeniable that it brought, at least partly, upon the issue of ethical norms to bear. A whole epoch, audiences, recognized their distress and uncertainty about the future addressed in that book. Later, under the Vichy government, the program of *Man, The Unknown* was drawn up.

Compared to the first wave of reception before the war, the various responses to the book afterward allow to examine the reaction of the various audiences to the norms at work in it. I shall focus here on the reception in the 50s. At that time, in both institutions of science related to the book, historiography was the mood. Indeed, whether at the Rockefeller Institute or INED, histories of institutions or the discipline itself were being written. Notably, the conduct of doctors during the war was criticized in order to separate contemporary practices from such behavior, which was attributed to an outburst of irrational thought, and, thus, fundamentally unlike the rationality of science. In addition, and perhaps concomitant with this enthusiastic reaffirmation of beliefs in the scientific adventure, there is a great "production" within the field of medical ethics. In 1946, 32 national medical associations convened in London to create the World Medical Association in response to the horrendous crimes perpetrated by Nazi doctors. In 1948, the World Medical Association issued the Oath of Geneva and then published in 1949 the first *International Code of Medical Ethics*. The world Congress of Medical Morals also met in Paris in 1955 and 1966. This "production" of ethics, ever so directly linked with what happened in Nazi Germany, merits further investigation. At first glance, it seems to have rested on the traditional foundation of the Hippocratic deontology. One question, however, remains: who were these ethical codes for medicine supposed to reassure, patients or members of the medical profession themselves?[16] On this issue, the Nuremberg Code stood in contrast to the traditional deontology. In reality, in the ten principles worked out in the course of the trials against the Nazi doctors, it is the right of the patients that is affirmed. On the other hand, the Hippocratic Oath is quite clearly intended to be taken as a code of honor marking the appearance of a profession, and thus insuring that it will be run honestly.

One last aspect of the link between norms and historical events needs to be addressed: what are we to make of the fact that the Code of Nuremberg went almost unnoticed until recently. It was only one element in the sentencing of the criminal physicians; today, in light of all the ethical norms edicted after the war, the Code serves even a largely symbolic function besides its actual content. Along the same lines, the work of Alexis Carrel which has fallen out of favor with a large part of the public, has raised another question: how was this book able to become such a literary success back then when it is so far from the norms of ethics we have today? Does this mean that the norms themselves have changed? The hermeneutic difference in the reading of such a work suggests that we are not reading the same book in 1935 as in 1995.

Conclusion

We must look at the way the need to experiment of living beings went from being tied up fundamentally in the work of Claude Bernard with ethical considerations to being bereft of such considerations in the experiments carried out at Auschwitz. The historical conditions of the development, which has been relatively well exposed by historians, do not clearly explain another historiographical dilemma: the uniqueness of the Holocaust or the possibility to compare it with other genocides. It has been argues that the move from Auschwitz to Nuremberg would help clarify, to some extent, this dilemma. Indeed, Nuremberg represents the arrival of the crimes committed by the Nazis in the public domain. In order to judge these people, the notion of "crimes against humanity" had to be invented. In the field of medicine, at the moment of the trials, ten principles of ethics concerning experiments on humans had to be drawn up. It was also the first time that the rights of the patient were so clearly affirmed. Thus, at Nuremberg the Hippocratic deontology prescribing the rules for the profession gave way to ethical principles questioning the practice of this profession. Finally, in tracing back the history of the reception of a medical work contemporary to these events, the extent of this shift in emphasis has become clear: a modification took place in our ethical norms, of which Nuremberg has become the symbol. This tells us something about what ethical norms dealing with conduct should be. Not a law, but perhaps linked to the law, something whose link with history raises questions, something, finally, that - as Paul Ricœur said of the symbol - makes us think.

Notes

1   Canguilhem, G. (1959), Thérapeutique, expérimentation, responsabilité. *Revue de l'Enseignement Supérieur.* Adopted in: (1968) Etudes d'Histoire et de Philosophie des Sciences, Vrin, Paris.

2   Bernard, C. (1927), An Introduction to the Study of Experimental Medicine. Macmillan, New York.

3   Ibid.

4   Ibid.

5   For a recent look at the "social significations" involved in surgery cf. Hirschauer, S.(1991), 'The Manufacture of Bodies in Surgery', *Social Studies of Science*, Vol 21: 279-319; or also Fox, N.J. (1992), *The Social Meaning of Surgery*, Open University Press, Milton Keynes; Collins sums it up in: Collins, H.M. (1994), 'Dissecting Surgery: Forms of Life Depersonalized', *Social Studies of Science*, Vol 24: 311-333, and the responses by S. Hirschauer, N.J. Fox, M. Lynch, and H.M. Collins in the ensuing sections of the same edition.

6   Wiezental, S. (1989), *Justice n'est pas vengance*. Robert Laffont, Paris.

7   Müller-Hill, B. (1988), *Murderous Science*. Oxford Univ. Press, Oxford.

8   Kater, M. (1987), 'The Burden of the Past: Problems of a Modern Historyography of Physicians and Medicine in Nazi Germany'. *German Studies Review.* Vol 10: 31-56.

9   Rütten, T. (in press), *Hitler with - or without - Hippocrates?* Korot, Jerusalem.

10 For more on the American Military Tribunal, cf. the article by Dominique Sprumont and Pascal Arnold in this book.

11 Celse. *De Medicina*, Proemium § 23-26.

12 Carrel, A. (1935), *Man, the Unknown*. Harper & Bros., New York.

13 Cf. Khül, S. (1994), *The Nazi Connection, Eugenics, American Racism, and German National Socialism*, Oxford Univ. Press, New York, Oxford, p. 101.

14 Lewis, S. (1925), *Arrowsmith*. Brace, Hartcourt, New York.

15 Dooley, D.J. (1967), *The Art of Sinclair Lewis*. The University of Nebraska Press, Lincoln, pp. 110.

16 On the ambiguities of the work of the World Medical Association since its creation, cf. Seidelman, W. (1995), 'Whither Nuremberg?: Medicine's Continuing Nazi Heritage', *Medicine & Global Survival* Vol 2: 148-157. This article, in my opinion, judiciously sheds light on the conclusions drawn in G. Herranz's study of the evolution of ethical norms after Nuremberg (in the present volume).

4 The Nuremberg Code in Light of Previous Principles and Practices in Human Experimentation

David J. Rothman

In the fifty years since the issuance of the Nuremberg Code, the ethics of human experimentation has assumed such centrality in social thought and public policy that it requires an act of imagination to recall just how novel this event was. Nuremberg represented the first attempt to set forth and enforce an explicit set of principles, literally a code, in the conduct of human experimentation. Whatever weaknesses commentators would later identify, and whatever refinements marked the content of successor codes, Nuremberg was the pioneer effort to implement standards that clinical investigators were required to observe.

Its originality as a code notwithstanding, Nuremberg was certainly not the earliest effort to analyze the ethics of human experimentation. Already in the thirteenth century, the English philosopher Roger Bacon had explained that progress in medicine would never come as quickly as in the natural sciences because scientists could "multiply their experiments till they get rid of deficiency and errors". The physician, on the other hand, was unable to do this "because of the nobility of the material in which he works".[1] Over the years, many individuals proposed appropriate standards for investigators to follow and decried particular abuses in practice. But until Nuremberg, there was practically no professional or public governance of human experimentation.

Thus, to appreciate the degree to which Nuremberg built on the past precedents and the degree to which it represented a novel departure, it is necessary to examine the state of clinical research and ethics in the pre-1947 period. First, in terms of principles, what obligations did the investigator owe the subject? What information was to be shared? What degree of consent, if any, was necessary? Second, in terms of practice, were the principles respected by investigators? Did they live up to the standards? Finally, to the extent that practice diverged from principle, what efforts were made at enforcing standards? Were penalties levied on errant researchers, either by legally constituted bodies or professional organizations?

50

All of these questions are of obvious relevance to the history of medicine. But no less important, particularly as we observe its fiftieth anniversary, they are essential to framing the contribution of the Nuremberg Code itself. At the trial of the Nazi doctors, defense attorneys claimed that before World War Two the ethics of human experimentation were undeveloped, both in the United States and Germany. Principles of voluntariness and of consent, they argued, were poorly understood and usually ignored. American physicians, no less than German ones, paid no heed to consent and frequently carried out experiments on ignorant and unwilling subjects. These points certainly establish Nuremberg's novelty, but at the price of finding a fatal flaw in the prosecution of the Nazi doctors. Nuremberg becomes an exercise in ex post facto punishment, setting new standards and then imposing them on the defendants. To be sure, the conviction and punishment of the offenders could easily be justified by ruling that their acts were so horrendous that they constituted a crime against humanity. They had committed war crimes, including the murder of innocent civilians; indeed, the Nuremberg court offered this very judgment: "the record clearly shows the commission of war crimes and crimes against humanity". But instead of stopping there it continued on to address the issue of "Permissible Medical Experiments". Ultimately, it condemned the Nazi doctors for unethical research; they were guilty as physicians, not as civilians, of "violating moral, ethical and legal concepts", not in a more straightforward sense, of murder. Precisely why the court eschewed war crimes and addressed human experimentation as such has never been satisfactorily explained. But whatever the reason, the court's posture brought unprecedented attention to the ethics of human experimentation.

Ethical Principles in Human Experimentation before Nuremberg

The modern history of the ethics of human experimentation begins with Claude Bernard's 1865 book, *An Introduction to the Study of Experimental Medicine*. No one more cogently than Bernard delineated the potential contribution that clinical research could make to medicine. So vital was it that Bernard regarded human experimentation as the third pillar of medical knowledge. As he traced it, physicians first based their treatments upon findings made through their senses, that is, what they saw and heard through direct and intimate encounters with the patient. They felt the pulse, noted the color of the face, examined the urine, and listened to the chest, initially by putting their ear to it, later by using a stethoscope. Physicians, Bernard continued, learned to do more than rely upon their senses. They also "observed", by which he meant that they grouped facts together and formulated hypotheses; they made predictions about treatment outcomes and then studied whether they proved right. In this way, observation was essential to determining which interventions were effective. From Bernard's perspective, however, this exercise was essentially passive. The physician stood back and collected data, wisely and shrewdly, but from a distance.

It was the third form of knowledge that Bernard celebrated, what might be called "active observation". To clarify its meaning and implications, Bernard invoked the French naturalist, Georges Cuvier: "the observer listens to nature; the experimenter questions [nature] and forces her to unveil herself". In his own terms:

> Experimenters must be able to touch the body on which they act, whether by destroying it or by altering it, so as to learn the part which it plays in the phenomena of nature...It is on this very possibility of acting, or not acting, on a body that the distinction will exclusively rest between sciences called sciences of observation and sciences called experimental.

The very language with which Bernard describes experimentation establishes its potency, not only in terms of its ability to create knowledge but to generate ethical problems as well. Bernard's experimenter "touches" parts of the body, not gently, but to destroy it or alter it so as to learn more about its biological function. In this way, the investigator forces nature to "unveil herself", and in the process, he himself becomes an aggressor, indeed, something of a sexual molester as he strips nature of her secrets.

Had Bernard stopped his analysis of clinical research there, the development of human experimentation in the nineteenth century would appear as an exercise in the ruthless accumulation of knowledge, one that was deaf to the decencies of humanity or principles of ethics. But Bernard went on, and after exploring the epistemology and methods of clinical research, he declared in passages now famous:

> Experiments, then, may be performed on man, but within what limits? It is our duty and our right to perform an experiment on man whenever it can save his life, cure him or gain him some benefit. The principle of medical and surgical morality, therefore, consists in never performing on man an experiment which might be harmful to him to any extent, even though the result might be highly advantageous to science, i.e., to the health of others.

Bernard provides a frank and full recognition of the power of human experimentation to do good and to do harm. And with this double-edged potential in mind, he insists that research must always be in the best interests of the subject. If an experiment has the potential to cure, it may be carried out. But if it has no therapeutic potential and may injure the subject, it must not be conducted, regardless of how important the findings might be for others.

Obviously, Bernard's maxims are not fully in accord with contemporary principles, particularly given the scant attention he paid to the idea and meaning of consent. But others among his contemporaries not only echoed his insightful judgments but on occasion went beyond them, incorporating principles of consent into their own frameworks.

This was certainly true of the great American clinician, William Osler. Properly credited with bringing scientific methods into medical education and clinical practice, Osler, as would be expected, was fully appreciative of the vital role of human experimentation. In 1907, he addressed "The Evolution of the Idea of Experiment in Medicine", sounding very much like Claude Bernard, and when it came to consent, superseding him.[2]

Like Bernard, Osler emphasized both the enormous capacity of clinical medicine to generate new knowledge and its highly invasive characteristics. In his formulation, "Man can interrogate as well as observe nature", and through this process, lighten many of "the burdens of humanity." Even more consistently than Bernard, Osler believed that experimentation was part and parcel of the conduct of clinical practice: "Every dose of medicine given is an experiment as it is impossible in every instance to predict what the result may be". Even so he, too, insisted on setting limits on human experimentation. First, experiments on man must never be carried out before they had been tried on animals. Second, and here departed from Bernard, Osler not only ruled out non-therapeutic research but required investigators to obtain the consent of the subject:

> For man absolute safety and full consent are the conditions which make such tests allowable. We have no right to use patients entrusted to our care for the purpose of experimentation unless direct benefit to the individual is likely to follow. Once this limit is transgressed, the sacred cord which binds physician and patient snaps instantly.

In effect, Osler enunciated the principles of consent well in advance of this proposition in the Nuremberg Code.

The viewpoints expressed by Bernard and Osler were shared widely. In 1886, a less prominent Boston physician, Charles Francis Withington, published an essay entitled, *The Relation of Hospitals to Medical Education*. The position he advocated were regarded as so important that his contribution won the prestigious Boylston Prize from Harvard University. Withington posed the ethical question in terms of the "possible conflict between the interests of medical science and those of the individual patient, and the latter's indefeasible rights". He was not at all confident that investigators satisfactorily resolved the conflict, and in truth, he himself had some trouble drawing boundaries between the needs of science and the "rights" (his term) of patients. But in the end, he came down staunchly on the side of rights, to the point of suggesting a remedy of a patient "Bill of Rights" which would not be adopted for another 90 years:

> In the older countries of Europe especially, where the life and happiness of the so-called lower classes are perhaps held more cheaply than with us, enthusiastic devotees of science are very apt to encroach upon the rights of the individual patient in a manner which cannot be justified. In this country, we

are less likely to fall into this error than those living under monarchical institutions, but even with us it may be well to draw up, as it were, a Bill of Rights which shall secure patients against any injustice from the votaries of science.

Withington insisted that patients had "a right to immunity from experiments merely *as such*, and outside the therapeutic application. This right is one that is especially liable to violation by enthusiastic investigators". Researchers who wished to try a new drug had to rely upon volunteers. In his view, "They had no right to make any man the unwilling victim of such an experiment".[3] He then concluded with a sentence that encapsulated the core principals of medical ethics: "The occupants of hospital wards are something more than merely so much clinical material during their lives and so much pathological material after their death".[4]

Although other texts reiterating these same principles could be easily marshalled, these three make apparent that the ethical dimensions of clinical research were recognized by physicians who advanced the development of modern medicine. Such a conclusion ought not to be surprising, for the bedrock principle on which they rested their analyses was as old as medical ethics itself: do not harm, neither to the patient nor to the subject. Experimentation was bound by the ethics of the doctor-patient relationship, which, as we shall see, was a useful starting point, although not an altogether adequate model upon which to base the regulation of human experimentation.

All these writings drew a sharp distinction between therapeutic and non-therapeutic research, and were far more concerned with the latter than the former. They had little difficulty in condemning non-therapeutic research, especially when it placed the subject-patient at risk. But what was almost completely absent from their analysis was a discussion of the ethical principles that should govern experiments with a therapeutic potential. What was the physician obliged to tell the patient about an experiment that might benefit him? Was consent required? Who was to make the calculus of risk of harm versus benefit of cure? By ignoring this set of issues and focusing so exclusively on non-therapeutic research, these commentators make the intent and motive of the physician-researcher the critical determinant. Were he seeking new knowledge and not attempting to benefit the patient, then he was obliged to share information with the subject and obtain consent. But were his intentions to cure or to treat, then apparently he did not have to divulge the facts or obtain the patient's acquiescence to the procedure. Thus, the position adopted (which would remain intact for many decades) was consistent with the tradition in medical ethics of trusting to the integrity of the physician, not requiring formal collegial oversight or consultation or the patient's agreement. So long as the researcher's self-styled purpose was to benefit the patient, he enjoyed an ample discretion unfettered by colleagues or patients. In brief, the mindset of the physician, not the autonomy of the subject, drove the ethical analysis.

The Practice of Human Experimentation before Nuremberg

The uniformity that marked the discussions of the ethical principles in research disappears when one examines the actual practices of investigators, and the reactions to them by the medical profession and the public. Here one finds countless examples of research conduct that blatantly violates the prevailing ethical norms. In a similar vein, one finds some observers outraged by the transgressions and others far more complaisant. The one generalization that can be offered is that no matter how grievous the ethical misconduct in research, professional disciplinary action or some collective expression of censure or disapproval almost never occurred. With a handful of exceptions, investigators who freely disobeyed all the norms set forth by a Bernard or an Osler paid no price for it.

The historical record, particularly as explored by Susan A. Lederer, makes abundantly clear that many investigators demonstrated scant regard for the rights or well-being of subjects. They conducted non-therapeutic research on unknowing or incompetent persons, putting them at risk and causing direct and serious harms. In 1904, a southern physician, Claude Smith, purposefully infected blacks with hookworm to study the transmission of the disease and did not give them the slightest hint as to what he was actually doing. "The patient", Smith stated in his published report, "seemed to have an idea that it was some medicine preparatory to the operation, as nothing was said to him about it".[5] In 1883, George Fitch, resident physician at an Hawaiian leper colony, purposely infected some unknowing 18 leprosy patients with syphilis to prove the similarities between the two diseases.[6] Another of his colleagues infected relatives of leprosy patients who themselves were free of the disease with the leprosy organism to study transmission. "A splendid field for experimental work was at hand", he candidly wrote, "and stretching all questions of professional ethics, I did not hesitate to avail myself of the opportunities afforded me for testing the inoculability of leprosy".[7]

Some research protocols inflicted such egregious harm on subjects as to earn the condemnation of other investigators. The research by the Italian bacteriologist Guiseppe Sanarelli was a case in point. To prove that he had isolated the bacillus that caused yellow fever, he infected five Montevideo hospital patients with it and claimed (mistakenly) that he had produced the disease in them. William Osler led the attack on the ethics of his research: "[T]o deliberately inject a poison of known high degree of virulency into a human being, unless you obtain that man's sanction, is not ridiculous, it is criminal".[8] In a later and fuller elaboration of this point, Osler explained:

> The limitations of deliberate experimentation upon human beings should be clearly defined. Voluntarily, if with full knowledge, a fellow-creature may submit to certain tests, just as a physician may experiment upon himself. Drugs, the value of which has been carefully tested in animals and are found harmless may be tried on patients, since in this way alone may progress be made, but deliberate experiments such as Sanarelli carried on with cultures of

known and tested virulence, and which were followed by nearly fatal illnesses, are simply criminal.[9]

In much these same terms, Osler, and many other colleagues as well, condemned the cancer research that had been conducted by two German surgeons, both of whom took malignant cells from the diseased breast of a patient and injected them into the other, healthy, breast, to study the transmissibility of cancer cells. *The Journal of the American Medical Association* reported the incidents, applauding the subsequent refusal of a French medical academy to discuss the findings because they were obtained in so unethical a fashion. It hoped that "the storm of indignation which has been aroused, shall deter others who might have in view, in their zeal for science, [conducted] similar unjustifiable experiments".[10]

The roster of non-therapeutic research on uninformed subjects could be extended almost indefinitely. In 1911, Hideyo Noguchi injected several hundred residents of a New York orphan asylum with an experimental substance, Luetin, to learn whether it might serve to indicate the presence of syphilis. Other researchers used orphans to test the efficacy of tuberculin as a vaccine against tuberculosis as well as to trace the development of such dietary deficiencies as scurvy. So too, researchers subjected black infants at an Atlanta, Georgia hospital to lumbar punctures without the permission of their parents. One investigator even went so far as to infect an infant with the herpes virus for experimental purposes. As with orphans, prisoners were used as subjects in non-therapeutic and harmful protocols, including one protocol that imposed a diet designed to cause pellagra, and another that injected ameba in order to study the course of dysentery. Finally, investigators in the 1920s used prisoners in San Quentin, California to study the effects of implants of testicles taken from executed prisoners and rams.[11]

The Disparities between Ethics and Practice

The research protocols that so flagrantly violated the existing ethical precepts in human experimentation were not carried out covertly or kept hidden from view. To the contrary, the findings were published in the major and widely read medical journals. Nevertheless, the conduct did not incite professional criticism, let alone discipline, except in a handful of cases. To be sure, Osler and several colleagues forcefully condemned some of the protocols described here, including the yellow fever and breast cancer examples. But these were individual reactions and the occasional efforts made to move beyond that to a more official condemnation or censure failed.

Why this professional passivity before these violations of ethics? First, such bodies as the American Medical Association had little authority or organizational standing. Well into the opening decades of the twentieth century, when the profession had managed to impose some standards on medical education and medical licensing, it still did not yet enjoy sufficient status or cohesion to act in concert in the arena of human experimentation. Second, and closely related to its lower status, the profession was unwilling to draw greater attention to ethical misdeeds for fear of arming its critics, particularly the outspoken members of anti-vivisection societies. To concede that some investigators acted irresponsibly was to give ammunition to those who thought that all investigators acted irresponsibly, and thereby subvert the entire research enterprise. Commenting on a recent discussion in the German parliament on research which purposefully infected prostitutes with syphilis, the *Journal of the American Medical Association* joined in the condemnation of the research but, apprehensive about lay reactions, added: "If laymen would divert their attention to charlatans...the world would be benefited, while these attacks on the regular profession tend to impair the confidence of the public in trained physicians and thus they fall easy prey to unscrupulous quacks".[12] The contention was by no means ill-founded. There was a popular and widespread suspicion about what went on in medical laboratories. Even so, the professional response to the violations was exceptionally timid.

Third, the absence of collective action may reflect the fact that the human subjects put at risk and harmed were almost always marginal to the society. They were poor Southern blacks, or prison inmates, or residents of orphan asylums, themselves vulnerable in all so many ways to abuse but outside the net of public concern. To mount a campaign on their behalf would have been extraordinary, and a reluctance to do so - particularly if it might lower the prestige of medical research - is not altogether surprising. The researchers, in the end, were abusing *other* peoples's bodies.

Human Experimentation in the United States, 1940-1945

The record that we have explored here provides the context for understanding the conduct of human experimentation in the United States during World War Two. The challenges that military needs posed for American medicine were pressing, including how to protect soldiers against malaria, particularly when the Japanese controlled the supply of quinine; how to protect them against influenza, especially in the wake of the 1919 pandemic; and how to protect them against dysentery. Investigators diligently attempted to develop vaccines or antidotes and to these ends, human experimentation was vital. There were few useful animal models available and to compound the difficulties, malaria was not naturally occurring in the United States, dysentery was rare, and influenza unpredictable. For obvious reasons, the diseases could not be researched where they were found, that is, under battlefield conditions. This meant that researchers had to create the very conditions that they had to study. Put more directly, they had to infect subjects with the disease organisms and test their preparations against them for efficacy.

How did the investigators recruit subjects for their research and were they respectful of the norms of consent and do no harm? In the overwhelming majority of cases, the answer is no. The subjects were typically made up of institutionalized mentally disabled persons (suffering from mental illness or mental retardation), institutionalized orphans, and prisoners. None of them were truly capable of giving consent, certainly not the mentally incompetent or the orphaned children, and (although this point has been debated) not convicts deprived of liberty, living in conditions of severe deprivation, and under total state control. Thus, the researchers violated long-standing ethical norms by carrying out non-therapeutic experiments that were dangerous and lacked subject's consent.

In specific terms, researchers conducted their studies on dysentery in state institutions for the retarded. Indeed, government research grants favored investigators who had "access to various state institutions where facilities for study of dysentery are unexcelled", precisely because hygienic conditions were so primitive. Researchers also carried out their investigations in orphan asylums; the boys at the Ohio Soldiers and Sailors Orphanage, were injected with "killed suspensions for various types of shigella group of bacteria", to see whether the compounds would protect against dysentery. Unfortunately, the preparations proved highly toxic, causing fevers on the average of 104 degrees Fahrenheit and leaving the boys exhausted.

The influenza research used subjects residing in state facilities for the retarded, in correctional centers for juvenile offenders, and in state hospitals for the chronic mentally ill. The protocols divided the residents in two - one group received the trial vaccine, the other a placebo, and then both were challenged with influenza virus. The vaccines proved to be of varying efficacy, but all the control group and for many of the active agent group contracted high fevers and suffered aches, pains, and debilitation.

The bulk of the malaria research went on in state mental hospitals and prisons. In one series of experiments, psychotic, backward patients were infected with malaria through blood transfusions and then given experimental anti-malarial therapies. A psychiatrist was a member of the team, but his function was not to determine the subjects' competency to give consent but to explain their symptoms to the investigative team.[13]

Thus, the marked disparity between the principles of research ethics and the reality of laboratory practices prior to the issuance of the Nuremberg Code confirms the import of promulgating a formal code. In its absence, individuals cogently and persuasively defined the rules of conduct that should govern human experimentation, but their precepts lacked formal standing or authority. What was so crucial, then, about the Nuremberg Code was not so much its content as its form. Its authors correctly insisted that the guidelines expressed well known and established values. Its uniqueness lies in the fact that these principles were formally endorsed by a court and presented as a code.

Thus, to understand the history of human experimentation immediately after Nuremberg, it must be remembered that this codification of principles owed little to organized medical bodies. The prosecutors called physicians as witnesses and used them as consultants, but the document stood as the work of judges and its stipulations were realized through a court, not through professional medical bodies. In essence, the initial regulatory effort in human experimentation was external to medicine - which helps to account for both its weaknesses and strengths in the post-World War Two period. This circumstance enables us to understand, on the one hand, why Nuremberg exerted so little impact on the practice of human experimentation. In the United States, for example, the Code seemed aimed at Nazis and madmen, not at bone fide physicians and researchers. But on the other hand, the Code helped to bridge the gap between medicine and other disciplines, initiating a concern for medical ethics among legal scholars, religious ethicists, and philosophers. Finally, the Code set an example that eventually influenced the policies of medical organizations. Nuremberg was the critical precedent for the formal and collective pronouncements of such bodies as the American Medical Association and the World Medical Association. What began outside the domain of medicine came, in time, to be integrated into medicine.

Notes

1   Quoted to Bull, J.P. (1959), 'The Historical Development of Clinical Therapeutic Trials', *Journal of Chronic Diseases*, 10, p. 222.

2   *Transactions Cong. Am. Phys. Surg.*(1907), 7, 1, pp. 7-8.

3   Withington was also alert to the possibilities of non-therapeutic experiments on terminally ill patients. An investigator, he insisted, "has no right to take advantage of the patient's extremity to *recommend* a procedure which can have no other advantage than to enhance the operator's reputation for boldness".

4   Withington, Charles Francis. (1886), *The Relation of Hospitals to Medical Education*, Boston, Cupples, Upham, p. 15.

5   Smith, Claude A. (1904), 'Uncinariasis in the South with Special Reference to Mode of Infection', *JAMA*, 43, p. 596.

6   Lederer, Susan E. (1995), *Subjected to Science: Human Experimentation in America before the Second World War*, New York, Oxford University Press, pp. 17, 16.

7   Mouritz, A. A. St. M. (1951), 'Human Inoculation Experiments in Hawaii including Notes of Arning and Fitch', condensed, arranged and annotated by W. Wade, *International Journal of Leprosy*, 19, p. 205.

8   Sternberg, George M. (1898), 'The Bacillus Icteroides (Sanarelli) and Bacillus X (Sternberg)', *Transactions of the Association of American Physicians*, 13, p. 71 (discussion of paper by Osler).

9   Quoted by Lederer. (1995), *Subjected to Science*, p. 63.

10   'Grafting Cancer in the Human Subject'. (1891), *JAMA*, 17, p. 234.

11   Lederer, Susan E. (1995), *Subjected to Science*, pp. 110-111.

12   'Experiments on Human Beings' (1900), *JAMA*, 34, p. 1359.

13   For further details of the American wartime research see, David J. Rothman. (1991), *Strangers at the Bedside*, New York, Basic Books, chapter two.

5 The Medical Experiments in Nazi Concentration Camps

Bernard Kanovitch

On October 26, 1946 an American military tribunal was formed to judge those responsible for the medical experiments that had been conducted under the National Socialist regime.

The doctors' trial (from November 21, 1946 to August 21, 1947) was the first of twelve trials called "Subsequent Proceedings" or "Proceedings Involving Various Groups of Professionals" that took place in Nuremberg following the trials of Nazi war criminals who had been brought before the International Military Tribunal. Of the 23 defendants, 20 were doctors, the highest ranking among them being Karl Brandt, the Reich Commissioner of Health. Found guilty of war crimes, crimes against humanity, and membership in a criminal organization, seven of them were sentenced to death and executed in 1948; nine others received ten to twenty years' imprisonment or were given life imprisonment. All motions for appeal were dismissed. The defendants pleaded not guilty, *nicht schuldig*, as did nearly all the Nazis brought to court after the war.

These proceedings brought to light some of the most horrifying atrocities of human history, as expressed by the inconceivable suffering and solitude of those deported, those who had become victims of the experiments and who thus became enmeshed in events that Hanna Arendt[1] described during the Eichmann trial as the experience of human guinea pigs being "radically extirpated from society". Most of them were Jews, but there were also Gypsies, Poles, Russians, clergy, and others, all without regard to whether they were men, women, or children. The atrocities committed against these human who had not been previously informed about the experiments, that had not been conducted for their benefit and for which they would not have given their consent anyway, were a nagging disgrace for those doctors responsible and for the regime that had permitted and even fostered such experiments. The authorization to use human beings for research experiments had been given by none other than Himmler himself, the senior Chief of Police and *Reichsführer* of the SS. Those responsible had veiled these events in a curtain of utmost secrecy.

Despite the problems this may engender, a distinction must be made between medical experiments and murders, the latter referring to what R.J. Lifton calls "medicalized killing".[2] The greatest possible number of people are killed thanks to highly refined technological advancements, with

60

doctors actively or passively present to give the procedure its scientific legitimization.

Medicalized killing primarily involved the euthanasia and sterilization programs. Euthanasia is a chapter of its own in the history of National Socialism. In general, all whose lives were deemed by the medical commissions as being "unworthy of life" were killed. Among these individuals were the mentally disturbed, the incurably ill, all Jews with chronic or other illnesses, all ill foreigners, mentally disturbed criminals, children and adults with handicaps or degenerative illnesses both with and without psychoses, even World War I invalids. Sterilizations were performed either via surgical intervention or by means of X-rays in various blocks of the concentration camps, especially in Auschwitz.

As far as the medical experiments are concerned, it is worthy of note that eye-witness testimonies confirm their reality. These witnesses were deportees, who had become victims of such practices, and deported physicians, who became direct eye-witnesses to these events, at times even being forced into committing acts of cruelty, performing surgical intervention, or giving injections and diverse inoculations themselves.[3] Their testimonies were further supported by the documents of the Nuremberg Medical Trial[4] and the copious correspondence between Nazi doctors, the directors of the concentration camps as well as between Himmler and Hitler. Despite this abundance of sources that corroborate each other, there are still certain difficulties in describing in clinical terms the misdeeds that had been perpetrated. The documents which would have normally been kept in the hospital wards or the *Reviers* of the concentration camps were deliberately destroyed. Also, very often the obligation to maintain secrecy was respected by the camp physicians and the responsible political agents in the Nazi hierarchy. After all, the "experiments" were for the most part carried out without the slightest therapeutic intention, often even without having the desire to further knowledge. The actual goal of these experiments was to cause suffering, humiliation, and death. The following list of experiments, which is by no means complete, provides some insight into what took place.

The Experiments Performed by Nazi Doctors[5]

Experiments on altitude

This was a series of experiments that were conducted from February to July of 1942 in a mobile hypobaric chamber set up inside the Dachau concentration camp with the full support of Himmler, the doctors of the *Luftwaffe*, and the SS. There were two different groups of subjects overseen by two different scientific teams. One team, headed by Drs. Ruff and Romberg of the "German Institute of Aeronautic Research" in Berlin, studied the problem of "rescuing people from high altitudes". The 10 - 15 inmates involved, termed "exposed experimental subjects", were volunteers with German citizenship. They were well treated and survived these experiments unharmed.

The second series of experiments focussed on the ability of humans to withstand high altitudes and was overseen by the *Stabsarzt* (Captain in the Medical Corps), Dr. Rascher of the *Luftwaffe*, who was initially an *SS-Untersturmführer* as well and had direct connections to Himmler. Seventy to 80 of those 150-200 tested, deportees who had been selected at random from among the camp inmates, died in these experiments.

Studies on Exposure to Cold

At the outset of 1942, in view of the large number of pilots who had been shot down over the North Sea and the sufferings of the German troops who had been caught by surprise by the Russian winter, the Inspectorate of the *Luftwaffe* Medical Corps entrusted Dr. E. Holzlöner, a professor and physiologist at the University of Kiel, with the task of studying the effect of the cold on warm-blooded animals. Upon Rascher's suggestion, the project was extended to include human beings and was conducted again under Holzlöner's direction in the SS facilities at Dachau. Rascher supported the project with Himmler's approval and began to carry out research himself pertaining to dry and damp cold from August of 1942 to May of 1943. He would make naked subjects stay outdoors in the freezing cold or make deportees stay submerged in vats of iced water either in the nude or partly clothed in some manner. Once the subjects' central body temperature had been lowered, Rascher tested various methods of re-warming and resuscitating the individual. He had recruited 200 to 300 individuals from the ranks of the political prisoners and prisoners of war for the 300 to 400 experiments. Eighty to 90 of them died in the process.

Experiments on Making Sea Water Potable

As of May 1944, Dachau became the setting for experiments with sea water. They were overseen by Dr. W. Beigelböck, Senior Physician and Professor at the First Medical University Hospital in Vienna and a *Stabsarzt* of the *Luftwaffe*. The decision to carry out this research program had come from both the *Luftwaffe* and the Navy. Of the approximately 60 healthy gypsies who had been enlisted for the experiments in Buchenwald with the prospect of being transferred to a better work crew, 44 had served effectively as experimental subjects. The goal of the experiment was to compare two well-known methods of desalinating sea water: Schaefer's method, with which salt water can be fully transformed into potable water through a complicated and costly process, and Berka's method, which eliminated the salty taste without actually removing the salt.[6] None of the subjects died during these experiments.

Experiments on Mustard Gas ("Lost") and Phosgene

For nearly the entire duration of World War II, experiments were conducted in the concentration camps of Sachsenhausen and Natzweiler-Struthof, the latter near Strasbourg, to find methods for treating casualties resulting from chemical warfare. Those involved with these and the same type of experiments previously conducted on animals were the full professor of anatomy of the "Reichsuniversity of Strasbourg", Dr. A. Hirt, who was also a *Hauptsturmführer* of the SS, Dr. K. Wimmer, a private docent, as well as Dr. O. Bickenbach, a professor and the head of both the Medical Polyclinic there and his own "medical research institute".

Experiments with mustard gas *("Lost")* were conducted on approximately 150 individuals all of whom suffered absolutely unbearable agony and many of whom died. Experimental subjects were Germans, Gypsies, Czechs, and Russian and Polish prisoners of war as well as inmates of the Sachsenhausen concentration camp who had been brought to Alsace. Two sets of experiments were conducted pertaining to phosgene: one set was under the sole direction of Bickenbach, apparently without the loss of human life, the other was under the direction of a research team comprising two other SS doctors beside Bickenbach and Hirt. According to Bickenbach's testimony, the latter set of experiments had provoked at least four deaths and had induced severe pulmonary problems among the survivors.

Pharmacological Experiments

With the approval of Himmler, the SS *Reichsarzt* (approximately equivalent in rank to a surgeon general), the police, Dr. E. Grawitz, and the head of the Hygiene Institute of the *Waffen-SS*, namely the professor Dr. J. Mrugowsky, new medications were tested on camp inmates. This was done primarily in the "Department for the Research of Typhus Fever and Viruses" in the concentration camp at Buchenwald under the direction of the camp physician and *SS Hauptsturmführer*, Dr. E. Ding-Schuler. In reality, however, this was the SS division for human experiments. Despite the little information that we have about these highly classified experiments, we do know that diamine phenylsulfone, then a newly synthesized sulfa drug, was tested in 1944 on deliberately infected typhus patients. In addition, in 1944 and 1945 synthetic hormones were implanted in the Buchenwald infirmary under the guidance of the Swedish physician, Vernet.

In 1942 or at the beginning of 1943, the Jewish chemist and Dachau inmate, R. Feix, discovered a hemostatic agent with which Rascher wished to conduct experiments. He called it Homlag, then Polygal, and finally Styptoral.

On October 7, 1943 Grawitz obtained Himmler's permission to test an ointment for treating phosphorus burns on "disabled" inmates of the Sachsenhausen camp. The Reich Commissioner's Office for Health headed by Brandt had sent him the ointment. The experiments were underway again in November under Ding-Schuler. The experiment consisted in inflicting burns in the forearm of inmates and then applying said ointment at varying intervals. Since in most cases the inflicted burns were highly severe, it is questionable whether they healed completely. It goes without saying that the experimental subjects suffered immensely.

Experiments Using Anti-gangrene Serum

At the end of 1942, a number of cases of septicemia that had been caused by an anti-gangrene serum containing phenol led the military authorities and official medical agencies to study the effect of phenol on the human body in greater detail. Phenol had been known since the 1870s as an antiseptic, i.e. an agent against wound infection. Upon Mrugowsky's behest, Ding-Schuler injected phenol in the bodies of the deportees in his department in Buchenwald.

In the presence of these two men, an experiment was performed there on September 11, 1944 using poisoned projectiles. Under the pretext of looking for an antidote, five Russian prisoners of war who had been sentenced to death were shot in the leg with bullets containing aconitine. Three of them died after two hours of agony because the bullet had become lodged in the flesh.

Other prisoners of war from the Sachsenhausen camp had to serve as guinea pigs in experiments intended to enhance the action of potassium cyanide tablets. These experiments were given the support of high-ranking SS officials as a preparation for their eventual suicide. However, it is not certain as to why - whether for the purpose of suicide or homicide - these experiments with poisons, which were either added to food or administered directly *per os*, were needed.

The experiments to decontaminate water that had been contaminated by ostensibly harmless gases served in developing a water purification process in the event of chemical warfare.

The Typhus Experiments

From December 1941 to nearly the end of the war, large-scale trials were conducted in Buchenwald and Natzweiler-Struthof to test various inoculations against a number of diseases, especially: typhus, yellow fever, smallpox, paratyphoid fever A and B, cholera, and diphtheria. The typhus fever experiments were extremely horrible. Test subjects were always inoculated with the test vaccine and later infected. The controls were infected without having been previously vaccinated. In the case of the typhus fever experiments, the subjects were only infected in order to have enough bacterial carriers available in the camp. Yet another medical professor from Strasbourg, Dr. E. Haagen, was the director of the experiments in Natzweiler; in Buchenwald Dr. Ding-Schuler and Dr. Mrugowsky were among those in charge. All told, there were still at least ten other doctors involved in the experiments.

The Experiments with Sulfa Drugs

These crucial experiments had been performed in the Ravensbrück concentration camp between July 1942 and August 1943. Among the troops stationed on the Russian front in the winter of 1941/42, gas gangrene had led to major losses and a crisis in confidence with regard to the troop physicians. For this reason, the authorities intended to improve treatment for this disease, most likely with sulfa drugs. However, just before the experimentation program could begin, the high-ranking SS dignitary, Heydrich, died from his wounds and gas gangrene in June of 1942. Dr. K. Gebhardt, a professor and chief physician of an Orthopedic Hospital near Ravensbrück as well as advisory surgeon for the *Waffen-SS* had not been able to save Heydrich. He now wished to "show that wound infections could not be healed with sulfa drugs and that in order to do so both the seriously ill and the deceased were [needed]".[7] Hence, prisoners were deliberately infected to induce gas gangrene. One group of these subjects served as a control and was not treated with sulfa drugs. The subjects were misled into believing they would be pardoned. They suffered severe pain and several even died. Grawitz was also involved in this program.

Experiments on Bones and Muscles

These experiments were conducted in Ravensbrück concomitantly with or following those with sulfa drugs and were directed by the *Stabsarzt*, Dr. Stumpfegger, a friend of Himmler's who had also become Hitler's attending physician after Brandt had fallen from favor. The experiments consisted of first breaking bones, generally the tibia, and then immobilizing them with splints or clamps. If the leg had been put in a plaster cast, the cast was removed before the fracture had properly healed. In addition, after the deliberate surgical removal of bones, a number of bone transplants was performed for purely experimental purposes. Professor Gebhardt had also been involved in these experiments. Incisions had been made on the tibia for the purpose of removing bone fragments at a later date. Following muscle operations, the victims suffered from atrophy of the muscles (myatrophy) in the leg region.

Experiments Pertaining to Phlegmons and Various Bacterial Infections

As early as August of 1942, Grawitz and the *SS-Standartenführer*, Dr. T. Lauer, who was an advocate of the alternative form of medicine referred to as "biochemistry", sent a report to Himmler, who was just as much an opponent of mainstream medicine as they were, about the first experiments using "biochemical" and homeopathic treatment methods on phlegmons.

Further experiments parallel to these took place up until 1943 in Dachau under the direction of Grawitz together with another "biochemical" physician, Dr. Kiesewetter of Magdeburg and three SS physicians of the camp. First, the inmates were artificially infected with pus. Pus was removed from the abscesses that frequently developed among the deportees and injected in others either intravenously, intramuscularly or intradermally. Sometimes the skin would also be scratched, pus would then be distributed in the wound which was then stitched/sutured. Primarily Catholic clergy and friars served as the subjects in these experiments.

The effects were terrible. The director of these experiments waited until huge abscesses the size of a dish formed only to then treat them either with sulfa drugs by incision, or with medical preparations according to "biochemical" indications (potassium phosphate), or with a homeopathic agent. The result was a mortality rate of about 20%. Each of the ten deportees who had died in this manner was carefully autopsied and the organs that were removed were subjected to microscopic examination. The likely purpose of such a procedure was to prove how the intravenous injection of pus infected the body and led to death by forming multiple abscesses.

Experiments Pertaining to the Treatment of Malaria

Long-term experiments on malaria immunization and treatment were conducted in Dachau under the direction of Dr. C. Schilling, a professor. About 1,100 healthy individuals of various nationalities, including Catholic clergy again, were inoculated with malaria. Gebhardt also informed Himmler about the purpose of such particularly infamous series of experiments: they were simply designed to cultivate human carriers of the infectious organisms so that these organisms could be removed for inoculating other individuals with the ultimate goal of finding a protective serum. The inoculations were protocolled with the utmost of care. Afterward, the ill were allegedly treated with quinine, a malarial agent that had been known for a long time, as well as with the antipyretics Pyramidon and Antipirin, with chemotherapeutic agents (Neosalvarsan), as well as various combinations of these medications. Viewed under these conditions, the purpose of these trials was clear. Thirty individuals died of malaria, while 300 to 400 died of complications due in part to excessively high doses of the medications.

Dr. Mengele's "Studies"

Of all the Nazi doctors, none is as well known as Dr. J. Mengele, a doctor in Auschwitz and an assistant to Dr. O. von Verschuer, a professor who was a radical advocate of racial hygiene. Mengele's "speciality" was his research on the anatomy and pathology of monozygous twins, dwarfs (based on a study about different cases of chondrodystrophy) and, as it seems and so he says himself, the noma, a relatively rare form of canker sore that appears primarily among the neglected and undernourished. It is well known that Mengele himself went to the ramp in Auschwitz and selected the twins for his experiments on the study of heterochromia (the different color) of the iris. According to the testimony of some witnesses, he had them play on his knees before killing them and removing their eyes which he then sent to the Frankfurt Institute for Hereditary Biology and Racial Hygiene that was run by Verschuer.

Collecting Jewish Skeletons

At the outset of 1941, Hirt told Himmler of his idea of setting up a collection of skulls of "Jewish Bolshevik Commissioners" together with other members of the "Society for Genealogical Ancestry": "Detailed skull collections are available of nearly all races and peoples", Hirt explained, "only not enough skulls of Jews are available for science so that no certain findings can be obtained about them. The war in the east now provides us with an opportunity to make up for this lack. The Jewish Bolshevik Commissioners who characterize a repulsive yet typical sub-category of human being, make it possible for us to obtain a tangible scientific document by seeing to it that we obtain their skulls".[8] Those who would come in question were taken prisoner alive on the Russian front, brought to Auschwitz, and transferred from there to Natzweiler-Struthof where they were gassed in August of 1943. Eighty-six bodies were then immediately brought to the Strasbourg Institute of Anatomy where they were preserved. As the Allied Troops advanced in September of 1944, some of the cadavers were burned, yet others were still in vats where they were later discovered.

Experiments and Medical Ethics

The issue of experimenting on humans had already been raised by Kant and Bernard.[9] How can experiments be conducted on human beings without harming them? How can the threshold for risks be stipulated in an experiment that is deemed necessary for the common good? Who bears the responsibility for medical acts ordered by the authorities? Death is an even more sensitive issue, since it concerns the philosophy of life and brings up the question of the value of human life and death such that placing less value on the one necessarily devalues the other as well. How could things be allowed to go so far that in our Western civilization doctors and biologists would help in setting limits that would stipulate when human life was no longer worthy of life, hence making it legitimate to destroy it? For the Nazis killing was considered a "merciful death" and not murder; the eradication of all "pathogens" was permitted for reasons of empathy, as in the struggle for survival.

And yet there are still people who point out the scientific significance of some of the experiments conducted by the National Socialists, particularly the experiments on hypothermia mentioned above. As of 1984 over 45 scientific publications have made reference to these experiments although they have been proven to be useless in the strict scientific sense, because the methods were dubious and the information inaccurate, even contradictory. In many cases the findings seem to have been fabricated and do not in any way coincide with what we now know about hypothermia.[10]

In May of 1988, a controversy ensued as Dr. Robert Pozos, the Director of the Hypothermic Research Laboratory of the University of Minnesota, used some findings from the Nazi experiments for his own papers. This researcher was of the opinion that the experiments of Dachau would be able to further the status of modern-day research, since they had gone beyond anything that we would ever expect of experimental subjects today. Regardless of the context in which these experiments had taken place, for Dr. Pozos they had become a scientific legacy to humanity. His decision to publish the papers of the Dachau doctors that had already been published in English in 1945 in a newly revised and corrected edition raised a storm of protest among scientists[11] and the heads of Jewish organizations throughout the United States, because to them the mere scientific aspect of experiments is no argument for publishing the findings of programmed crimes.

The unscientific nature of the Nazi experiments is all the more surprising in that they pursued a goal that was directly associated with the war. The experiments were supposed to help rescue German pilots who had been shot down over the North Sea. Rascher, the doctor whom Himmler entrusted with supervising these experiments was not only a repugnant sadist but also a notoriously incompetent swindler. The fact that he was entrusted with this task proves, if at all necessary, that the mixture of ideological fanaticism, cruelty, and incompetence is inherent to totalitarian systems. In addition, Rascher was an ingratiating flatterer, always eager to support the hypotheses of Himmler who liked to boast of his scientific knowledge. After all, the reason for the lax methodology of the experiments was that they were intolerable. Some of those in charge of the experiments deliberately falsified results in order to save lives. Conversely, the sadism of the torturers precluded any scientific objectivity whatsoever.[12]

The major research work of Eduard Wirths, chief physician in Auschwitz, about precancerous growths in the cervix is another significant example for the undependability of Nazi experiments. In this research project, the colposcope, a then-new experiment for observing the cervix, was being tested along with certain substances (acetic acid and an iodized compound). If certain changes were observed in the cervix, Wirths would remove it and send it to his brother's laboratory in Hamburg, although the examination with the colposcope was known to be unreliable. Also, it was not at all necessary to extirpate the entire cervix; it would have been enough to do a biopsy. The overall poor state of health of the camp inmates in Auschwitz fostered a number of complications, including infections and hemorrhages, which either led to death or left the victims in such poor condition that they were sent to the gas chamber.

This chapter is dedicated to the memory of those men, women, and children who became the victims of the worst acts of violence in the history of medicine and it should call to mind their loneliness and their suffering. It also intends to show the senselessness of these acts that were committed without the consent of the subjects and without the intend to heal or nurture, the only goal being to exert power and perpetrate suffering.

Today, 50 years after these horrible events, it is our duty to subject these facts, the immediate circumstances, those responsible as well as the decision-making authorities to even closer scrutiny. It is the obligation of historical research to carry out further investigations toward this goal, for many questions still remain to be answered.

How should one assess the most recent papers that lay claim to being scientific while being based on the experiments of Nazi doctors? The worthlessness and shocking nature of these so-called experiments should cause one to refrain from such a practice in all cases and to develop a strict ethical stance in the field of therapy and research on humans.

In addition, the Nazi doctors should not be regarded as mere executioners. The charges brought against them along the lines of moral and ethical violation of professional ethics weigh all the more heavily in view of the knowledge that they possessed and the possibility they had of conducting research programs on their own and of their own volition.

Last of all, the expression "medical experiment" poses problems in the context of the experiments described here. Naturally, all progress in medicine and biology requires preliminary experiments. But should that which occurred during World War II in the concentration camps of the National Socialists continue to be termed "experiments"? Certainly not. Yet this semantic problem will be difficult to resolve. What other term can be found that would make it possible to distinguish between experiments that further medical progress and those that, as we have seen, only have suffering, humiliation, and ultimately death as their goal?

Notes

1 Arendt, H. (1984), *Les origines du totalitarisme*, Le Seuil, Paris, pp. 226-227.

2 Lifton, R.J. (1986), *The Nazi Doctors and the Nuremberg Trial*, Paris, p.7.

3 Nyisl, Adélaide (1960), *Auschwitz: A Doctor's Eyewitness Account*, New York.

4 Cf. the trials of the major war criminals, particularly the publication of the French Scientific Committee on War Crimes headed by François Bayle entitled *Croix gammée contre caducée - les expériences humaines en Allemagne pendant la Deuxième Guerre Mondiale*.

5   Ibid. and the writings of Ternon, Y. (1969), *Histoire des médecins SS*, Casterman, Paris; Ternon, Y. (1971) *Le massacre des aliénés*, Castermann, Paris; Ternon, Y. (1973) *Les médecins allemands et le national-socialisme*, Casterman., Paris.

6   As a result it was concluded that Schaefer's method provides potable water while Berka's method is of no benefit.

7   Bayle, F., opt.cit., p. 1095.

8   Quoted in Mischerlich, A. and Mielke, F. (1960), *Medizin ohne Menschlichkeit*, Fischer, Frankfurt, p. 174.

9   Kant, Immanuel (1994), *Grundlegung zur Metaphysik der Sitten*, Meiner, Hamburg. Bernard, Claude (1966), *Introduction à l'étude de la médecine expérimentale*, Garnier-Flammarion, Paris. Cf. A.M. Moulin's chapter in this publication.

10   Berger, R. L. (1990), 'Nazi Science: The Dachau Hypothermia Experiments', *NEJM*, 330, pp. 14-40. See also Angell, M. (1990), 'The Nazi Hypothermia and Unethical Research Today', *id.*, 322, pp. 1462-1464.

11   Its title: "The treatment of shock caused by prolonged exposure to cold".

12   Berger, R. L. op.cit.

6 The Nuremberg Code: The Proceedings in the Medical Case, the Ten Principles of Nuremberg and the Lasting Effect of the Nuremberg Code

Erwin Deutsch

> Und also sei zum Schluß, was wir bisher betätigt,
> Für alle Folgezeit durch Schrift und Zug bestätigt!
> (Faust II "Des Gegenkaisers Zelt" 10970)

The Medical Case and the Ten Principles of Nuremberg, the So-called Nuremberg Code

In the years 1946 and 1947 at the palace of justice in Nuremberg took place the first of the so-called secondary war crime tribunals.[1] Three American state justices were sitting as judges in a military court. Indicted were 23 German doctors and high functionaries of the German health system. The indictment cited the crimes of conspiracy, war crimes and crimes against humanity as well as membership in criminal organizations. Of the 23 accused seven received the death penalty, seven more were sentenced to life, two of the accused got limited jail terms, and seven were acquitted. In normal terms the charges were murder as well as assault and battery against persons who were inmates of concentration camps. Since the injury was performed under the guise of medical interventions, the accused raised the defense of permissible medical experimentations. In order to distinguish between criminal assault and battery on the one hand and allowed medical research on the other the court formulated the ten principles of Nuremberg or the Nuremberg Code.[2]

The Nuremberg Code reads as follows:

1. The voluntary consent of the human subject is absolutely essential. This means that the person involved should have legal capacity to give consent; should be so situated as to be able to exercise free power of choice,

71

without the intervention of any element of force, fraud, deceit, duress, over-reaching, or other ulterior form of constraint or coercion; and should have sufficient knowledge and comprehension of the elements of the subject matter involved as to enable him to make an understanding and enlightened decision. This latter element requires that before the acceptance of an affirmative decision by the experimental subject there   should be made known to him the nature, duration, and purpose of the experiment; the method and means by which it is to be conducted; all inconveniences and hazards reasonably to be expected; and the effects upon his health or person which may possibly come from his participation in the experiment. The duty and responsibility for ascertaining the quality of the consent rests upon each individual who initiates, directs, or engages in the experiment. It is a personal duty and responsibility which may not be delegated to another with impunity.

2. The experiment should be such as to yield fruitful results for the good of society, unprocurable by other methods or means of study, and not random and unnecessary in nature.

3. The experiment should be so designed and based on the results of animal experimentation and a knowledge of the natural history of the disease or other problem under study that the anticipated results will justify the performance of the experiment.

4. The experiment should be so conducted as to avoid all unnecessary physical and mental suffering and injury.

5. No experiment should be conducted where there is an *a priori* reason to believe that death or disabling injury will occur; except, perhaps, in those experiments where the experimental physicians also serve as subjects.

6. The degree of risk to be taken should never exceed that determined by the humanitarian importance of the problem to be solved by the experiment. Proper preparations should be made and adequate facilities provided to protect the experimental subject against even remote possibilities of injury, disability, or death.

8. The experiment should be conducted only by scientifically qualified persons. The highest degree of skill and care should be required through all stages of the experiment of those who conduct or engage in the experiment.

9. During the course of the experiment the human subject should be at liberty to bring the experiment to an end if he has reached the physical or mental state where continuation of the experiment seems to him to be impossible.

10. During the course of the experiment the scientist in charge must be prepared to terminate the experiment at any stage, if he has probable cause to believe, in the exercise of the good faith, superior skill, and careful judgment required of him that a continuation of the experiment is likely to result in injury, disability or death to the experimental subject.

The Judgment and the Medical Case: Reactions

The judgment by the military court in the Medical Case had different follow-ups: the proceedings established beyond any doubt that many and considerable cruelties had been committed by doctors on patients/prisoners and that these cruelties had been supported by their superiors in the medical hierarchy. On the other hand there are relatively few analysis and scientifically based discussions during the last 50 years concerning the ten principles of Nuremberg[3] which should not only serve as a basis of convicting the accused, but which should lead the medical researches in the future as well. The immediate reaction as far as the creation of new legal rules concerning medical experimentation is concerned, was twofold. Ethicists and some doctors agreed that the judgment established the Nuremberg Code as a unique legal instrument. On the other side there were positions that can only be described as trying to put some distance between the judgment and the medical profession or to acknowledge the Medical Case and leave it alone.

The early backers of the Nuremberg Code were naturally the chief of the prosecution, Telford Taylor, and Dr. Leo Alexander, the medical expert of the prosecution. Speaking on a symposium in 1976 in Hastings upon Hudson, Taylor has judged the proceedings in the Medical Case and its result as necessary.[4] In 1970 Alexander judged the Nuremberg Code as a useful guide concerning the limits of experimental research on human subjects.[5] In his comprehensive text book, *Experimentation with Human Beings*, Katz reserved much space for the opening statement by Telford Taylor in the Medical Case.[6] The opening statement is impressive, especially because Taylor stresses that the accused doctors violated the relationship of trust that has to exist between doctor and patient. On the other hand his personal notion of "Thanatology" seems to be somewhat misplaced. Turning to Germany the book by Mitscherlich and Mielke, *Doctors in Infamy (Medizin ohne Menschlichkeit)* was published first in 1948 and has been reprinted many times. In his memoirs, however, Mitscherlich has shown that leading doctors turned to the daily routine after the judgment in Nuremberg and did not like to be reminded of it.[7] The two most recent publications by Ginsburgs and Kudriavtsev on the one hand and Annas and Grodin on the other hand treat the Medical Case as a necessary criminal procedure and an established international precedent in criminal law.[8]

At least immediately after the Medical Case the American medical establishment regarded the Nuremberg Code not uncritical. Two eminent doctors show us their attitude. Beecher contradicts Taylor who had demanded that doctors in clinical research follow the ten principles of Nuremberg as standard rules. Firstly, Beecher does not concede the binding nature of the Nuremberg Code. According to his opinion the researches would follow these rules just under the condition that they knew how to do it.[9] Moore - like Beecher a professor at the Harvard Medical School - went even further. In 1969 Moore discussed the Krebiozen-scandal in which Dr.

Ivy, vice-president of the University of Illinois and main expert witness for medical ethics in the Medical Case, became involved. A substance called Krebiozen, an alleged wonder drug against all kinds of carcinoma, had been handed over to Dr. Ivy by someone who claimed to have distilled it from the blood of hundreds of horses. Moore then went on, Dr. Ivy administered the medication to a dog, then he tried it out on himself (as provided by the Nuremberg Code) and after three weeks on a patient.[10]

It may be of interest that in the late fifties a group of researchers and ethicists in the United States of America proposed to rewrite the Nuremberg Code. There was even a committee to work on a second edition of the Nuremberg Code. Main reason for the setting up of that commission were structural defects of the code, for instance that there was no distinction between therapeutical experimentation and purely scientific research, then far reaching personal conditions, e.g. that the experimental subjects had to have capacity, and finally that part of principle No. 5 that has been called bizarre by no less a man than Beecher himself as far as a higher degree of danger might be permissible if the researcher-in-chief participates in the experiment. The committee was of the opinion that the Nuremberg Code was still a valuable guide but needed further discussion. The members of the committee then proposed to change no less than five of the ten points of Nuremberg.[11] The work of the committee coincided with the first Declaration of Helsinki concerning biomedical research on human beings that was adopted by the World Medical Association in 1962. Here, we had a totally new set of ethical rules concerning experimentation on human beings. Nuremberg somehow became overshadowed by Helsinki. The discussion and a second edition of Nuremberg had become less urgent.

Although the Nuremberg Code was somehow overtaken by the 1975 Revised Declaration of Helsinki, in the interest of medical science and legal doctrine the Nuremberg Code will still be subject of discussion. It is especially interesting for the lawyer to reach over the taboo which surrounded the Medical Case so long and to discuss the validity of the ten principles of Nuremberg and to look at their basis in the actual proceedings 50 years ago.

Judges and Accused; Lawyers and Physicians

The Medical Case constituted the first subsequent proceedings after the International Case. Telford Taylor has revealed that the cruelties which had been committed by doctors or at least had been done under the guise of medicine, had a certain unity. Therefore they became subject to the first subsequent proceedings. The constitution of the bench was somewhat unusual, because it consisted of state justices only. The chief justice of the Supreme Court of the United States, Harlan Fiske Stone, did not give his permission anymore for federal judges to work in Nuremberg. One had to employ state judges, a good many of whom were already retired.[12] The bench in the Medical Case consisted of three state judges, a former Chief Justice of the Supreme Court of the State of Washington, a judge of the Supreme Court of the state of Florida and a state judge from Oklahoma.[13]

Accused were standing before these three American state justices a group of German doctors and high functionaries of the German health system. That scenario in itself led to many misunderstandings. Even under normal circumstances physicians and lawyers have totally different starting points and views of what has happened or is happening. The doctor looks ahead, the judge looks back; the physician looks at the overall result of his treatment, the lawyer measures every single one of the steps leading to it; the researcher longs for something totally new, he who writes a judgment looks for some secure basis. The prosecuting attorneys and the judges had at the beginning very little notion about clinical research; they learned it during the proceedings.[14] Nevertheless, it was obvious that the medical interventions charged were crimes recognized as such by the laws and courts all over the world. Unfortunately, the charges were not based on common crimes. Instead of charging the accused with murder, man-slaughter, assault and battery, etc., the indictment named war crimes and crimes against humanity as well as conspiracy. Because of that the Medical Case is subject to the same objection often raised against the international tribunal that it created crimes after the deed. At least for a continental European lawyer this contravened the basic principle in criminal law *"nulla poena sine lege"*.

Medical Experimentation Basically Crime?

The indictment at Nuremberg cited grave criminal acts which resulted in death and mutilations of the experimental subjects. The only recourse the defense had against these obviously irrefutable charges was to pass off nearly all of these cases as medical experimentations,[15] even if sometimes the crimes were just committed under the guise of scientific research. Unfortunately, the prosecution and to a lesser degree the court itself followed the approach by the defense, which can be only understood because, as Taylor has shown, the prosecution had to improvise and in large part follow the path taken by the defense.[16] Were medical experiments on human subjects regarded as something doubtful anyway? Or was the idea to treat all medical interventions charged as experimentation a way to forestall the expected defense?

Medical science has suffered from this basic approach until today. If someone talks about medical experimentations on human beings there is the shadow of Nuremberg. Recently all the newspapers of the big city of Hamburg carried the headline that there had been human experimentation at the university hospital as if something totally unexpected, maybe even criminal had happened there. Telford Taylor and others brought the indictment against the doctors not only because they had committed crimes but because they had betrayed the trust that patients usually have in doctors. Thus there were two reasons for bringing the medical case first. Unfortunately, clinical research as much as it has benefited mankind it has been drawn into the abyss. One may deplore that the indictment as well as the judgment in the Medical Case did not really distinguish between criminal cruelties without a valid scientific purpose and medical experimentation on human beings according to the rules of medical science even if the latter had been performed without informed consent. Medical research is basically different from cruel crimes without even a scientific pretext. There is a difference between the experimentation with inoculation against yellow fever performed by Prof. Rose and the killing of prisoners of war by deep freezing committed by Dr. Rascher.[17]

Break for the Defense: Medical Experimentation on Prison Inmates in the USA

The defense in the Medical Case first looked hopeless. The defense lawyers got some uplift from a piece in the periodical *LIFE* that reported experimentation on inmates in the Stateville prison in Illinois during the Second World War. Today we know even more about these experimentations because Nathan Leopold reported them in his bestseller *LIFE & 99 Years*.[18] Leopold had taken part in the preparations and on some tests concerning malaria and the use of inoculations against that illness. He tells us that the choosing of inmates in the Stateville Prison were performed carefully and the experimental subjects were treated with respect. All of them gave their informed consent, the experimentations were performed openly with the press present from the beginning. Leopold tells us moreover that the prisoners did not receive promises as to an earlier release and that there were no deaths among these probands. Nevertheless, in 1947 many of the experimental subjects were paroled, maybe some of them had hoped that their participation in the malaria experiment might help them with their parole.

Genesis of the Nuremberg Code

To distinguish between illegal crimes on the one hand and permissible medical experimentations on the other the court in the Medical Case established the so-called ten principles of Nuremberg or the Nuremberg Code. The ten principles appear in the first part of the judgment and are referred to in nearly every single case. All we know for certain is that the Nuremberg Code is prefaced by the judges' statement.

All agree, however, that certain basic principles must be observed in order to satisfy moral, ethical and legal concepts.[19] It is a tantalizing question to try to find out who formulated the ten points of Nuremberg. Up to now nobody knows for certain who had done it. There are different schools of thought for the origin of the ten principles of Nuremberg. There is Taylor who by personal observation came to the conclusion that judge Sebring formulated essential parts of the Nuremberg Code.[20] " [T]he judge who I think is primarily responsible for the famous ten principles in the opinion of the Medical Case, was judge Harold Sebring". Dr. Ivy, the vice president of the university of Illinois, was heard as expert witness in ethical matters by the court. He had formulated three principles and therefore many regard him as the author of the ten principles of Nuremberg. Dr. Ivy followed the guidelines established by the American Medical Association, though there is some doubt whether the American Medical Association did not in fact adopt the three principles of Dr. Ivy lateron as their guidelines.[21] But Dr. Ivy's testimony somehow fell short of what was expected of the author of the ten principles of Nuremberg. Here, there are the three principles by Dr. Ivy:

1. The voluntary consent of the individual upon whom the experiment is to be performed must be obtained.

2. The danger of each experiment must be previously investigated by animal experiments.

3. The experiment must be performed under proper medical protection and management.[22]

It is much more likely that the ten principles of Nuremberg originated from a memorandum that Dr. Leo Alexander prepared. Dr. Alexander was the medical expert working with the prosecution, a psychiatrist by profession. He has published about the Nuremberg case and medical experimentations on humans in general.[23] In 1970 Dr. Alexander revealed that he had submitted a memorandum to the United States chief council for war crimes and to the court on April 15, 1947. We do not know whether that memorandum was ever passed on to the defense. At least, there is no written record of it, and the defense counsels made no reference to it. Even the chief prosecutor Mr. Haney does not mention it in his closing argument on July 14, 1947. The ten principles suddenly appear in the judgment delivered by judge Beals on July 19, 1947.

Dr. Alexander shows that he had formulated six principles, which the judges had enlarged to ten. This happened by enlarging one principle into three and that two more principles had been added. Dr. Alexander regrets that the court omitted his reference to psychic illnesses and feels that this might have been done because the question of psychic illness did not come up in the Medical Case at Nuremberg. Moreover, Dr. Alexander is of the opinion that the ten principles of Nuremberg do not just deal with purely scientific research. Clinical experimentation with therapeutical aspects are covered by the Nuremberg Code according to his opinion. Here are his original six principles:[24]

1. Legally valid voluntary consent of the experimental subject is essential. This requires specifically:
a. the absence of duress; and
b. sufficient disclosure on the part of the experimenter and sufficient understanding on the part of the experimental subject of the exact nature and consequences of the experiment for which he volunteers to permit an enlightened consent. In the case of mentally ill patients, for the purpose of experiments concerning the nature and treatment of nervous and mental illness, or related subjects, such consent of the next of kin or legal guardian is required; whenever the mental state of the patient permits (that is, in those mentally ill patients who are not delirious or confused), his own consent should be obtained in addition.

2. The nature and purpose of the experiment must be humanitarian, with the ultimate aim to cure, treat, or prevent illness, and not concerned with methods of killing or sterilization (kienology). The motive and purpose of the experiment shall also not be personal or otherwise ulterior.

3. No experiment is permissible if the foregone conclusion exists, or the probability or the *a priori* reason to believe that death or disabling injury of the experimental subject will occur.

4. Adequate preparations must be made and proper facilities be provided to aid the experimental subject against any remote chance of injury, disability, or death. The provision specifically requires that the degree of skill of all those who are taking an active part as experimenters, and the degree of care which they exercise during the experiment, must be significantly higher than the skill which is considered qualifying, and the care which is considered adequate for the performance of standardized medical or surgical procedures, and for the administration of well-established drugs. American courts are very stringent in requiring for the permissible use of any new or unusual technique or drug, irrespective of whether this use is experimental or purely therapeutic, a degree of skill and care on the part of the responsible physician, which is higher than that required for the purpose of routine medical or surgical procedures.

5. The degree of risk taken should never exceed that determined by the humanitarian importance of the problem to be solved by the experiment. It is ethically permissible for an experimenter to perform experiments involving significant risks only if the solution, after thorough exploration along all other lines of scientific investigations, is not accessible by any other means, and if he considers the solution of the problem important enough to risk his own life along with the lives of his non-scientific colleagues, such as was done in the case of Walter Reed's yellow fever experiments.

6. The experiment to be performed must be so designed and based upon the results of thorough thinking-through, investigation of simple physico-chemical systems and of animal experimentation that the anticipated results will justify the performance of the experiment. That is, the experiment must be such as to yield decisive results for the good of society and should not be random and unnecessary in nature.

If one compares open-mindedly the three principles by Dr. Ivy and the six points by Dr. Alexander, it is easy to establish who is the father of the famous Nuremberg Code. To name Dr. Ivy in this respect gives him too much honor.[25] Clearly, Dr. Alexander is the prime architect of the Nuremberg Code which is foreshadowed in the closing argument by the chief prosecutor.[26] Nevertheless there is the problem under which a psychiatrist would have to labor for a long time: the Nuremberg Code does not distinguish between purely scientific experimentations and therapeutical trials; moreover, it declares necessary that the experimental subject has to have capacity and give its free informed consent, which bars experimentation on children and mentally ill persons.

Valid Principles of the Nuremberg Code

The Nuremberg Code established a good many recognized principles of medical ethics in human experimentation. Most important is the principle of informed consent that serves as starting point for the Nuremberg Code. The extraordinary importance which the informed consent had in the United States even at that time made it one of the main bases of the international instrument called the Nuremberg Code. This is explained in detail in principle 1 of the Code. Principle 3 of the principles contains the rule that the anticipated results will justify the performance of the experiment. Thus, the necessity of a scientifically valid research protocol appeared on the scene, something that concerns Institutional Review Boards (IRB) until today. No IRB should positively review a research protocol, that is not scientifically valid.

Another very valuable rule is expressed in the first part of principle 5. According to that principle no experiment should be conducted when there is a reason to believe that death or disabling injury will occur. One would have wished that other codes, e.g. the Revised Declaration of Helsinki or the German Pharmaceutical Act, would have contained a similar absolute prohibition against those experimentations. Finally, even today, the principles 9 and 10 are valuable because they emphasize the liberty of the experimental subject to end his involvement in the experimentation any time. Likewise, the scientist in charge has to terminate the experiment if it is likely to result in injury, disability or death of the experimental subject. It has become common practice by the IRBs to request that the experimental subject is informed that he or she can stop participation in the experiment any time without giving reasons or having to fear the consequences.

Obsolete Parts of the Nuremberg Code

On the other hand it should not be overlooked that one main structure and some specific rules of the Nuremberg Code appear obsolete today. Again, it has to be emphasized that the ten principles do not distinguish between purely scientific experimentation on the one hand and therapeutical experimentation on the other. In 1947 this distinction had already become common knowledge. Even the German guidelines for new forms of treatment and scientific experimentations issued in 1931, which were well known to the court, started out with that distinction already. It is not easy to follow Leo Alexander, the probable author of most of the Nuremberg principles, that both types of medical experimentations are covered by the Nuremberg principles.[27] Even if we follow Alexander, all the ten principles apply without exception to both types of medical experimentation, which does not make their interpretation easier.

Principle No. 1 which requires that the person involved should have legal capacity to give consent seems to bar experimentation on children and the mentally ill. The prohibition made sense as far as purely scientific experimentation was concerned. But it would be regrettable if the prohibition expressed by the first principle, which does not name any exceptions, would make all therapeutic research in psychiatry and pediatrics impossible. Taken literally the Salk-experiments concerning poliomylitis would have been unlawful, even criminal.

The second part of principle No. 5 has been called by Beecher a bizarre rule. According to principle No. 5 an experiment where death or disabling injury could occur, should not be conducted: "except, perhaps, in those experiments where the experimental physicians also serve as subjects".[28] Today we know that the really dangerous experimentations are performed first by the researcher on himself or herself. Forssmann used the first catheter to reach the heart on himself.

The Nuremberg Code and the Revised Declaration of Helsinki

Now most Institutional Review Boards use the Revised Declaration of Helsinki promulgated by the World Medical Association as basis for reviewing research protocols. Rarely are the ten principles of Nuremberg referred to by an Institutional Review Board. I personally have witnessed it just two times in more than twenty years of membership in IRBs. This shows that for today's structured and complicated research protocols the modern instrument of the Revised Declaration of Helsinki is more adaptable than the strict ten principles of Nuremberg. But even immediately after the adoption of the Declaration of Helsinki Alexander held the Nuremberg principles still applicable because they were much more specific.[29]

Recently the question whether the Nuremberg Code is a living and applicable precedent or should be just used as a collection of principles has been discussed in more detail.[30] In my opinion the Nuremberg Code was a necessary step into the right direction. Many of its principles still stand today. Others have fallen by the wayside as experimentation became better known. Even the expressions used today are different from the ones we find in the ten principles of Nuremberg. This is partly due to the fact that the defensive language of the Nuremberg Code shows that it served as a basis for a criminal conviction. So, instead of speaking about informed consent, we read that the voluntary consent is absolutely essential. The first principle then goes on: the human subject should be so situated as to be able to exercise free power of choice, without intervention of any element of force, fraud, deceit, duress, over-reaching or other ulterior form of constraint or coercion, etc. Moreover, the Declaration of Helsinki has been revised many times to confront new developments, a chance the Nuremberg Code never had. Finally, the Revised Declaration of Helsinki has established two means of enforcing the Declaration and its principles. The first one is the establishment of Institutional Review Boards or ethics committees. The other one is the prohibition that research results should not be published if the research is not in conformity with the standards set up by the Declaration. This includes the prior evaluation by an Institutional Review Board.

Finally a caveat by the lawyer: the ten principles of Nuremberg might have gained in adaptability if all of them had been discussed in open court. But even if this had been the case, they still would have been mainly the instrument for the conviction of grave crimes. Since the criminal offenses charged, i.e. crimes against humanity, war crimes and conspiracy, were not specific in themselves, it was almost inevitable, that the ten principles should address specific parts of the experimentation that were brought before the court. Few, if any of the criminal acts before the court in Nuremberg constituted typical research. Hence, it was not to be expected that the judgment could regulate all experimentations in the time to come.

If we look at today's theory and practice, as it is administered daily in Institutional Review Boards or ethics committees, the Nuremberg Code does not just contain ten principles. It is a principle. The rules applied today may have their origin in some of the principles of the Nuremberg Code, but they are expressed in the Revised Declaration of Helsinki or in special national laws.

Notes

1   U.S. v. Brandt et al. (1948), Trials of war criminals before the Nuremberg military tribunal, vol. I and II: *The Medical Case*, Washington D.C., U.S. government printing office. A short German description is to be found in Mitscherlich and Mielke (1960), *Medizin ohne Menschlichkeit, Dokumente des Nürnberger Ärzteprozesses.*, Fischer, Frankfurt.

2   Telford, T. (August 1976), 'Biomedical ethics and shadows of nazism', *Hastings Center Report, Special Supplement*, p. 6, is of the opinion that judge Sebring, justice at the Supreme Court of the state of Florida, insisted that the court established standards concerning clinical research.

3   More recent exceptions are Ginsburgs and Kudriavtsev (1990), *The Nuremberg Trial and International Law*; Annas, G.J. and Grodin, M.A. (1992), *The Nazi Doctors and the Nuremberg Code. Human Rights in Human Experimentation*. New York, Oxford University Press

4   Telford, T., *Hastings Center Report*, op. cit. p. 4 et seq.

5   Leo, A. (1970), 'Psychiatry: Methods and processes for investigation of drugs', *Annals of the New York Academy of Science*, 169, p. 344, p. 347.

6   Katz, J. (1972), *Experimentation with Human Beings*, p. 294 et seq.

7   Mitscherlich, A. (1982), *Ein Leben mit der Psychoanalyse.*

8   Ginsburgs and Kudriavtsev (1990), *The Nuremberg trial and international law.*
    Annas, G.J. and Grodin, M.A. (1992), *The Nazi doctors and the Nuremberg Code.*

9   Beecher, H. (1970), *Research and the individual*, p. 234.

10 Moore (1969), Therapeutic invention: Ethical boundaries in the initial clinical trials of new drugs and surgical procedures, *98 Daedalus*, p. 502, p. 515.

11 Ladimer and Newman (1963), *Clinical investigation in medicine*, pp. 140 et seq. Even Taylor (1976) acknowledged that the ten principles and the proceedings were "all quite hasty and improvised", *Hastings Center Report*, p. 6.

12 Harlan Fiske Stone was very bland concerning the international case in Nuremberg: "Jackson is away conducting his high grade lynching party at Nuremberg. I don't mind what he does to the nazis, but I hate to see the pretense that he is running a court and proceedings according to common law". Bosch. (1970), *Judgment on Nuremberg*, p. 133.

13 Mitscherlich, A. and Mielke, F. (1960), *Medizin ohne Menschlichkeit*, p. 275.

14 Telford, T., *Hastings center Report*, op. cit., p. 6, "... we were educated in large part by our opponents".

15 Cf. Telford, T., Opening statement of the prosecution, reprinted in Annas & Grodin. (1992), *The Nazi doctors and the Nuremberg Code*, pp. 67 et seq.; The term "Thanatology" used in this context usually describes something else.

16 Taylor, T. *Hastings Center Report*, op. cit. p. 6 .

17 Prof. Rose who had been sentenced to a prison term was later acquitted. The retrial took place in 1963 and 1964, cf. Mitscherlich, A. and Mielke, F., *Medizin ohne Menschlichkeit*, p. 282. In a strange twist of justice Dr. Rascher and his wife were charged before a SS-court with abduction of children and falsifying birth certificates. Both were condemned to prison terms which they did not survive. This is at least the story told by the father of Dr. Rascher as reported by Countess Kalnoky in *The Guest House, A Nuremberg Memoir*, The Bobbs-Merrill Co. Inc. Indianapolis/New York, pp. 222 et seq.

18 Leopold Nathan F. (1958) *Life & 99 years*, pp. 305 et seq.; cf. in this respect Taylor,

T. (August 1976), *Hastings Center Report special supplement*, p. 10.

19 Military Tribunal, Vol. II, pp. 181 et seq.

20 Telford, T., *Hastings Report*, op. cit., p. 6.

21 Grodin, M.A. (1992), *Historical Origins of the Nuremberg Code in the Nazi doctors and the Nuremberg Code*, p. 134.

22 *Journal of the American Medical Association*. (1946), 132, p.1090. Taken at face value it seems improbable that Dr. Ivy and his three principles could have been the sole source for the ten principles of Nuremberg.

23 Alexander, L. (1949), 'Medical Science under Dictatorship' *New England Journal of Medicine*, 241, p. 39.

Alexander, L. (1966), 'Limitations and experimental research on human beings', *Lex et Scientia*, 3, p. 8.

Alexander, L. (1970), Psychiatry: Methods and processes for investigation of drugs, *Annals of the New York Academy of Science*, p. 344.

24 Alexander, L. (1970) Psychiatry: Methods and processes for investigation of drugs, 169, *Annals of the New York Academy of Science*, p. 344, pp.346 et seq.

25 Grodin, M.A. op. cit. feels that Dr. Ivy and Dr. Alexander are both responsible for the ten principles of Nuremberg.

26 Cf. Grodin, M.A., op. cit., p. 137.

27 Alexander, L. (1970) Psychiatry: Methods and processes for investigation of drugs, 169, *Annals of the New York Academy of Science*, p. 344, p. 346.

28 Beecher, H. *Research and the individual*, p. 233.

29 Alexander, L. (1970), Psychiatry: Methods and processes for investigation of drugs, 169, *Annals of the New York Academy of Science*, p. 346: "But it is my opinion that the Nuremberg Code covers all these contingencies in a much more specific manner than subsequent formulas such as the Helsinki resolution".

30 Especially in Annas, G.J. and Grodin, M.A. (1992), *The Nazi Doctors and the Nuremberg Code, Human Rights and Human Experimentation*, by Drinan, The Nuremberg principles in international law; Glantz, The influence of the Nuremberg Code on U.S. statutes and regulations; Annas, G.J. The Nuremberg Code in U.S. courts, ethics vs. expediency.

7 The "Nuremberg Code": Rules of Public International Law

Pascal Arnold and Dominique Sprumont

Introduction*

To understand the "Nuremberg Code's" significance in public international law, it is necessary to analyze the post-World War II trials at Nuremberg. They can be divided into two groups, the trial at the International Military Tribunal (IMT) of those persons most culpable for the war in Europe and the 12 additional trials before American military tribunals which tried war criminals based on their professions. The "Nuremberg Code" was elaborated during the "doctor's trial", the first of the 12 additional trials. This occured contemporaneously with the development of fundamental public international law principles, labeled the "Principles of Nuremberg", based on the case before the IMT.

In Part One of this article, we will discuss the IMT trial and the "Principles of Nuremberg". Part Two will explore the influence of these principles on the doctor's trial, as well as the trial's international character. In Part Three, we will narrow the focus to an evaluation of the legal valence of the "Nuremberg Code" in public international law. The conclusion will assess the relationship between the "Nuremberg Code" and codes of medical ethics, in particular the Helsinki Declaration.

The Trial Before the International Military Tribunal and the Principles of Nuremberg

Genesis of the International Military Tribunal and the Trial

During the war, the Allied Forces made several official declarations expressing their determination to punish war crimes. For instance, during a meeting of the Great Powers in London on 13 January 1942, representatives from nine governments in exile - Belgium, France, Greece, Luxembourg, Norway, Netherlands, Poland, Czechoslovakia, and Yugoslavia - declared that one of their principal objectives was "to punish the persons guilty or responsible of these [war] crimes during an ordinary procedure".[1] Later, the United Kingdom, the United States and the Soviet Union confirmed that intention in the Moscow Declaration. They announced on behalf of the 32 Allied Nations that: "At the time of the granting of any armistice to any government which may be set up in Germany, those German officers and men and members of the Nazi party who have been responsible for, or have taken a consenting part in the [war] atrocities... [will be] punished according to the laws of these liberated countries". The major criminals "whose offenses have no particular geographical localization... will be punished by the joint decision of the Government of the Allies".[2]

On 8 August 1945 the United States, France, the Soviet Union and the United Kingdom set forth the constitution of the International Military Tribunal in the London Agreement.[3] Ratification by 19 additional nations[4] confirmed its international significance. Those crimes over which the IMT could exercise jurisdiction were enumerated in Article Six of the IMT Charter (which was annexed to the London Agreement) and divided into three categories - crimes against peace, war crimes and crimes against humanity.[5] Concerning the approach to be taken by the court, the IMT itself declared in its final judgment that: "The Charter is not an arbitrary exercise of power on the part of the victorious nations, but in the view of the Tribunal, as will be shown, it is the expression of international law existing at the time of its creation; and to that extent is itself a contribution to international law".[6]

The four major Allied Powers[7] were represented on both the court and the prosecution. Among the accused in the trial lasting nearly a year were individuals who played key roles in ordering and committing war crimes. Of the 22 accused, 12 were sentenced to death, most of them leaders of the Nazi government such as Göring, von Ribbentrop, Keitel, Rosenberg, Frank, Frick, Streicher, Jodl and Seyss-Inquart. Three were acquitted, while the remainder were sentenced to imprisonment of between ten years and life.

The Principles of Nuremberg

The principles articulated in the London Agreement and judgment of the IMT were confirmed by the General Assembly of the United Nations[8] in a resolution which also directed the International Law Commission (ILC) to reformulate them. Known as the "Principles of Nuremberg", the ILC's seven principles were published in 1950 as a Resolution of the UN General Assembly.[9] (See Appendix.)

Before discussing the principles further, it is useful to briefly recall the primary sources of public international law. First, there is conventional public international law established through bi- and multilateral treaties between countries. Then, there is customary public international law derived from practice by states over time (*usus*) out of a sense of legal obligation (*opinio juris sive necessitatis*). A third source consists of those legal principles common to all civilized countries.[10] Some are so deeply rooted in the international legal conscience that they are applied in the common interest of all nations. These rules are defined as peremptory norms of public international law or *ius cogens*.[11]

The practice of public international law in the post-IMT era has in large part confirmed the validity of the Principles of Nuremberg. Direct punishment of individuals for crimes breaching the standards of public international law has clearly been accepted. The fact that the actor was exercising official functions is no defense to criminal charges. Similarly, the order of a superior to commit a wrongful act does not free an actor from responsibility under international law. Most of the Nuremberg Principles, most notably the first four, have been codified in conventional public international law. Additionally, numerous rules of international humanitarian law, the violation of which was condemned at the Nuremberg trial, have become peremptory norms of international law (*ius cogens*).

The judgment of the International Military Tribunal has also contributed to the development of several conventions for the protection of war victims. In 1948 the Convention on Genocide was drafted (it has yet to be ratified by Switzerland). The following year the four Geneva Conventions which constitute the core of international humanitarian law were completed. Indeed, since 1945 over 20 conventions designed to further the international protection of human rights have come into effect.

A further effect of the Nuremberg trials was to reinforce domestic prosecution of war crimes under the principle of universality. Thus, the obligation to suppress war crimes, regardless of where and by whom the crimes are committed, has been adopted by many national criminal codes. Furthermore the Principles of Nuremberg have been introduced in many military law codes and manuals.[12] These constitute a direct contribution to public international law by the Nuremberg trial and the Principles of Nuremberg.

The Importance of the Nuremberg Trial

The greatest contribution of the Nuremberg trial was that for the first time war criminals were condemned before an international tribunal under rules of public international law. Therefore the Nuremberg trial is a cornerstone of international criminal and conflicts law.[13] The trial was conducted by lawyers of international reputation under fair procedures. Even if the criticism that it constituted victor's justice may not be completely dismissed, the principles drawn from the Nuremberg trial have had a fundamental influence on the recent evolution of public international law.

Shortly after the Nuremberg trial, the UN drafted statutes for an international criminal court of justice. However, it took nearly half a century before the international community set up an international tribunal to punish war criminals involved in horrors such as the ones of Rwanda and Yugoslavia. Unlike the IMT, the legal basis for the Tribunal for Yugoslavia and Rwanda is found in UN Security Council resolutions. Based on the fact that these two conflicts constitute a threat to international peace (Art. 39 of the United Nations Charter), the Security Council created these ad hoc tribunals as a UN Charter Art. 41 measure. It is important to note that the action was taken pursuant to Chapter VII of the Charter, which governs threats to peace, breach of peace and acts of aggression. The law they apply is based in large measure on rules elaborated during the Nuremberg trial. To prevent any breach of the principle *"nullum crimen, nulla poena sine lege"*, their statutes refer directly to the rules of existing international conventions (the Hague Regulations, the Geneva Convention and the Genocide Convention).

It must also be noted that in 1993 the ILC completed work preparatory to establishment of a Permanent International Criminal Court ("Draft Statute for a Permanent International Criminal Court").[14] Thus, the likelihood that an entity possessing international criminal jurisdiction will once again be created seems to be growing.[15]

The Nuremberg Doctor's Trial

The Trial

The doctor's trial (United States v. Karl Brandt et al.)[16] was the first of the 12 additional trials before the American tribunals at Nuremberg. During these trials, 185 accused were tried.[17] The trials against the lawyers and doctors have garnered the greatest attention. In the lawyer's trial[18] the Nazi apparatus' leading lawyers, as well as the president of the third Reich's tribunals of exception, were tried for their total lack of respect for, and deliberate violation of, the fundamental principles of law and justice.[19]

During the doctor's trial, 23 doctors, physicians and high ranking officials of the Ministry of Health in the Nazi government were brought before the court. Accused of barbaric and often deadly experiments on prisoners of war, concentration camp prisoners, and others, 15 of the defendants were declared guilty of war crimes and of crimes against humanity.[20] The human experimentation was judged to have been performed in "complete disregard of international conventions, the laws and customs of war [and] the general principles of criminal laws of all civilized nations and the Control Council Law N° 10".[21] The tribunal pronounced seven death sentences, including that of Karl Brandt. The other accused were sentenced to ten years to life imprisonment.[22] Though conducted by an American military tribunal composed of American judges and prosecutors, the doctors trial remains of great significance in public international law due both to its legal basis and the rules on which it based its judgments.[23]

Legal Basis of the Doctor's Trial

Initially, the intent was to prosecute other war criminals before the IMT. Yet, with the onset of the Cold War it quickly became difficult for the Four Powers to cooperate.

Nevertheless, Art. 10 and 11 of the IMT Charter provided for the possibility of punishing war criminals before national tribunals, whether in military or occupation courts. Under this provision, the Control Council for Germany that had been formed by the Military Commanders of the four occupation zones enacted Control Council Law N° 10 of 20 December 1945.[24] It gave each Zone Commander the authority to set up tribunals to judge Nazi war criminals.

The Military Commander of the American zone adopted Regulation N° 7 on the "Organization and Powers of Certain Military Tribunals",[25] which created American military tribunals to try Nazi war criminals. These were the only tribunals other than the IMT which operated at the international level. The 12 additional judgments are in that sense of a different nature than other war crimes trials which were held before national tribunals, such as that of Eichmann in Israel,[26] or more recently the trial of Barbie in France.[27]

In summary, while the doctor's trial was conducted in an American military tribunal, it was based on rules of delegation found in the London Agreement that had been signed by the Four Great Powers and ratified by 19 nations besides the US. Its validity in public international law was later confirmed, in particular by the General Assembly of the United Nations. This recognition is important evidence of the international character of the tribunal's decisions.

The Legal Nature of the Rules Applied During the Doctor's Trial

The doctor's trial applied the same rules as the International Military Tribunal. For instance, the crimes charged were identical: crimes against peace, war crimes and crimes against humanity.[28] Their legal descriptions were essentially the same as those found in the Charter of the International Military Tribunal and the Principles of Nuremberg.[29] The American military tribunal which judged the doctors was also bound to respect the Nuremberg principles; the principle of individual responsibility of the war criminals had to be followed and a doctor could not resort to the defense of superior orders. Art. 10 of Ordinance N° 7 also stated that "the determination of the IMT in [its] judgment shall be binding on the tribunals established hereunder... Statements of the IMT in [its] judgment constitute proof of the facts stated, in the absence of substantial new evidence to the contrary".[30]

The rules applied during the doctor's trial are therefore rules of public international law. If their international character could have been contested at the time of the judgment, the issue has now been put to rest. We can therefore conclude that the doctor's trial before the Nuremberg Court inbreed belongs to public international law.

The "Nuremberg Code" in Public International Law

As mentioned above, the American military tribunal did not operate under new rules, but rather applied public international law found in international conventions and the Principles of Nuremberg developed by the IMT. In its judgment, the Tribunal refers expressly to the laws and customs of war, general principles of law, international conventions and provisions of Control Council Law N° 10. The judges applied general rules of public international law on war crimes and on crimes against humanity in the field of research on human beings and formulated specific rules in that regard. The text of Art. 6 of the IMT Charter and Art. 2 of Control Council Law N° 10 was indeed too general to define the basic conditions to follow while doing human experimentation. Therefore, the judges elaborated ten specific rules concerning war crimes and crimes against humanity committed in connection with research on human beings. Known as the "Nuremberg Code", these specific rules distinguish between authorized and non-authorized research.[31]

After setting forth the "Nuremberg Code's ten principles", the Court added that "of the ten principles which have been enumerated, our judicial concern, of course, is with those requirements which are purely legal in nature - or which at least are so clearly related to matters legal that they assist us in determining criminal culpability and punishment. To go beyond that point would lead us into a field that would be beyond our sphere of competence. However, the point need not be labored. We find from the evidence that in the medical experiments which have been proved, these ten principles were much more frequently honored in their breach than in their observance".[32] Thus, the Court recognized the possible existence of ethical norms which could go further than the law, but found that in the present case such a distinction did not occur. It is also important to note that when introducing its ten fundamental principles the Court stated that "certain basic principles must be observed in order to satisfy moral, ethical **and** legal concepts".[33] Thus, the Tribunal expressly recognized that the basic principles of the "Nuremberg Code" possess legal character.

Many countries have adopted the basic rules of the "Nuremberg Code" in national legislation,[34] thus reinforcing their legal impact. Furthermore, at the beginning of the Cold War the American Department of Defense acknowledged the legally binding character of the "Nuremberg Code" in several long classified documents, the existence of which was cited in the Report of the Advisory Committee on Human Radiation Experiments appointed by President Clinton.[35] The legal importance of the "Nuremberg Code" was also reaffirmed in a recent case: "*In re Cincinnati Radiation Litigation*".[36] "[E]ven were the Nuremberg Code not afforded precedential weight in the courts of the United States, it cannot be readily dismissed from its proper context in this case". Provisions concerning research on human beings were also adopted in several international conventions. Among those to be noted are Art. 7 of the International Covenant on Civil and Political Rights,[37] as well as Art. 12 of the 1st and 2nd[38], Art. 13 of the 3rd[39] and Art. 32 of the 4th 1949 Geneva Conventions.[40,41] The "Draft Convention for the Prevention and Suppression of Unlawful Human Experimentation"[42] offered in 1980 by Cheriff Bassiouni, a world expert in international criminal law, is also in large measure based on the "Nuremberg Code".

Due to its continuing and uniformed application (usus) by a majority of countries, as well as the general recognition of its binding nature (opinio juris), these basic principles have become rules of customary international law.[43] In fact, they are applied in the common interest of all Nations and are so deeply rooted in the international legal consciousness that they constitute peremptory public international law (ius cogens).[44] This means that they can not be modified by any State or professional organization, either by statute or ethical guidelines.

The "Nuremberg Code" is undoubtedly a set of public international law rules.[45] The only provision that merits revision is Art. 5 of the "Nuremberg Code", which allows an investigator to conduct research where "there is an a priori reason to believe that death or disabling injury will occur" if "the experimental physicians also serve as subjects". Nevertheless, the structure of the "Nuremberg Code" should be revised[46] and the wording of certain outdated provisions should be adapted to the needs of modern society. This criticism in no way diminishes the fundamental role of the "Nuremberg Code" in public international law. On the contrary, it is important to emphasize the fact that the most recent international conventions and codification projects concerning research on human subjects, far from weakening their content and significance, tend to reinforce the rules expressed in the "Nuremberg Code" and offer an ever more detailed and specific legal framework for human experimentation (depending, of course, on the nature of the studies regulated and the subjects population to be protected). Therefore, the importance of the "Nuremberg Code" as the core of public international law research regulation appears even greater.

An often made criticism of the "Nuremberg Code" may deserve somewhat closer attention. It concerns the rule of freely given informed consent. Few are the texts which express in such strength and precision the principle of freely given informed consent by human subjects. It is interesting to note that the "Nuremberg Code" is often criticized on that basis, with some authors asserting the idea that a restrictive understanding of this Code rule prohibits all research using incompetent persons. Such an interpretation seems inappropriate. It is necessary to avoid interpreting this rule in abstracto, but rather to view it in light of general principles of law, in particular those of equality and proportionality. To prohibit, without exception, any research on persons incapable of giving informed consent is equivalent to restricting access to better health care and treatment for the same group. The result of such a protective measure would be to create unjustified inequality of treatment. Application of the principle of proportionality seems even more appropriate in this case for it is expressly recognized in several provisions of the "Nuremberg Code" concerning the favorable balance between risks and benefits, specifically Arts. 4 - 6.

Conclusion

Recognizing the essentially legal character of the "Nuremberg Code" leads directly to questioning the role and place of medical ethics codes in regulation of human research generally. Indeed, it is striking that until very recently physicians enjoyed a quasi monopoly in this matter, there being few legal provisions specifically concerning medical activities.

The fact that doctors quickly characterized the "Nuremberg Code" as a code of medical ethics is not without consequences. By denying, or rather ignoring, the legal nature of the document, doctors have retained control over human experimentation. If the "Nuremberg Code" is but a code of ethics without binding character, violation of its principles will not be subject to social sanctions other than that doctors impose on themselves, namely the prohibition on publishing the results of research not conducted in accordance with the Helsinki Declaration. It is important to emphasize that lawyers and legislators have long tolerated this situation. Their forty year silence can be understood in light of the principle of subsidiarity on which Western legislative activities are based. According to this principle, the State does not intervene in a field which is regulated in a satisfactory way by private initiative. The guidelines of medical ethics have long been considered as sufficient regulation in the field of human research, as well as organ transplantation and medically assisted reproduction.

Under this model, a weakening of the protection of the human subjects until the seventies is apparent. The first version of the Helsinki Declaration, adopted in 1964 by the World Medical Association and claiming a relationship with the "Nuremberg Code", does not mention the rule of informed consent among the basic principles of research ethics. Furthermore, though it provides that the informed consent of human subjects should be obtained before starting a study with no direct therapeutic benefit, the Helsinki Declaration only requires that "if at all possible, consistent with patient psychology, the doctor should obtain the patient's freely given consent after the patient has been given a full explanation".[47] This wording seems to admit the possibility of applying the therapeutic privilege in the field of clinical trials. Such an interpretation contradicts the first principle of the "Nuremberg Code". It has been partly abandoned in the later versions of the Helsinki Declaration.[48]

In fact, the first goal of the Helsinki Declaration was not to protect the freedom and rights of the human subjects, but rather to allow the continuation of human experimentation: "Because it is essential that the results of laboratory experiments be applied to human beings to further scientific knowledge and to help suffering humanity, the WMA has prepared the following recommendations...".

We agree with Dr. Leo Alexander when he states that: "The Nuremberg Code covers all these contingencies in a much more specific manner than subsequent formulation such as the Helsinki Resolution".[49] By enacting codes of medical ethics, the medical profession created a barrier against misplaced intervention by law in medical practice and research. Doing so, they have given themselves greater room to maneuver than they would have been allowed by specific legal provisions. Though the ethical dimension of ethical guidelines and their important role in preventing abuses for some 30 years (or even 40 years after World War II) are unquestionable, it is important not to forget that they were also important tools of professional policy for doctors. Thus, Prof. Otto Gsell, while president of the Central Ethical Commission of the Swiss Academy of Medical Sciences, declared in 1980: "From an ethical point of view, respect for the guidelines specifically requires a strong sense of self-discipline and a high sense of responsibility; it also prevents the enactment of criminal or legislative measures, which is one of the goals of the guidelines of medical ethics".[50]

A careful observer of the medical world is bound to recognize that such a statement definitely belongs to the past. Indeed, many national laws have been adopted in fields originally regulated strictly by medical ethics guidelines. A similar evolution is ascertainable at the international level. This is particularly true in the field of human research, a field which has drawn growing attention from national legislative bodies since the beginning of the 1970s. As the law intervenes in an ever more detailed way in these matters, we believe that the importance of codes of medical ethics will diminish, or at least that their role will be deeply modified. Medical ethics should therefore abandon in large part its normative nature in order to take on a new, still to be defined, form.

Appendix

The generally accepted principles of international law, recognized in the statutes and the sentence of the Nuremberg Tribunal (compiled by ILC), YBILC 1950 II 374, UN Doc. A / 1316 (1950)

I   Any person who commits an act which constitutes a crime under international law is responsible therefore and liable to punishment.

II   The fact that international law does not impose a penalty for an act which constitutes a crime under international law does not relieve the person who committed the act from responsibility under international law.

III   The fact that a person who committed an act which constitutes a crime under international law acted as Head of State or responsible Government official does not relieve him from responsibility under international law.

IV   The fact that a person acted pursuant to order of his Government or of a superior does not relieve him from responsibility under international law, provided a moral choice was in fact possible to him.

V   Any person charged with a crime under international law has the right to a fair trial on the facts and law.

VI   The crimes hereinafter set out are punishable as crimes under international law:

    a)   Crimes against peace:

        i)   Planning, preparation, initiation of waging of a war of aggression or a war in violation of international treaties, agreements or assurances;

        ii)   Participation in a common plan or conspiracy for the accomplishment of any of theacts mentioned under (i).

    b)   War crimes:

    Violations of the laws or customs of war which include, but are not limited to, murder, ill-treatment or deportation to slave-labour or for any other purpose of civilian population of or in occupied territory, murder or ill-treatment of prisoners of war, of persons on the seas, killing of hostages, plunder of public or private property, wanton destruction of cities, towns, or villages, or devastation not justified by military necessity.

    c)   Crimes against humanity:

    Murder, extermination, enslavement, deportation and other inhumain acts done against any civilian population, or persecutions on political, racial or religious grounds, when such acts are done or such persecutions are carried on in execution of or in connexion with any crime against peace or any war crime.

VII   Complicity in the commission of a crime against peace, a war crime, or a crime against humanity as set forth in Principle VI is a crime under international law.

Notes

*   The authors wish to thank Lieutenant Colonel Michael Schmitt (JD, LL.M) of the United States Naval War College's Department of Law for his friendly and critical support in editing the English version of this paper.

1   Allied Declaration of the governments in Exile at London of 13 January 1942 on the Punishment of War Crimes, reproduced in Heinze/Schilling, p. 309 (translated by the authors).

2   Moscow Declaration on German Atrocities of 1 November 1943, reproduced in Annas/Grodin, *The Nazi Doctors and the Nuremberg Code*, Oxford 1992, p. 8

3   London Agreement of 8 August 1945 reproduced in Annas/Grodin, *The Nazi Doctors and the Nuremberg Code*, Oxford 1992, p. 9.

4   Abyssinia, Australia, Belgium, Denmark, Greece, Haiti, Honduras, India, Yugoslavia, Luxembourg, the Netherlands, Norway, New-Zealand, Panama, Paraguay, Poland, Czechoslovakia, Uruguay and Venezuela.

5   a) *Crimes against Peace*: planning, preparation, initiation or waging of a war of aggression, or a war in violation of international treaties, agreements or assurances, or participation in a common plan or conspiracy for the accomplishment of any of the foregoing.

    b) *War Crimes*: namely, violations of the laws or customs of war. Such violations shall include, but are not limited to, murder, ill-treatment or deportation to slave labor or for any other purpose of civilian population of or in occupied territory, murder or ill-treatment of prisoners of war or persons on the seas, killing of hostages, plunder of public or private property, wanton destruction of cities, town or villages, or devastation not justified by military necessity.

c) *Crimes against Humanity*: namely, murder, extermination, enslavement, deporta-
tion and other inhumane acts committed against any civilian population, before or
during the war, or persecutions on political, racial or religious grounds in execution or
in connection with any crime within the jurisdiction of the Tribunal, whether or not in
violation of the domestic law of the country where perpetrated.

6　International Military Tribunal, Opinion and Judgement, p. 48, sec (E), The Law of
the Charter.

7　France, the United Kingdom, the United States and the Soviet Union.

8　Resolution adopted by the General Assembly, Affirmation of the Principles of International Law recognized by the Charter and Judgment of the Nuremberg Tribunal, G.
A. Res. 95, UN Doc. A/64/Add. 1, p. 188 (1946).

9　YBILC, II, 1950, p. 374 ff; UN Doc. A/1316 (1950); See Jescheck, *Die Entwicklung
des Völkerstrafrechts nach Nürnberg*, Revue Suisse de Droit Pénal 72 (1957), p. 221
ff.

10　Art. 38, Statute of the International Military Tribunal; see also Verdross/Simma, *Uni-
verselles Völkerrecht*, 3. Aufl., Berlin 1984, Kap. 3; Brownlie, *Principles of Public
International Law*, 4th ed., Oxford 1990, p. 1 ff.

11　The Vienna Convention on the Law of Treaties of 22 May 1969 defines a peremptory
norm of public international law in article 53: "For the purposes of the present Convention, a peremptory norm of general international law is a norm accepted and recognized by the international community of States as a whole as a norm from which no
derogation is permitted and which can be modified only by a subsequent norm of general international law having the same character." See also Verdross/Simma (note 10),
p. 328 ff.; Brownlie, (note 10), p. 512 ff.

12　The United States, the United Kingdom and other States. See Drinan, *The Nuremberg
Principles and Intentional Law*, p. 176, 178 f., in: Annas/Grodin, *The Nazi Doctors
and the Nuremberg Code*, Oxford 1992.

13　See Triffterer, *Dogmatische Untersuchungen zur Entwicklung des materiellen Völkerstrafrechts seit Nürnberg*, Freiburg i. Br. 1966, p. 3; Woetzel, *The Nuremberg Trials
in International Law*, New York 1962, p. 244; Taylor, *Die Nürnberger Prozesse, 50
Jahre danach, Hintergründe, Analysen und Erkenntnisse aus heutiger Sicht*, 2. Aufl.,
München 1994, p. 722 ff.

14　United Nations, Report of the International Law Commission on the Work of its 46th
Session, 2 May-22 July 1994, GAOR, 49th Session, Suppl. No. 10, A/49/10.

15　See Nill-Theobald, *Anmerkungen über die Schaffung eines Ständigen Internationalen
Strafgerichtshofs*, in: ZStW 108, (1996), Heft 1, p. 229 ff.

16　United States v. Karl Brandt et al., The Medical Case, Trials of War Criminals Before
the Nuremberg Military Tribunals under Control Council Law No 10., Vol. I and II,
Washington D. C., U. S. Government Printing Office, 1948.

17　Of 185 accused, four persons committed suicide or had their trial deferred for health
reasons. Twenty-four persons were sentenced to death or imprisoned, of whom 12
were executed. Nineteen were condemned to jail for life, 18 for a period of 20 years
and less, and 35 were freed, Taylor, *Nuremberg Trials, War Crimes and International
Law*, New York 1949, p. 277 ff.; see also Lediakh, *The Application of the Nuremberg
Principles by other Military Tribunals and National Courts*, in: Gins-
burgs/Kudriavtsev, *The Nuremberg Trial and International Law*, Dor-
drecht/Boston/London 1990, p. 268.

18　U.S. v. Altstoetter et al. (The Justice Case), Case 3, III Trials of War Criminals Before
the Nurnberg Military Tribunals (Wash: GPO, 1950-51), also in VI Law Reports of
Trials of War Criminals (London: HMSO, 1948).

19 For more details of the consequences of the Nuremberg trial, see Jung, *Die Rechts-
    probleme der Nürnberger Prozesse*, Tübingen 1992; Lediakh (note 17), p. 263 ff.;
    Taylor (note 17), p. 272 ff.

20 Furthermore, one accused received a sentence of ten years for belonging to the SS
    while knowing the criminal practices of this group.

21 United States v. Karl Brandt et al., (note 16), Vol. II., Judgment, p. 182.

22 Taylor (note 17), p. 280 ff.

23 By contrast, Jescheck considers the American military tribunal as a jurisdiction of oc-
    cupation, having no relationship to public international law (Jescheck, *Die
    Verantwortlichkeit der Staatsorgane nach Völkerstrafrecht*, Bonn 1952, p. 156). An-
    nas also speaks of the primarily American character of this Court: "[T]he Doctors'
    Trial was conducted by U.S. judges under the authority of the U.S. military, U.S. pro-
    cedures were followed, and U.S. lawyers acted as prosecutors." Annas, *The Nurem-
    berg Code in U.S. Courts: Ethics versus Expediency*, in: Annas/Grodin, *The Nazi
    Doctors and the Nuremberg Code*, Oxford 1992, p. 201.

24 Reproduced in Annas/Grodin, *The Nazi Doctors and the Nuremberg Code*, Oxford
    1992, p. 317.

25 Ibid., p. 322.

26 Attorney General of Israel v. Adolf Eichmann, printed in AJIL 56 (1962), p. 805 ff.

27 Cass. (Ch. Crim.), 6 October 1983, Receuil Dalloz Sirey, Jr.,1984, p. 113 ff.

28 See art. 2 of the Control Council Law N° 10 (note 24).

29 The definition of the crimes is found in the Sixth Principle of Nuremberg.

30 See Lediakh (note 17), p. 268 ff.

31 See Deutsch, *Die zehn Punkte des Nürnberger Ärzteprozesses über die klinische For-
    schung am Menschen: der sog. Nürnberger Codex*, p. 74; Wille, *Grundsätze des
    Nürnberger Ärzteprozesses*, in: NJW 10 (1949), p. 377.

32 United States v. Karl Brandt et al., (note 16), Vol. II., Judgment, p. 182.

33 Ibid.

34 Concerning the influence of the "Nuremberg Code" on American legislation and ju-
    risprudence, see Glantz, *The Influence of the Nuremberg Code on U.S. Statutes and
    Regulations* and Annas, *The Nuremberg Code in U.S. Courts : Ethics versus Expedi-
    ency*, in : Annas/Grodin, *The Nazi Doctors and the Nuremberg Code*, Oxford 1992, p.
    183 ff, 201 ff.

35 See Advisory Committee on Human Radiation Experiments, Final Report, October
    1995, p. 101 ff.

36 In re Cincinnati Radiation Litigation, 874 F. Supp. 796 (S. D. Ohio 1995) of 11. Janu-
    ary 1995, p. 819 ff.

37 "No one shall be subjected to torture or cruel, inhuman or degrading treatment or
    punishment. In particular, no one shall be subjected without his free consent to medi-
    cal or scientific experimentation."

38 Treatment of the wounded, sick and shipwrecked: "Any attempts upon their lives, or
    violence to their persons, shall be strictly prohibited; in particular, they shall not be
    murdered or exterminated, subjected to torture or to biological experiments; they shall
    not willfully be left without medical assistance and care, nor shall conditions exposing
    them to contagion or infection be created."

39 Treatment of prisoners of war: "In particular, no prisoner of war may be subjected to
    physical mutilation or to medical or scientific experiments of any kind which are not
    justified by the medical, dental or hospital treatment of the prisoner concerned and
    carried out in his interest."

40   Treatment of civilian persons: "The High Contracting Parties specifically agree that each of them is prohibited from taking any measure of such a character as to cause physical suffering or extermination of protected persons in their hands. This prohibition applies not only to murder, torture, corporal punishment, mutilation and medical or scientific experiments not necessitated by the medical treatment of a protected person, but also to any other measures of brutality whether applied by civilian or military agents."

41   See Perley/Fluss/Bankowski/Simon, in Annas/Grodin, *The Nazi Doctors and the Nuremberg Code*, Oxford 1992, p. 152 ff.

42   Reproduced in: Revue Internationale de Droit Pénal 51 (1980), p. 419 ff.

43   In the same sense, see also Perley/Fluss/Bankowski/Simon (note 41), p. 149 ff.

44   See Bélanger, Droit International de la Santé, Paris 1983, p. 43. Bélanger rightfully acknowledges the fact that rules of international medical law, among them the Nuremberg Code, are peremptory rules of public international law.

45   Jay Katz underlines the legal character of the "Nuremberg Code", in Katz, *The Nuremberg Code and the Nuremberg Trial*, in: Journal of the American Medical Association 276 (1996), 1662. See also Annas/Grodin, who denies the fact that the "Nuremberg Code" is solely a code of ethics. Medicine and Human Rights: Reflections on the Fiftieth Anniversary of the Doctors' Trial, in: Health and Human Rights, Vol. 2, No. 1, 1996, p. 7 ff.

46   See Deutsch (note 31), p. 77.

47   Cf. Annas/Grodin (note 45), p. 11 ff.

48   Tokyo 1975, Venice 1983 and Hong Kong 1989.

49   Alexander Leo, *Psychiatry : Methods and Process for Investigation of Drugs*, in: Annals of the New York Academy of Science 169 (1970), p. 344, 346, cited by Deutsch (note 31), p. 74.

50   Gsell Otto, *Einführung in die "Richtlinien zur Aerztlichen Ethik" der Schweizerischen Akademie der medizinischen Wissenschaften*, in: BMS 36 (1980), p. 351 (translated by the authors).

8 The Disturbed Equilibrium Between Science, Myths and Medicine: Towards a New Rationalism?

Maurice A.M. de Wachter

An Intricate Web: Science, Myths, Medicine

It is difficult to grasp the complex relations evoked by the title I was given for this paper on 'Science, Myths and Medicine after Nuremberg'. On the one hand, it may seem possible to put science and medicine (at least to the extent that medicine is a science) under a common denominator and thus bring some logic and order in both the fields of science and medicine. On the other hand, such harmonization seems hardly possible with science and myth. However, a closer look at historical and even contemporary writings on the relationship between myth and science will reveal that the link between them is not uncommon. As for the link between myth and medicine, today's vast literature on the miracles of medicine, certainly, displays numerous examples of mythical language. For instance, hormone replacement therapy reminds one of the medieval myth on the rejuvenating waters of the 'source de jouvence'. The same goes for several techniques which assist human reproduction and for genetic engineering. These techniques provoke dreams of perfect offspring and longevity with great quality of life. Amongst the many such myths of health and medicine I have chosen 'death with dignity'.

Given the complex, if not chaotic rapport between myths, science and medicine we ought to raise, amongst others, the following questions: Are myth and science like water and fire? Are they rather like brothers and sisters, albeit sometimes quarreling siblings? Should perhaps one of them prevail over the others? Should it then be science and, certainly, medicine that prevails over myth? Or, should we turn the question around and ask if it is perhaps our despair with abusive science which has sprung upon us the last hope hidden in the box of Pandora that might save us? And last but not least, should we not clarify the words, especially the word 'myth', in order to allow for some focus in the debate? But, to begin with, let us look at today's state of the *ars moriendi* in our Western culture.

The State of Ars Moriendi

The myth of death with dignity is alive and well in our Western societies. While collecting notes for this paper, pertinent material was provided by media such as *Time Magazine* and the London *Sunday Times*. *Time* (April 15, 1996) reported on the US Courts (of New York State and of San Francisco) that opened the way to physician-assisted suicide. To follow suit the American Medical Association (AMA) announced plans to revisit the current policy of frowning upon doctors who participate in patient suicide. The *Sunday Times* (April 14, 1996) made front page news of an upcoming ruling by a High Court Judge regarding decisions not to use artificial feeding. The newspaper put the issue in the context of "fears that people were being pointlessly subjected to painful cardiopulmonary resuscitation (CPR) instead of being allowed **to die with dignity**" (boldface print added by the author).

Sherwin Nuland, a surgeon and medical historian at Yale University, recently wrote about the way we die:

> We compose scenarios that we yearn to see enacted by our mortally ill beloved, and the performances are successful just often enough to sustain our expectations. Faith in the possibility of such a scenario has ever been a tradition of Western societies, which in centuries past valued a good death as the salvation of the soul and an uplifting experience for friends and family and celebrated it in the literature and pictorial representation of **ars moriendi**, the art of dying. Originally, **ars moriendi** was a religious and spiritual endeavor, described by the fifteenth century printer William Caxton as 'the craft for to deye for the helthe of mannes sowle.' In time it evolved into the concept of the beautiful death, truly the correct way to die. But **ars moriendi** is nowadays made difficult by the very fact of our attempts at concealing and sanitizing - and especially preventing - which result in the kinds of deathbed scenes that occur in such specialized hiding places as intensive care units, oncology research facilities, and emergency rooms. The good death has increasingly become a myth. Actually, it has always been for the most part a myth, but never nearly as much as today. The chief ingredient of the myth is the longed-for ideal of 'death with dignity'.[1]

This passage well illustrates the troubled relationship between myth, science and medicine. It shows indeed today's poor state of the **ars moriendi**, and how it is a counterfeit to call the way we mostly die a 'death with dignity'. Yet that death with dignity was explicitly claimed by the newspaper reporter in the Sunday Times, when he said: '...instead of being allowed to die with dignity'. This same death with dignity was also mentioned by Sherwin Nuland but without him approving when he spoke of 'the longed-for ideal of "death with dignity", hinting that this would mean a death without loss of dignity. This death without loss of dignity is considered by Nuland as the chief ingredient in the myth of the good death.

In 1983 Michel Vovelle, a French historian in the school of 'l'histoire des mentalités', published his book 'La mort en Occident de 1300 à nos jours'. Roughly the book reflected positions we knew well from Philippe Ariès' expositions on the efforts of our medicalized society to hide death and dying from the public eye. Vovelle summarily sketched the last four decades as follows: 'médicalisation de la mort dans le système hospitalier, acharnement thérapeutique surtout, conduisant par une réaction en chaîne à formuler les problèmes de l'euthanasie - passive et active - d'où sort la revendication de la **"mort dans la dignité"**' (boldface print added by the author).[2] Vovelle also highlighted the reaction in society against the power of doctors and hospitals. People do not always want heroic measures to be taken. Moreover, people 'fear' pointless and painful treatments such as cardiopulmonary resuscitation (CPR).

During those same four decades, more particularly starting off with the first court case (1974) and a near acquittal of a physician who had terminated her own mother's life, the Netherlands has become a leader in the field of death and dying. Often an explicit appeal is made for the patient's quasi absolute rights of self-determination. One cannot but confirm that the myth of 'death with dignity' is alive and well in the Netherlands. One striking phenomenon, though, which I wish to mention is that 65% of all deaths do occur at home, and that about 75% of all euthanasia cases and assisted suicides take place at home under the supervision of a family physician. Death and, even more, the process of dying are not hidden by Dutch society. Sometimes dying becomes a public event that can be seen on television. It seems, then, correct if we say that the Dutch have led the way: the new attitudes toward death and dying appearing since the 1970s have gradually been incorporated into the Dutch health care system. When commenting about these changes in 1989, I wrote that 'Time will reveal the wisdom or folly of this experience in medical ethics'.[3] Today it is clear that many countries worldwide are striving to go through the same if not identical experience. However, Dutch physicians and policymakers are mostly appalled by this, because they are convinced that a number of special conditions have to take hold before any society can be deemed ripe for the practice.[4]

The above description of the myth of 'death with dignity' shows that our contemporaries evaluate it in either one of the two following ways. Either people will call the myth of 'dying with dignity' a lie. They might even say that here is a denial of any form of good death. Or, they will say that 'death with dignity' is no myth at all but the missing piece of truth in the way we die. For them it is, in actual fact, the only way of dying without loss of dignity.

By now it has become clear that accepting the challenge of undoing the knots evoked by the title of this paper can only be faced by elucidating some concepts, in particular the concept of 'myth'. This we shall try to do by offering a definition of myth and by, subsequently, applying it to science and medicine.

A Definition of the Word 'Myth'

Most language dictionaries provide three different definitions for the word 'myth': one refers to stories about human origins, another to untruths or lies, and a third to social and cultural symbols.

First there is 'myth' in terms of basic stories about the beginnings, about the origins of man, of creation, of disease and many more human situations. These beginnings came about through superhuman or divine intervention. A modern version of this use of the word is given by Michel Serres in his wonderful story called 'Angels. A modern myth':

> In the old days, the immortals only bothered about men - who were anyway condemned to an early death - in order to hand down cruel orders or to lecture them on morality. Armed with Zeus' atomic thunderbolts, they sat round their tables, laughing and drinking pharmaceutical liquors of immortality, and entertained themselves with complex love affairs, in mountain hideaways, defended by the power of fire and separated from mortals who, for their part, were deemed to live a life of implacable necessity... Do you recognize these Olympian figures?[5]

Another example is the myth of Pandora telling us how disease was sent to us mortals by the gods. The best known version of Pandora's box is the one given by Hesiod in his Works and Days. Hesiod tells us that, after Prometheus had stolen fire from heaven and bestowed it upon mortals, Zeus determined to counteract the blessing. Zeus accordingly commissioned Hephaestus to fashion a woman out of earth, upon whom the gods bestowed their choices gifts. She had or found a jar, the so-called 'Pandora's box', containing all kinds of misery and evil. Zeus sent her to Epimetheus, who, forgetting the warning of his brother Prometheus to accept no present from Zeus, made her his wife. Pandora afterward opened the jar, from which all manner of evils flew out over the earth. According to the version given in Hesiod, Hope alone remained inside, the lid having been shut down before she escaped.[6] And in the words of Hesiod himself:

> But all the other numerous evils roam around amongst the humans. Indeed, the earth is filled with evils, and so is the sea. The diseases move around as they please. By night and by day they bring suffering to the mortals.[7]

A second use of the word 'myth' denotes stories of ill-founded beliefs that are held uncritically. Sometimes 'myth' is used in this sense to condemn opinions as lies, e.g. in the debate on euthanasia the notion of 'death with dignity' is rejected by some as being an outright lie. Paradoxically, some of the greatest anthropologists have used the word 'myth' in this sense. Sir James Frazer, for instance, 'assumed that humanity's progressive evolution could be measured by the degree to which it had cast off the myth and magic of primitive religion'.[8] The second use of the word 'myth' is mainly a question of semantics. To call something 'a myth' is not what matters in the user's mind. What does matter is the negative slant with which the word 'myth' is imbued, making it synonymous with the lie. For our debate this second use is only of minor interest.

A third use of the word 'myth' denotes a set of symbolic representations that influence social life. 'Myth', according to Dumézil, fulfills three functions in society. First, there is the function of the sacred as a source of all creativity represented in the role of seers, priests and kings. Second, there is the function of the warrior in protecting communal existence and vital energy. Third, there is the function of productivity embodied in the roles of workers, artists and craftsmen, including for instance, physicians. Such myths serve to unfold a world view or to explain, possibly even justify and legitimize a certain practice. Some[9] believe that western society is suffering from a serious imbalance of the three functions of myth. This is due to the fact that the myth of progress, particularly its economic version, has come to justify affluent society as the main goal of our existence, even at the expense of the two other vital functions that are needed to strike a balance.

In this paper we shall mainly focus on myths according to the first and the third meaning. Scientists trying to reintegrate science in its humane context will mainly refer to the first meaning. Historians and anthropologists will rather work with myths and mythology in the third sense. Schama, for instance, as we shall illustrate shortly, accepts the idea that myths may be highly complex systems of understanding with the power to generate and determine social behavior.

"Pour une nouvelle rationalité"

Patrick Trousson, a physicist and computer specialist, currently in charge of scientific projects at the European Commission, wrote a book called *Le recours de la science au mythe. Pour une nouvelle rationalité*. In it he argues that classical science, in particular physics, needs myth. He holds that myth makes whole again what science (epitomized by its rationalistic and analytic approach) has taken apart. Mythical wholeness heals the brokenness of scientific fragmentation. Trousson acknowledges today's misuse of the word myth. Instead of referring to the foundation of culture, myth has become obsolete and expendable.

True myth, however, has for centuries had a connotation of sacredness and of the highest levels of knowledge and wisdom. It was the prime vehicle for expressing the mysteries of our world. Nowadays 'le beau mot "mythe" en est venu évoquer, dans le langage courant, quelque chose d'imaginaire, d'irréel, de faux, de mensonger'.[10] Instead of explaining the origins of our being, it is now a children's tale, a moralizing story, a fantastic 'utopia'.

Nevertheless, Trousson highly values mythology in the first meaning of the word as we described previously, viz. the story of how things, all things (heaven and earth, man and woman, life and death) occurred at the beginning. He agrees with Kerboul who says that mythology explains by directly referring to origins, rather than by concatenation of proximal causes, which is the way classical science used to explain things.[11]

The new rationality, according to Trousson, has taken its initial steps through the systemic thinking in physics. Having abandoned the mechanistic model and having accepted the model of indeterminacy in physics (such as Heisenberg's admission that ultimate precision is impossible), today's scientists should have no major objections against the holistic thinking of mythology. By definition myths acknowledge the impossibility of ultimate precision, yet by using symbols they are able to impart information in a more general and more global sense, though admittedly do so more vaguely. Myths grasp the meaning intuitively, whereas classical science wants to grasp reality rationally. Our efforts today should be at bridging both modes of knowledge: analytic reasoning and intuition.[12]

The task which the Freiburg Project set out to achieve will find encouragement in Trousson's concluding sentence: 'Restons fidèles à cette Europe au sein de laquelle se sont développés à la fois les mythes et les sciences et gardons cette vision large en alliant la lumière de la raison et la clarté du mythe'.[13]

Beyond Medicine: Myth and Memory

The historian Simon Schama is equally convinced of the persistence of myth and of the vital role myths play in culture and in the value choices nations make. Schama does not want 'to concede the subject by default to those who ... apprehend myth not as a historical phenomenon but as an unchallengeable perennial mystery'.[14] Where Trousson seeks a new rationality and new myths, Schama wonders what can be wrong with the old ones. In a context of today's concern about ecology Schama wants to 'suggest the strength of the links that have bound (nature and culture) together' by excavating beneath the hidden layers 'to recover the veins of myth and memory that lie beneath the surface'.[15] For Schama "it is clear that inherited landscape myths and memories share two common characteristics: their surprising endurance through the centuries and their power to shape institutions that will still live with".[16]

The mythical facets of the forest, for instance, were portrayed in Anselm Kiefer's 'Die Hermannschlacht' in 1977. In this 'portrait gallery of the physiognomy of natural destiny' Kiefer wishes to illustrate the German cultural revival since Napoleon times. The gallery displays such German authors as Arminius, Fichte and eventually Heidegger. 'What they all share is a fateful implication in national, tribal myth: a force hard to resist, but which leads up the forest path, to a wooden grave'.[17] Schama's powerful interpretation of Kiefer's paintings must be quoted in full:

> Evidently, Kiefer did not share the view, popular among empirical historians in the 1960s, that the Third Reich was a historical aberration that owed little or nothing to long traditions of German militarist authoritarianism. It would be convenient, of course, if the violent myths of blood and soil could be safely pigeonholed as peculiarly Nazi, and leave it at that. But Kiefer is too conscientious a cultural historian to tolerate such tidy classifications. Democracy, he seems to say, averts its face from these myths at its perils. To exorcise their spell means, to some extent, understanding their potency at close quarters, even, perhaps, within contamination range.[18]

Thus Schama shows what disasters befall us when myth dominates science and reason, when myth and magic take over from the Enlightenment the skepticism about them. Although myths may be universal in nature, it depends of course on particular nations to make a particular myth such as the one of 'blood and soil' a dominant folk model for a given 'Volk' under Nazi dictatorship.

A further remark Schama makes about myths concerns not so much the user as the student of myth. 'To be sure, he says, myths are seductive things. A truly disconcerting number of those who have spent their lives codifying, narrating, and explicating them have not gone unbewitched by their spell'.[19] The names of Mircea Eliade and Joseph Campbell are frighteningly close to our days. Schama extends the line to Jung, of course, and Nietzsche, even to the French anthropologist Dumézil and many more 'whose embrace of myth fired their hostility to natural-rights individualism, and the democratic politics that protects it'.[20]

Ambivalence: The Janus-head of All Myth

Both rational thinking and mythical thinking are instruments with which our mind tries to master and organize the world we live in. Whereas rationality walks the ever narrowing path of empirical analysis and logic, myth walks the ever widening road of analogy and experimental symbolism. Rationality is reductionist. Myth is holistic. Each rivals with the other in attempting to control the way we view our world. Twentieth century history reveals the disaster that follows when one outweighs the other. Before Nuremberg, when Nazis myths outlawed rationality, the world became the sad witness of what happens when 'democracy averts its face from these myths at its peril'.[21] Should we then join the doomsday prophets who say that after Nuremberg the Western World is still learning its lessons the hard way from the potentially destructive scientific applications in nuclear and medical technologies? Despite the fact that science nowadays increasingly admits the need for images and symbols which it formerly rejected (e.g. the contraction of space) it keeps on dreaming of a rational way of controlling all being.

Western medicine reflects the reductionist trend of science, thereby often loosing the original experience of health and illness. True, a few efforts have been made to introduce a holistic approach into medicine and thus to rebuild the original all-encompassing complexity of health and illness. But could this be all that myth is supposed to do for medicine? If this were the case, Fritjof Capra's critique of the false 'myth' in medicine is more valid than ever. He says that the biomedical model is generally accepted, that its basic principles are so thoroughly ingrained in our culture that 'it has even become the dominant folk model of illness. Most people do not understand its intricacies very well, but they have been conditioned to believe that the doctor alone knows what made them sick and that technological intervention is the only thing that will get them well'.[22] We want of course to emphasize the words '**dominant folk model of illness**' as well as '**they have been conditioned to believe**'. And we hear an echo from Schama's statement about the dangers to democracy when violent myths (e.g. the one of blood and soil) dominate a given society.

But, then, we should ask if this is the only plausible way of looking at myth. Is the rapport between rationality and myth perhaps a dialectical one? Are rationality and myth perhaps two sides of one coin? Should we, therefore, ever resist the temptation of letting one outdo the other. Both Schama and Trousson seem to come to this constructive view. Schama wonders: 'how much myth is good for us? And how can we measure the dosage?'[23] As for Trousson, he advocates 'une nouvelle rationalité'. This new rationality combines the clarity of myth with the light of reason. Schama pleads for myth cautiously and gives early warning signals. To quote him: 'The real problem is whether it is possible to take myth seriously on its own terms, and to respect its coherence and complexity, without becoming morally blinded by its poetic power'.[24] Trousson pleads for myth rather uncautiously. To quote him: 'La science et le mythe répondent tous deux à une rationalité',[25] viz., science through analysis and myth through intuition.

In this best of world interpretations, where myth and medical science are not necessarily seen as conflicting but possibly as partners in harmony, there remains, however, a more fundamental ambivalence that needs to be faced. It is perhaps the same situation that some agencies had perceived before Nuremberg and had tried to bring under control by means of guidelines for medical experimentation.

... After Nuremberg

Would it be too much 'hineininterpretiert' if we were to read the presence of both myth and rationality in the Reich Minister's guidelines? Although issued in 1931, the guidelines fell back upon a directive issued on December 29, 1900, by the Prussian Minister of Religious, Educational and Medical Affairs. Take article 13 of the Reich Minister's which reads:

> While physicians and, more particularly, those in charge of hospital establishments may thus be expected to be guided by a strong sense of responsibility toward their patients, they should at the same time not be denied the satisfying responsibility (Verantwortungsfreudigkeit) of seeking new ways to protect or treat patients or alleviate or remedy their suffering where they are convinced, in the light of their medical experience, that known methods are likely to fail.[26]

The very word 'Verantwortungsfreudigkeit' added by the translator could suggest that, next to it being somewhat unusual, the word might carry a particular message which has been only in part rendered by his translation as 'satisfying responsibility'. More importantly, the light which both Trousson and Schama have shed upon our exploration of myth in connection with our Nuremberg commemoration may help us to perceive the meaning of the guideline. The 1931 guidelines are for physicians who, according to Dumézil's theory of myth, contribute to the third role of myth, viz. society's productivity, welfare, and the maintenance of its well-being. The myth of progress could be at work in the legitimizing by official political instances of 'new ways to protect or treat or alleviate or remedy their (i.e. the patients') suffering'. We find ourselves, therefore, in doubt as to how to read article 13: is it meant as a warning signal coming from an authority which draws lines to permissible experiments, or as the encouragement by a public authority to experiment at all levels of medicine 'where physicians are convinced, in the light of their medical experience, that known methods are likely to fail?' The latter is, of course as we all know, what most methods then meant for most diseases.

Conclusion and Further Exploration

Any society that has lived through Nuremberg, be it as defendant or as prosecutor, ought to be alert and watch out for a possible disturbance of the balance amongst the three functions of myth: sacredness, self-defense, and productivity. Focusing more on medicine and its role in the field of 'productivity' of life, its generation, maintenance, protection and restoration, three further avenues can be sketched for further exploration.

First, we need to explore the notion of human dignity and its diversity in a multicultural society.[27] Official documents, such as the European Convention on Bioethics, want to make this notion a fundamental one. But, how universal is the notion of human dignity? Acute problems arise when biomedical technologies indiscriminately invade individuals, families and groups in society. Lately, Western countries have become aware of the decomposing influence which some forms of health care may have upon minorities and vulnerable individuals. Predictive medicine, in particular, seems to reclassify individuals out of the boundaries of their natural belonging, out of the social fabric of their origins. We cannot but notice that 'reclassification' of the others is an age old effect of mythical thinking. Some transplantation practices and the transcultural problems they raise are forms of reclassification.

Second we need to explore the ancient myth of humans as female and male. In doing so, we may restore a long lost balance in the duties of healing and caring. The elaboration of feminist ethics may be one appropriate way of building the bridge between intuition and reason in the field of medicine. But little has been done.

Finally, we need to continue our evaluation of 'informed consent' in a society which perceives information and knowledge as power.

The aim of the informed consent requirement is double: patients ought to know what they consent to, and they ought to be capable of consenting to what they know. It not only protects against possible abuse by physicians but also against hypertrophy of patient autonomy. We need not too readily submit to an absolutized exercise of self-determination, to the point that only our poets dare to ask if perhaps 'the choice itself creates the value?'[28]

Summary

I have tried to illustrate that the myth of dying with dignity is alive and well in today's medical practice and in decisions regarding the end of life. I have illustrated Trousson's plea for a new rationality which would combine in his own words 'la lumière de la raison et la clarté du mythe'. I have borrowed from Schama the viewpoint that certain societal myths may dominate science and reason, which leads to terrible catastrophes. I pointed out that the relationship between science and myth seems always to be an ambiguous one. At the commemoration, fifty years after Nuremberg, this ambivalence should be part of our approach to bioethical questions today as well as then. Early warning signals about permissible experiments with humans can be formulated on the basis of our renewed understanding of myth. The most important question raised by Schama also applies: 'So how much myth is good for us? And how can we measure the dosage?'[29]

Notes

1   Nuland XVI
2   Vovelle 79
3   Wachter 1989
4   Wachter 1996

5   Serres 191
6   Rose 55
7   Hesiod Part I vv 100-13
8   Schama 208
9   Trousson 191
10   Trousson 34
11   Kerboul 55
12   Trousson 264
13   Trousson 266
14   Schama 134
15   Schama 14
16   Schama 15
17   Schama 133
18   Schama 133
19   Schama 133
20   Schama 134
21   Schama 133
22   Capra 161
23   Schama 134
24   Schama 134
25   Trousson 265
26   Grodin 131
27   Taylor et al.
28   Heany 51
29   Schama 134

References

Capra F. (1982), *The Turning Point. Science, Society, and the Rising Culture*. Toronto, Bantam Books.

Dumézil G. (1969), *Mythes et épopées I. L'idéologie des trois fonctions dans les épopées des peuples européens*. Paris, Gallimard.

Annas G. and Grodin M.A. (1992), *The Nazi Doctors and the Nuremberg Code*. New York/Oxford,1992.

Heany S. (1987), 'The Riddle', *The Haw Lantern*. London, Faber and Faber, p. 51.

Hesiod. (1978), *Works and Days* (ed. M.L. West), Part I. Oxford.

Kerboul C. (1980), *L'homme du verseau, essai sur l'avenir de notre civilisation*. Paris, Dervy Livres.

Nuland S.B. (1993), *How we Die. Reflections on Life's Final Chapter*. New York, A A Knopf.

Rose H.J.(1957), *Handbook of Greek Mythology*. London.

Schama S. (1995), *Landscape and Memory*. Berkeley, University of California Press.

Serres M. (1995), *Angels. A Modern Myth*. Paris, Flammarion.

Taylor C. et al. (1992), *Multiculturalism. Examining the politics of recognition*. Princeton University Press.

Trousson P. (1995), *Le recours de la science au mythe. Pour une nouvelle rationalité*. Paris, L'Harmattan.

Vovelle M. (1983), *La mort en Occident de 1300 à nos jours*. Paris, Gallimard.

Wachter M.A.M. de (1989), 'Active Euthanasia in the Netherlands'. *JAMA*, 262, pp. 3316-3319.

Wachter M.A.M. de (June 1994), *Euthanasia and assisted suicide in The Netherlands and Europe. Proceedings of the European Conference, Report (EUR 16636 EN)*, European Commission DG XII, 1996.

9 Scientific Progress in Socio-Cultural Context: Natural Science, Medicine and Myth after Nuremberg

Dietrich von Engelhardt

The relation between science, myth and medicine is essential and complex; it depends on the meaning of these concepts as well as on the economic, political, social and cultural changes of our century. Without getting into a fundamental discussion, it will suffice here to understand a myth as representations, images and symbols guiding human beings in their thoughts and actions constituting no empirical or scientific rules or facts and no revealed truths either.

The idea of a sequence of myth, religion, philosophy and science in the course of history is common. Auguste Comte held this idea of succession with his concept of the three stages: religion, philosophy and science (Cours de philosophie positive, 1830). Hegel too says in his *Lectures on the history of philosophy* (1833):

> The mythical representation, as one of ancient times, is the representation of a locus where thought is not free... Myth belongs to the pedagogy of the human race. When the concept is adult, it then no longer needs the myth.

In the last years and decades, this view has been discussed on repeated occasions and declared as doubtful (Lévi-Strauss 1958). Obviously, the Christian religion as well as empirical sciences cannot fulfil the emotional and intellectual needs of modern man to the extent or in the way he wishes them to be. In this open space, myths have gained a new function - with consequences for both natural science and medicine and their relations. There is by no means any telling yet which will be the particular and general effects of these changes and movements. But we will undoubtedly come in this context to new evaluations of the Nuremberg Trials.

Nuremberg marks the end of an epoch and the beginning of a new one at the same time, not only for culture and the political world, but also for ethics in general and for ethics in the natural sciences and medicine especially.

In this perspective, Nuremberg means a twofold interrelation of connections: on the one hand the cause of, or direct and indirect condition for, new initiatives and, on the other hand, a horizon against which the postwar situation and contemporary developments can be appraised. The Code of Nuremberg (1947) is doubtless an example for the first type of connection. The same is equally true for the Declarations of Helsinki (1964) and Tokyo (1975). The recent discussions on the idea of health and disease, on the understanding of euthanasia and the concept of the physician-patient relation, as well as contemporary attempts to integrate ethics in medical training are examples of the second type of relation.

Nuremberg is therefore a cause of changes and the scene of their assessments. Certainly, not all developments discussed in the 1996 Freiburg forum can be derived from the Nuremberg Trial and the end of the Third Reich. However, these developments can be described, analyzed and assessed in the light of Nuremberg and the Third Reich. Nuremberg is also a comprehensive answer to the past. It is not only a reaction to the Third Reich, but, in addition to this, a reaction to the general tendencies of modern medicine since the Renaissance and above all since the 19th century marked by positivism.

In this perspective, we must include in our considerations the international trials of Tokyo and Le Havre for the crimes perpetrated in Asia during World War Two and in Bosnia Herzegovina in our days, and reflect about their consequences on natural science, myth and medicine in those parts of the world or in the world in general.

Nuremberg means an end and a beginning. At the same time, there are continuities in practice and in theory, in making both science and its critique something absolute, in the dangers for humanity in medicine and in the attempts to humanize and personalize medicine, in the destructive attitude towards Nature and above all towards animals and in the new search for ecology and bioethics.

Through a few examples, this short article will also go into these continuities or these traditions. In order to understand the uniqueness or the particularity of the topic "science, myth and medicine", it is necessary to draw a comparison with the times which preceeded Nuremberg.

Myths are observable in private and public life. Natural science and medicine themselves have turned into myths. Ancient myths still do mean something today: Apollo, Dionysos, Prometheus, Sisyphus, Cassandra, Oedipus. Apollo and Dionysos stand for reason and feeling, Prometheus for human power and hubris, Sisyphus for powerlessness or, after Camus (*Le mythe de Sysiphe*, 1942), for freedom, Cassandra for ignored prophecy, Oedipus for sexuality and sin. But there are also modern myths, negative and positive ones: progress, rapidity, growth, beauty, health, race, unlimited feasibility, inexhaustibility of Nature, unity between Man and Nature, solidarity, equality, humanity.

The myths of human omnipotence and of inexhaustibility of Nature have lost their force. The concept of Man as the "master and owner of Nature" ("aître et possesseur de la nature", advocated by Descartes (*Le discours de la méthode*, 1637)), with which he met a good response among scientists, physicians and philosophers and through which he secularized the representation of God or transferred it to earthly life, is being increasingly and generally criticized. We have understood that limits are set to human action and ability, that Nature is by no means inexhaustible, that it furthermore depends decisively on Man's responsibility and behavior, that Nature and culture are essentially interwoven in a common destiny.

The question whether the roots of modern science and technique, both in their positive and negative aspects, lay in the Judeo-Christian tradition (Krolzik 1979, White 1967) or in the spirit of Greek-Roman Antiquity (Snell 1946) has not yet been answered once and for all. The answer not only depends on the understanding of science, but also on the significance ascribed to the realm of ideas for the real course of history.

The debate on both myths of predisposition and of environment is characteristic and momentous for our century. One can easily unterstand that, after the pseudotheories of race and their corresponding barbarous experiences during the Third Reich, the weight put on the environment had been exaggerated. However, no one will be able to forget or to disregard the negative experiences our century has made in this respect too. With the increased possibilities of our times to link predisposition and milieu or to examine their specific interplay in the formation of intelligence and genesis of diseases, these two myths will disappear.

The secularization of Paradise - a central fundament of the modern situation and of the almost uncontrollable progress of the natural sciences and medicine - has given birth to powerful myths: to stay young and beautiful, to live without disease and pain till death and maybe even to overcome death. The idea of the prolongation of life stands between myth and science and dominates medicine as well as the population and public life.

The division of two or four cultures plays an essential role in this development and this mythological meaning of scientific and medical aims. C.P. Snow pointed out in his book entitled *The Two Cultures and the Scientific Revolution* (1959) that the differentiation between the natural sciences and humanities which no longer understand each other, brings forth negative consequences for both sides. Scientists consider humanities as unimportant; in the eyes of scholars of the humanities, natural sciences are cultureless.

> Between the two a gulf of mutual incomprehension - sometimes (particularly among the young) hostility and dislike, but most of all lack of understanding.

One must however add two further divisions to this division: arts and behavior. The culture of the natural sciences like the culture of humanities includes by no means the culture of literature, painting and music. Finally, culture can mean theory or practice. One can be a successful scientist and a great cognoscente in literature, but behave improperly or inhumanly. The German language differentiates between the formation of the heart

(*Herzensbildung*) and the formation of the mind (*Verstandesbildung*). Undoubtedly, this is an important differentiation, especially in the field of medicine, and for physicians in their relations and behavior toward sick and dying human beings.

In this perspective, today's comprehensive or cultural attempts make sense and are justified. These attempts are related to the understanding of health and disease, the concept of causality and that of the physician-patient relation. In the natural sciences, these trials apply to the scientists' responsibility for the consequences of their knowledge and research as well as for freedom or rationality of scientific progress (Meyer-Abich 1979).

An ecology which does not stand for a closet economy belongs in this context too. History and present times are rich in corresponding experiences, in theoretical approaches and general myths (Zirnstein 1996). With his cleaning out of Augias' stalls, demigod Heracles fights against environmental pollution. Roman law demanded air pollution control (*aerem corrumpere non licet*). The cultivation of Nature was a central task for monks in the Middle Ages. At the time of the Enlightenment, Voltaire ended his 'Candide' (1759) with the programmatic call to man not to make the changing of the entire world his goal, but rather to cultivate his own garden (*cultivons notre jardin*). This is a request reminding at the same time of the momentous biblical word according to which man had to subjugate Nature (*dominium terrae*) in the responsible and caring, and not adventurous, destructive meaning of the term. At the same time, the French natural scientist Buffon warned his contemporaries against the danger that man might misuse his might over Nature and destroy it. Nature in turn could rise up against man and drag culture to its end: "Tout rentre sous la main de la Nature: elle reprend ses droits, efface les ouvrages de l'homme, couvre de poussière et de mousse ses plus fastueux monuments, les détruit avec le temps" (*Epoques de la nature*, 1764).

Nature and Man belong together; in spite of all ontological and ethical differences - stones, plants and animals are not moral or legal subjects - both are linked together by a common fate in their genesis and future. For the philosopher Schelling, Nature is visible Spirit and Spirit is invisible Nature (*Ideen zu einer Philosophie der Natur*, 1797). In this perspective and in face of the destruction of Italy, the Romantic physician, natural philosopher and painter Carl Gustav Carus was confirmed in his conviction that "not only Man needs the Earth for his life and actions, but also the Earth needs Man" (*Von den Naturreichen*, 1820). In 1866, Ernst Haeckel coined the word 'ecology' in his *Generelle Morphologie*. But, in the researcher's conception, the term was first limited to the "physiology of the relations of the animal organism to the outer world."

Medical ethics not only as foundation of principles, but also as theory of the practical realization of these ethical principles or obligations is an essential example of new initiatives in a medical perspective; biology, psychology and sociology should be taken into consideration, and so-called "natural fallacies" be avoided (confusions between natural observations and ethical requirements) and therefore the individual's autonomy or freedom be respected in the first place. Autonomy does not generally mean arbitrarity, but reasonable will in the moral sense of the word. The concept of "autonomy" is made of both words "autos/self" and "nomos/law". The realization of ethical principles takes place in the world of affects and social interrelations. But ethics is at its core independent of biology, psychology and sociology. Kant rightly stressed the fact that "empirical principles are nowhere meant to be the basis of human laws".

The complex relation between ethics in medicine and psychology, sociology and jurisprudence can be illustrated on the concept of "informed consent", which is essential for medical ethics and medical research. According to the law in force therapy without beeing informed and without consent means bodily injury; this juridical view sets uneasiness and citicism off for physicians, because this view lacks humane motivation of physicians in their job, which in general is not denied by the legal profession. The need of beeing informed and consent emerge in social interaction and demand psychological abilities of the physician and the patient. Beeing informed and consent as such do not guarantee an ethical standard; both can be related with immoral and inhumane subject matter. Ethics in medicine come true in informed consent, only if physicians pay attention to the autonomy and dignity of the patient, the patient him- or herself and the society; therefore it better should be spoken of "moral and legal informed consent".

Nowadays, various movements in medicine deserving attention must be understood in this context: palliative medicine, euthanasia between life-shortening and giving aid during the process of dying, the hospice movement, "Medical Humanities".

Palliative medicine provides, beyond physical pain-relief, assistance to psychological, social and moral pains (Zielinski 1993). With his quotation from the poet Léon Bloy "to suffer passes by, to have suffered never passes by" (*souffrir passe, avoir souffert ne passe jamais*), the physician and anthropologist F.J.J. Buydendijk (1943) reminds us of the span between biology and culture in the understanding of what pain is - "to suffer" as a physical and present dimension, "to have suffered" as a psychological and historical dimension. Human medicine, which wants to be more than a technique for curing, will try, in its dealing with pain, to do justice to this spectrum. It will endeavour to relieve pain and to apprehend its cosmological and anthropological meaning at the same time.

Euthanasia does not have to mean therapy interruption or termination of life at all. There is a long tradition of euthanasia as assistance in the death process. Especially in the perversion of euthanasia as active homicide in absence of consent or even against the person's will during the Third Reich and in the face of the newest developments in the present, it is necessary to recall this tradition constantly. In Antiquity, euthanasia was synonymous with a pleasant and good death (*felici et honesta morte mori*). While active euthanasia was forbidden to the physician in the Hippocratic oath, Plato and Stoa justified passive and active euthanasia. In the Christian Middle Ages, euthanasia as the shortening of life and abortion were equally excluded. Unforeseen death - an ideal in people's opinion today - was considered as a bad death (*mala mors*). At the beginning of modern times, Morus (1516) and Bacon (1623) made the plea for euthanasia in their Utopian state outlines. Bacon differentiated between a *euthanasia exterior* as physical termination of life and a *euthanasia interior* as mental preparation for death. But physicians did not go along with the plea for active euthanasia. The physician C.W. Hufeland (*Enchiridion medicum*, 1836) warned firmly against the active ending of life by physicians, who would be among of the "most dangerous persons" in the state. Things changed around 1900 in medicine, in natural sciences and humanities, in arts and among the population. Oaths and declarations must prevent in present times a "medicine devoid of humanity" (Mitscherlich and Mielke 1948) as it became reality during the Third Reich. Active euthanasia - always under the requirement of consent - is made possible or is accepted nowadays in the legislations of a few countries. The consideration of the different types of euthanasia and above all their importance as a mental and physical assistance during the dying process are essential in today's debates.

The hospice movement (Saunders et al. 1981), taking up the term "hospice" in its original medieval sense, tries to overcome the separation between hospital and the outside world (*Lebenswelt*). This division can be overcome in two ways: through bringing disease and death back into the family or community or inversely through integrating outside life into the hospital, through rooming-in in obstetrics and pediatric wards as well as in intensive care units and any rooms where people die.

"Medical humanities" apprehends the therapeutic power of arts and sees medicine itself as an art and not only as a natural or applied science. The accurate concept of medicine as a science of action should not let us forget that medical action refers to persons who have a conscience and feelings, a language and social contacts, and not to machines or inorganic or organic objects. In this view, diseases are by no means conceived of only as physical, but also always as social, psychological and mental phenomena. Culture presents, with its representations and interpretations, a fundamental contribution to our ways of dealing with birth, health, disease and death. Medicine for its part exerts an essential influence on culture, theology, philosophy and arts. At the same time, culture goes beyond medicine and psychotherapy - in the sense of Kafka's word on literature as being the "ax for the frozen sea in us" (Letter 27.1.1904). "Medical humanities" transcend medical ethics and offer important contributions to its theory and practice.

Natural science and medicine have developed, were tested and supported not only by natural scientists and physicians, but also by the general public and politicians. Culture as a whole has changed as far as birth, health, disease, death and human relations are concerned. The difficulties in understanding the natural sciences and their results have led to a paradoxical or ambivalent position: we meet natural sciences with skepticism or we even reject them, but we want to enjoy their fruits. Apollo and Dionysos face each other as enemies or as contrary principles. According to an empirical study, the character of Frankenstein (Shelley 1820) is more well-known in the United States than any other dead or living natural scientist (Holton 1974).

The economic crisis gave new impulses to ethical debates in medicine and society - debates on the quality of life, on work and leisure, on the relations between the generations. Herbert Marcuse (1964) criticized the dominating principle of utility: "We live and die rationally and productively". We know today that being put out of one's work can result in a lost of personal contacts and of self-respect. The apotheosis of work is as equally unsatisfying as the apotheosis of leisure.

The demographic changes in Germany, Great Britain and France as well as in other European countries will cause serious political and economic problems. The younger generation will have to pay for the elder and their diseases.

The myth of youth, for its part, proved to be threatening for handicapped and older people. But each stage in life has both its positive and negatives sides. In his *Speech on age* (1860), Jacob Grimm discussed in detail those advantages and disadvantages and drew the general conclusion "that aging does not represent a mere decline of virility, but much more a power of its own which has developed according to its particular laws and conditions." As Romano Guardini emphasized in his study *The ages of life* (1967), the active responsibility of older people is one element of these conditions and laws: "What is the use of all gerontology and all provisions of social care if the older person himself or herself does not reach at the same time a conscience of his or her own?"

In addition, Germany faces here another important consequence: the immigrants necessary for further developments - one finds here the most important number of them in Europe - cannot live in the full consciousness of the Nuremberg tradition like the normal German population does. But what do the words "collective guilt" mean to the new generations and, most of all, to people who come from other countries and have become German citizens?

Numerous sociological and psychological surveys, and anthropological and philosophical analyses have emphasized a more comprehensive understanding of what health, disease and the physician-patient relation are, than it had previously been viewed in established medicine, and furthermore still is. These articles, especially those coming from philosophy, arts and anthropological medicine, were mostly written regardless of Nuremberg. But they gain special significance in the perspective of the Third Reich.

The introduction of the subject in medicine, according to Viktor v. Weizsäcker, holds for the patient, the physician and science. In the therapeutical relation, a subject in pain encounters a helping subject, and not a defective machine a repairing technician. "The real essence of the state of being sick is a distress and it is expressed as a call for help. I call sick the person who visits me as a physician and in whom I as a physician recognize as distressed" (1926). Objectivity is not only related to physical appearances; there are also facts of conscience of supra-individual or general validity. The concept of science is no privilege reserved to the natural sciences.

With the dualism of methods of explaining and understanding, medicine joins natural sciences and humanities together, as the philosopher and psychiatrist Karl Jaspers has shown in the tradition of Vico, Schleiermacher and Dilthey: explaining as the method of the natural sciences and understanding as the method of the humanities. The physician-patient relation stands in this perspective under the ideal of an existential or metaphysical communication lending all empathy its real contents. At the same time, Jaspers not only warns against the banalization, but also against the overappreciation of the concept or idea of the physician: "The physician is neither technician nor Savior, but existence for existence, a transitory human being who realizes with the other, in the other and in himself dignity and liberty, and recognizes them as standards" (1932).

Such representations were and are by no means developed only in Germany. The Spanish physician and anthropologist Pedro Laín Entralgo (1964) differentiated between four dimensions in the physician-patient relationship: the diagnostic recognition relationship, the operational therapy relationship, the affective partner relationship and the ethical religious relationship. The French philosopher Gabriel Marcel (1953), too, opposed the existential relationship between physicians and patients to the technicized relation or to that exclusively fixed on the body. "This relation cannot be functionalized without the being becoming sclerotic."

The well-known definition of health given by the World Health Organization (WHO) as a "state of complete physical, social and mental well-being and not merely the absence of disease or infirmity" (1948) is impressive by its taking into account the social and mental dimensions of health. But it cannot, on grounds of its utopianism and its equating normatively health with the positive and disease with the negative, be satisfying anthropologically speaking. To be able to live with diseases and a handicap can equally be understood as health. It can express psychological and moral force and arouse sympathy and produce social support.

Quality of life is not limited to what an individual is worth for society, to his or her ability to work or to love (Schölmerich 1990). In the Middle Ages, the terms of "salutary disease" (*infirmitas salubris*) and of "pernicious health" (*sanitas perniciosa*) were commonly used. Montaigne, likewise, spoke in his Essays (1580/95) of the *maladies salutaires*, and after Novalis, chronic diseases could become "years of apprenticeship in the art of living and the formation of emotional life" (*Lebenskunst und Gemütsbildung*, Fragmente 1799/1800). It is necessary for us to regain these normative and cultural dimensions of health and disease in medicine and in our personal lives.

There is no doubt about the fact that the general public opinion influences the natural sciences and their progress. It is deplorable that a decline of the natural sciences has taken place, most of all in Eastern European countries. The economic crisis and the end of the myth of communism have reduced by half the number of dissertations in Russia. They are a threat to basic research. There is fear that research in natural sciences in these countries will fall down to the level of that of developing countries.

In Western countries, one must also fear the anti-scientific and antirational currents. Myths do not only have an irrational, but also an irreal component. The dangers inherent to science must be recognized and limited. But we cannot dispense with science; the survival of humanity is endangered without its contribution. One must draw more forcefully politicians' and people's attention to these relations and connections. Scientists too must engage themselves publicly for sciences, for research and academic education.

With the integration of ethics and of psychology, sociology and history in medicine, the possibilities to accept the limits of individual life and of medicine become more important. In the same way, conceptional ways are being opened which make it possible to reconcile the autonomy of the individual with the rights of society.

The economic crisis, and more especially the structural crisis of our times, compels us to develop or to activate new forms of social relations which will have an influence on the natural sciences and on medicine. These in turn will be able and must look for new answers to those changes. In his book *Der moderne Konflikt* (1991), Ralf Dahrendorf discusses the essential "ligatures" or places which link the individual with society: family, community, neighborhood initiatives, values, myths. Communitarianism (Zahlmann 1994) is also an answer to this challenge: private commitment when states have no money. In Seattle (USA), for example, citizens have organized private financing of emergency assistance for acute heart and circulatory diseases.

Our century experienced the parting from two political myths: Nazism and communism. It should also take leave of other myths or illusions in the natural sciences and in medicine. But to live without ideas and myths is impossible. Living so paralyses social responsibility and limits individual zest for life. We must have perspectives and concepts in regard to health and disease, birth and death, loneliness and solidarity, the relation to nature, the link between science and art, between history, present and future in order to lead both an active and contemplative life, to fulfil oneself personally in a social context, to provide a cultural, and not only an egoistical, technical or practical education for the next generation.

In view of the immediate history and the destructive ideologies of our century, which have by no means lost any of their force and attraction, liberty and human dignity, as well as truth and beauty of nature should guide the natural sciences and medicine and be defended inwardly and outwardly by their representatives.

References

Buytendijk, F.J.J. (1948), *Over de Pjin*, Utrecht 1943, germ. Bern.

Dahrendorf, R. (1991), *Der moderne soziale Konflikt*, Stuttgart.

Engelhardt, D.v., and H. Schipperges (1980), *Die inneren Verbindungen zwischen Philosophie und Medizin im 20. Jahrhundert*, Darmstadt.

Eser, A., M. v. Lutterotti and P. Sporken, (Eds.) (1992), *Lexikon Medizin, Ethik, Recht. Darf die Medizin, was sie kann? Information und Orientierung*, Freiburg i. Br.

Furet, F. (1995), *Le passé d'une illusion*, Paris, German (1996), München.

Grimm, J. (1860), *Rede über das Alter*, in: *Kleinere Schriften*, Bd. 1, Berlin 1864, pp. 188-210.

Guardini, R. (1967) *Die Lebensalter*, Würzburg.

Haeckel, E. (1866), *Generelle Morphologie der Organismen*, vols. 1-2, Berlin.

Holton, G. (1974), 'On being caught between Dionysians and Apollonians', in: *Daedalus* 103, pp. 65-81.

Jaspers, K. (1973), *Ein Beispiel: ärztliche Therapie*, in: Jaspers: *Philosophie*, vol.1, Berlin 1932, Heidelberg 4.ed., pp. 121-129.

Krolzik, U. (1979), *Umweltkrise – Folge des Christentums?*, Stuttgart.

Kuhn, T.S. (1962), *The Structure of Scientific Revolutions*, Chicago, 2.ed. 1970, German: Frankfurt a. M. 1976.

Laín Entralgo, P. (1964), *La relación médico-enfermo. Historia y teoría*, Madrid, German: Munich 1969.

Lévi-Strauss, C. (1958), *Anthropologie structurale*, Paris, German: Frankfurt a.M. 1967.

Marcel, G. (1956), *Bemerkungen über die Entpersönlichung der Medizin*, in.: J. Rolin, Ed.: *Was erwarten wir vom Arzt?*, Stuttgart.

Marcuse, H. (1965), *One-dimensional man. Studies in the ideology of advanced industrial society*, Boston, German: Neuwied 1967.

Meyer-Abich, K.-M. (Ed.) (1979), *Frieden mit der Natur*, Freiburg i. Br.

Mitscherlich, A., and F. Mielke (Eds.) (1948) *Medizin ohne Menschlichkeit. Dokumente des Nürnberger Ärzteprozesses*, Stuttgart, Frankfurt a.M. 1978.

Popper, K.R. (1984), *Logik der Forschung*, Wien 1934, Tübingen 8.ed., engl. London 1959.

Reich, W.T. (Ed.) (1995), *Encyclopedia of Bioethics*, vols 1-5, New York 2.ed..

Reiser, S.J.; A.J. Dyck and W.J. Curran (Eds.) (1977), *Ethics in medicine. Historical perspectives and contemporary concerns*, Cambridge/London.

Saunders, C., D.H. Summers and N. Teller (Eds.) (1981), *Hospice. The living idea*, London.

Schölmerich, P. (Ed.) (1990), *"Lebensqualität" als Bewertungskriterium der Medizin*, Stuttgart.

Snell, B. (1946), *Die Entstehung des Geistes. Studien zur Entstehung des europäischen Denkens bei den Griechen*, Hamburg.

Snow, C.P. (1964), *The two cultures and the scientific revolution*, London 1959, A second look, London.

Weizsäcker, V. v. (1926), *Der Arzt und der Kranke*, in: *Gesammelte Schriften*, Bd. 5, Frankfurt a.M. 1987, S. 121-129.

White, L., Jr. (1967), 'The historical root of our ecological crisis', in: *Science* 155, 1203-1207.

Zahlmann, C. (Ed.) (1994), *Kommunitarismus in der Diskussion. Eine streitbare Einführung*, Berlin.

Zielinski, H. (1993), *Palliative Medizin und Hospizbewegung in der BRD*, Dadder.

Zimstein, G. (1996), *Ökologie und Umwelt in der Geschichte*, Marburg.

10 Crimes against Humanity: The Forgotten History of Japan

Rihito Kimura

Introduction

One of the most important ethical norms which has been reconfirmed by the Nuremberg Medical Court was, of course, the principle of autonomy and the right of informed consent that belongs to the patient or research subject in a biomedical setting.

It is surprising that the Nuremberg court decision and it's ethical norms have not been implemented by the medical profession in Japan until very recently even though it was known by many clinical and experimental medical experts.

My premise is that the ethical "norms" of the Nuremberg trials had a great impact in ethics discourse, however they did significantly not change the stagnant situation of the physician-patient or researcher-subject relationship, which remains embedded in the traditional paternalistic hierarchy of biomedical professionalism in Japan. The ethical "norm" in biomedicine has not been radically changed by affirming the very important event of the Nuremberg decision. But change has come through the process of international social upheaval of the 1960s and 1970s challenging professionalism, authority and establishment before unquestioned. Various decisions recognizing the right of informed consent, together with various social movements in support of patients' rights, women's rights, and grass-roots commitments to health services for the poor and minorities, were mutually reinforcing phenomena that brought gradual changes in laws, medical practices and ethical norms[1]. And without these active social movements claiming justice in civil rights, equal treatment and opportunity between both sexes and various races, and actual social action in order to establish an institutionalized system for protection of human rights in various social infrastructures including academic, research and clinical settings, the ethical "norms" in biomedicine could not have been changed so radically during these twenty years.

And we have to carefully recognize the difference between practical application of ethical "norms" in ordinary and routine medical clinical

119

practice, and academic and theoretical efforts to analyze ethical "norms" in a more abstract way.

The "Ab"normal out of Normal?

There are many books on medical ethics in Japan. And almost all of them quote or mention the Nuremberg Code in some pages or chapter. However, they explain these principles in an abstract way; the actual reality of the normal clinical situation has been that physicians have unquestionable authority to which patients were usually obedient[2].

To make the situation worse, there are very few books of medical ethics in Japan referring to the War Crimes of the Japanese medical profession. During World War II Japanese physicians engaged in human experimentation on POWs, making biochemical, bacterial weapons used for battles and performing vivisection practices on living persons, etc.

Now, historical documentation together with several living witnesses in Japan has shown some horrifying human experimentation cases in China using human subjects captured from Chinese, Russian and some other peoples during World War II.[3]

According to the then classified report *Naval Aspects of Biological Warfare* (August, 1947), "The human subjects were used in exactly the same manner as other experimental animals, i.e., the minimum infectious and lethal dosage of various organisms was determined on them, they were immunized with various vaccines and then challenged with living organisms; and they were used as subjects during field trials of bacteria disseminated bombs and sprays".[4] One of the former staff members of this Unit 731 has mentioned that:

> "The experiment on human body at ANTA Experimental Laboratory was conducted in the following way: a bomb filled with bacteria was placed on the ground and about twenty Manchurians were tied to poles or made to sit down on the ground at a proper distance (that is, enough distance to prevent men's death) from the bomb, which were electrically exploded. By the bomb blast, which was caused by the explosion of the bomb, and its fragments, the plague bacilli and anthrax bacilli penetrated through the wound into human bodies. The wounded were kept in the laboratory until the symptoms of the disease appeared and when they were taken ill, they were given medical treatment and their cases were studies, but most of them died in agony. The experiment obtained results just as expected".[5]

The approach to the human subject was basically similar to Nazi experimentation in concentration camp. The Japanese military biomedical experts utilized the captured prisoners not only as experimentation material but also used as an anatomical vivisection material in performing demonstrations for autopsy training in causing death finally.[6]

Consent of the subject was never a part of this process. There was a great difference between the occupation policy of dealing with German and Japanese medical experts who were engaged in these kind of human experimentation. The occupation forces in Europe and in Asia-Pacific took different approaches to prosecution of war crimes in these two nations.

There were different standards of military codes of ethics to be applied to the occupied personnel accused of War Crimes before a military tribunal. Even though there were similar cases of medical crimes against humanity, the case of Japanese medical experimentation on human subjects should not be brought to the court, according to U.S. policy decision makers. In order to get all of the information relating to the results of experimentation, the interrogation was made extensively to the former staff members of the Unit 731 (official name is Water supply and Sanitary Corp. under General Shiro Ishii) who were exempted by the U.S. authority.

This was confidentially justified by the US. Military as a "National Security" matter which should be classified to the public as top secret. Now, after 40 years, due to the "Freedom of Information Act in the U.S.", I was able to verify the related documents at the U.S. National Archive in Washington D.C. The documents which I have searched have stated as follows:

"For all practical purposes an agreement with Ishii and his associates that information given by them on the Japanese BW program will be retained in intelligence channels is equivalent to an agreement that this Government will not prosecute any of those involved in BW activities in which war crimes were committed.

Such an understanding would be of great value to the security of the American people because of the information which Ishii and his associates have already furnished and will continue to furnish."

The last paragraph of this page stated that "In addition, there is a strong possibility that the Soviet prosecutors will, in the course of cross-examination of Umezu, introduce evidence of experiments conducted on human beings by the Ishii BW Group, which *experiments do not differ greatly from those for which this Government is now prosecuting German scientists and medical doctors at Nuremberg.*"[7]

Very few Japanese people knew of this whole process of investigation of Japanese medical professionals, including the actual happening of this incident during the war, while the Nuremberg medical court was known somehow widely among the international public.

The Japanese Military biomedical experimentation became known in 1970s by many people because of the publication of the book written by a leading contemporary writer Seiichi Morimura. The title of the book is *Akuma no Hoshoku* (The Devil's Gluttony) and it was a result of an intensive search for documents and a series of interviews.[8] When this semi-nonfiction book was published, the majority of the medical profession as well as the general public expressed feelings of shock and uneasiness to hear of such inhuman experimentations on human beings. And the incident was regarded as an "ab"normal event which occurred in the abnormal situation of War and was done by rather abnormal people.

Here, I would like to point out the most relevant comments also relating to Nazi medical experimentation and policies. These problems relate to the most fundamental issues of "norms" for normal person that should apply to a person in a particular specified situation. I know that some people would say that it is "unfair" to criticize the particular person's action and behavior out of context of a particular social and ethical "norm" of a particular age.

However, I must say, on behalf the dead and those experimented upon to say that what is "abnormality" in that era does not solve the issues nor immunize those involved from responsibility.

We are able to recognize common elements which penetrate the cases between Nazi-Germany and Imperial-Japan in relationship to human experimentation. That is to say even the "normal" people professionally trained with high motivation would do their service in the name of superior cause, such as in the name of Hitler (see the testimony of Mengele) or Emperor. In particular situation, it is easy to recognize the lacking of a sense of "norms" to fellow human being. One example can be seen in the notorious case of Tuskegee for the study of syphilis among the black population in the U.S.

The medical historian Dr. James Jones mentioned that

> There was a similarity between the Nazi experiments and the Tuskegee Study, one which went beyond their racist and medical natures. Like the chain of command within the military hierarchy of Nazi Germany, the Tuskegee Study's firm entrenchment in the PHP bureaucracy reduced the sense of personal responsibility and ethical concern. For the most part doctors and civil servants simply did their jobs. Some merely 'followed orders'; others worked for the glory of science.[9]

This is exactly the similar sort of expressions by some of the Japanese biomedical experts charged and sentenced at Soviet Russian Military Tribunal at Khabarovsk in 1949 (based on the Order of the Supreme Soviet of the USSR, 19th, April 1943)[10] . The human being could not be normal without ethical "norms" against killing and prohibiting experimentation on humans without consent, and these are the elements of the reaffirmation of the traditional human "norm" clearly mentioned in the decision of the Nuremberg Military court focusing on human dignity and autonomous decision making.

Ethics of Time-lag

Those researchers who know well what's happening in Germany have got a detailed information about Nuremberg Court Decision. However, I think, the general public has been less familiar with these kinds of new developments of principles in biomedical ethics. In relating to this gap between public and professional understanding, one of the recent examples of investigation in the U.S. could be mentioned here.

The Report issued in 1995 by the Advisory Committee of Human Radiation Experiments in the USA states that: "the actual impact of the Nuremberg Code on the biomedical community in the United States, both inside and outside of Government, is a matter of some disagreement".[11] For some medical professionals in the U.S., the principle of "consent" has a rather extreme connotation as bioethical standard for clinical trials.

An eminent medical researcher Dr. Henry Beecher, formerly at Harvard Medical School, expressed some sense of dissatisfaction of the medical profession with the idea of the Nuremberg Code. He mentioned that it is easy enough to say, that the subject should have sufficient knowledge and comprehension of the subject matter involved as to enable him to make an understanding and enlightened decision. Practically, this is often quite impossible".[12] Dr. Beecher says also that: "It is not my view that many rules can be laid down to govern experimentation in man. In most cases, these are more likely to do harm than good".[13]

One of his colleagues, Dr. Joseph W. Gardella observed in 1961 that:

> The Nuremberg Code was conceived in reference to Nazi atrocities and was written for the specific purpose of preventing brutal excesses from being committed or excused in the name of science. The code, however, admirable in it's intent, and however suitable for the purpose for which it was conceived, is in our opinion not necessarily pertinent to or adequate for the conduct of medical research in the United States.[14]

Faced with various revelations about human experimentation reported in the mass-media in the late 1960s and 1970s in the U.S. and elsewhere in the world, there were very drastic changes of ethical "norms" in clinical settings including hospitals and biomedical research institutions. The Japanese Declaration of the rights of sick persons in 1970, accusations of a hasty and failed transplantation failure by a surgeon Dr. Wada, AHA's patients' Bill of Rights in 1972, the National Research Act of 1974 mandating "Institutional Review Boards" are obvious results of growing acceptance of patients' involvement in medical decision making and commitment to the "Informed Consent" process.

The confirmed legal precedents particularly in the U.S. were also causing great effects in international medical research community giving enormous influence in supporting these institutional changes of ethical "norms" in clinical settings even though there were some "time lag" after the important event of the Nuremberg.

Ethics of Transcendence

The documents with full medical data and some of the photos are accessible to be investigated by the general public at the Holocaust Museum in Washington D.C. The subjects of experimentation - many of whom are unidentified - are dead, but the results of experimentation in signs, data, graph and statistics remain as living examples of the tragic violation of ethical "norms".

With deep empathy and vivid imagination to be identified with the experimented in these photos, I feel my strong sense of moral responsibility to advocate the necessity for ethical "norms" in the field of biomedical and clinical settings.

"Nuremberg" is still our starting point to recognize the lack of "norms" in the past, and our continuous effort to ensure autonomy and informed consent in the present and future.

Systematic and institutional efforts are a necessity for protecting human dignity and fundamental rights of the person in sickness. The admission of wrong doing by an entire professional group is, I think at least, a positive start in order to not repeat similar mistakes in the future.

We have heard that with many agonies and great regrets, the German medical community has gone through this hard process in organizing a special exhibition in 1989 in Berlin on the theme of The Value of Human Being: Medicine in Germany 1918-45.[15] This exhibition was also held at Kanagawa University in Japan.[16] By doing this, some elements of public accountability in the medical profession were regained; the common understanding between lay public and medical profession which is now totally different identity then existed under the Nazi regime. On the other hand, in Japan, the issues continue to be obscured and hidden. There have been no serious and official statements made by any biomedical professional body or group. Only very recently, the Japanese citizen's group investigating this matter of biomedical human experimentation focusing on Unit 731 has been organizing the special exhibition around the nation that caught the attention of the mass-media. In the process of investigating and tracing the work of Unit 731, we have recognized the continuation of blood research and it's application technology were utilized in one of the pharmaceutical corporation in Japan, Midori-Jyuji. It's late president was a former staff member of Unit 731. The company was producing blood supply by using imported material for the hemophiliacs without testing for HIV which caused around 2,000 HIV infected patients which 400 of them died of AIDS. All the necessary information was bared to the public and now the corporations and the Ministry of Health and Welfare officially admitted the total failure of blood supply policy in the beginning of 1980s.

All of these mistakes were just recently, a few weeks ago, opened to the public and this has shown the typical example of attitudes of medical experts and bureaucrats who were not admitting any wrongdoing until last moment. It is the responsibility of the Japanese public to level up the professional ethical standard from the peoples point of view using more political pressure.

The Japanese medical crime of the human vivisection cases in China and Japan are less talked about, and do not receive enough public attention. In writing fiction based on this fact, one eminent contemporary author, Shusaku Endo, in his novel titled as *Sea and Poison* dealing with the medical atrocity of vivisection cases on captured American POWs at Kyushu University Medical School during World War II, asks the question of "Absolute ethical principle" transcendent from "Time" and place.[17] The answer given by one of the members of the medical team who was going to be involved in this horrifying, inhuman vivisection, was saying that there are no transcendent values and all questions are relevant to the context. The meaning of Mr. Endo's story is very clear. There should be a "norm" that creates a boundary which any human being could not step out from in the realm of mutual respect for dignity and rights of persons. Mr. Endo challenged the still existent mentality of Japanese medical experts who are so eager to accomplish research oriented studies in order to write a paper and publish without confronting complicated ethical issues[18].

Nuremberg Tribunal (*Ex Parte Quirin*, 317 U.S. I, 63 S.Ct.2" [1942]) clearly stated that "Individuals have international duties which transcend the national obligations of obedience imposed by the individual state. He who violates the law of war cannot obtain immunity while acting in pursuance of the authority of the State if the State in authorizing action moves outside its competence under international law".[19]

Concluding Remarks

The narrow egocentric, and nationalistic orientation of the medical experts could be seen in some cases to be at the expenses of scientific progress to save a life of patient. International acceptance of bioethical principles is getting more and more important beyond cultural, historical and national differences among countries of the world today.

We have to avoid fostering any kind of milieu, such as war, or motivation to pursue innovative treatments leading into experimental "temptation" as biomedical and clinical scientists, and we have to not only deliver ourselves from that kind of opportunity but also create our sacred norms to engage and envisage new human hope in the true understanding of human dignity and human rights in our daily practice of medical services.

We should remember these medical tragedies of human experimentation in Japan, Germany, the U.S. and elsewhere by taking vows of our constant efforts to live by bioethical norms of "autonomy", "informed consent" and "institutionalized system of open and public scrutiny" to be guaranteed in the development of biomedicine in clinical and research settings now and towards the 21st Century.

Notes

1   Kimura, R. (1986), 'Bioethik als metainterndisziplinäre Disziplin', *Medizin, Mensch, Gesellschaft*, Band 11, Heft 4, Dezember (IV), Ferdinand Enke Verlag Stuttgart.

2   Kimura, R. (1991), *Fiduciary Relationship and the Medical profession: A Japanese Point of View.* In *Ethics, Trust, and the Professions: Philosophical and Cultural Aspects*, pp. 235-245. Ed., by E.D. Pellegrino, R.M. Veatch, and J. Langan. Georgetown University Press, Washington D.C.

3   Williams, P., and Wallace, D. (1996), *Unit 731: Japan's Secret Biological Warfare in World War II*, Free Press, New York, 1989 and Gold, Hal. *Unit 731: Testimony*, YENBOOKS, Tokyo.

4   USN. Naval Aspects of Biological Warfare, Appendix XIII, Biological Warfare in Japan, Aug. 1947, p.90, The National Archive, Washington D.C.

5   Hubbert, Cecil F., Memorandum for COMDR.J.B. CRESAP, 15 July 1947. pp. 4-5. and also Cresap, J.B., Commander, USN. State-War-Navy Coordinating Subcommittee for the Far East, 1 August 1947, p. 8 The National Archives, Washington D.C.

6   Ken Yuasa (1994), *Witness as a War Criminal: Engaging in Vivisections as a Military Physician"* (in Japanese), pp. 43-51, in 731 Butai (Unit 731), Azia no Koe (Voice of Asia), Vol. 8, Edited by Executive Committee for the Assembly in thinking and memorizing the War Victims in Asian and Pacific Region, Toho Syuppan.

7   Hubbert, Cecil F., op.cit., pp. 4-5. and Cresap, J.B. op.cit., p. 8.

8   Morimura, Seiichi (1981), *Akuma no Hoshoku* (The Devil's Gluttony), in Japanese, Kobun Sha, Tokyo.

9   Jones, James H. (1993), *Bad Blood, The Tuskegee Syphilis Experiment.* New and Expanded Edition, p. 180. The Free Press. New York.

10   Documents on Trial against the former military personnel prosecuted for the preparation and use of Bacteriological Warfare Weapon (in Japanese translation), Foreign Books Publishing Press, Moscow, 1950.

11   Advisory Committee on Human Radiation Experiments (ACHRE), *Final Report*, Washington D.C. 1995.

12   ACHRE, op.cit. p.157.

13   ACHRE, op.cit. p.157.

14   ACHRE, op.cit. p.158.

15   Ärztekammer Berlin (1991) *The Value of the Human Being: Medicine in Germany 1918-1945*, Druckhaus Hetrich, Berlin.

16   Editorial Committee of Kanagawa University Review Series, Medicine and War: Japan and Germany (in Japanese), Kanagawa University Review, Ochanomizu Shobo, Tokyo, 1994.

17   Endo, Shusaku (1958), *Umi to Dokuyaku* (Sea and Poison: English translation by Gallagher, Michael, Chales E. Tuttle Company, 1973), Bungei Shunju Co.Ltd., Tokyo.

18   Kimura, R. (1995), *Contemporary Japan; History of Medical Ethics*, in: *Encyclopedia of Bioethics* (ed., by Reich Warren, T.), vol.3, p. 1948, Simon & Schuster Macmillan, New York.

19   Hirsch, H. (1995), *Genocide and the Politics of Memory*, p.188, The University of North Carolina Press, Chapel Hill, London.

11 The Inclusion of the Ten Principles of Nuremberg in Professional Codes of Ethics: An International Comparison

Gonzalo Herranz

Introduction

How did the Nuremberg Code influence ethical-professional norms since 1947 in Europe (aside from the United Kingdom) and Latin America? The following description cannot cover all the material that would have been necessary for a complete study. In addition, the facts and commentaries that follow, though representative, are still provisional. It seems, however, that a conclusion can still be drawn: the Nuremberg Code's influence on ethical codes in medicine was late in coming and only partial.

Let us first investigate its late comings. From 1947 to 1975, the Nuremberg Code was practically ignored by both national and international medical organizations, including the World Medical Association (WMA)[1] And afterwards it seemed to be eclipsed by the Helsinki Declaration of 1975. In reality, it was through Helsinki II that the doctrine of Nuremberg found its way into codes of medical ethics. Only recently, in the last two decades, has the Nuremberg Code been rediscovered and begun to be considered a polar star of ethics in biomedical research.[2]

Second, the acceptance of the content of the Nuremberg Code was never complete: within the profession, deontological norms and guides to medical ethics have put certain components of the Nuremberg Code aside as though they were inaccessible ideals - components which, in my opinion, are among the most noble of ethical ideas: the assertion that both the researcher and the subject must be morally sincere, incorruptible, and dedicated.

127

Material and Methods

After contacting and recontacting 40 national medical associations in Europe (22 countries) and Latin America (18 countries), the author was able to collect and revise a total of 74 codes or regulations in the medical profession published after 1947 in 17 European and 15 Latin American countries. Table 1 a and b show the countries and the year of publication of the codes examined.

Table 1a   Countries and publication dates of the codes of ethics (before and after Nuremberg) in the analysis of Europe (excluding the United Kingdom)

Country	before Nuremberg	1948-57	1958-67	1968-77	1978-87	1988-96
Belguim		50		75		90,92
Denmark						89,91
Finland		56				88, 93
France	47	55			79	95
Germany	31	49, 56		70, 76, 77	83, 85, 88	90, 93, 96
Greece		55				
Iceland						92
Ireland					81, 84	89, 94
Italy		48, 54			78	89, 95
Luxembourg						91
Netherlands						93, 94
Norway			61			94
Poland						91, 94
Portugal	15, 39, 42	56			85	
Spain	45				79	90
Sweden				68		
Switzerland				71		96

Table 1b   Countries and publication dates of the codes of ethics (before and after Nuremberg) in the analysis of Latin America

Country	before Nuremberg	1948-57	1958-67	1968-77	1978-87	1988-96
Argentina			64			
Bolivia					86	93, 96
Brazil	31, 45	53	65		84, 88	
Chile					86	96
Colombia			58		81	
Costa Rica				70	81	
Cuba					83	
Equador						92
Guatemala				74	81, 84	93
Honduras			64			
Mexico					87	
Paraguay				77		
Peru				70		
Uruguay	24					95
Venezuela	24			71		

In order to detect and characterize the effect that the Nuremberg Code had on ethical norms that followed it, a very simple heuristic instrument was used: a schematic list of the ten precepts of the Code of Nuremberg that have been taken as markers of its influence. To facilitate the analysis, the markers were divided into two groups. The first group contains those which were incorporated, to a more or less great extent, into successive versions of the Declaration of Helsinki and, from there, passed on to codes of ethics of various medical associations, chambers, societies or colleges of physicians[3]. The second group comprises two ethical criteria not adopted by Helsinki and, in fact, abandoned by normative ethics afterwards.[4] These two types of "markers" are presented in table 2 (a and b).

Table 2a   Markers of the Nuremberg Code

MARKERS ADOPTED: **Criteria from the Nuremberg Code that were incorporated into the Declaration of Helsinki**

a. Voluntary consent of the subject.
b. An expected beneficial outcome of the experiment.
c. Prior experimentation on animals.
d. Avoidance of unnecessary pain and harm.
e. Avoidance of any risks of death or disablement.
f. The risks taken may not exceed the expected advantages.
g. Protecting against the possibility, however slight, of injury, disablement, or death.
h. Scientifically and technically qualified experimenters.
i. The subject's freedom to retract consent.
j. The experimenter's obligation to stop the experiment if it turns out that it is dangerous.

Table 2b   Markers of the Nuremberg Code

MARKERS ABANDONED: **Criteria from the Nuremberg Code that were not incorporated into the Declaration of Helsinki**

a. The personal, non-transferable responsibility of everyone involved in initiating and carrying out the experiment to assure the ethical quality of the subject's consent.
b. The right of the subject to quit the experiment if his condition seems to rule out the possibility of continuing.

Results and Comments

Chronology of the Reception of the Nuremberg Code in Professional Codes

Contrary to what is normally stated, medical associations remained oblivious to the Nuremberg Code for some two decades. Things didn't change much when the WMA published its Declaration of Helsinki I, which recapitulated the principle points of Nuremberg. Its impact on medical codes of ethics was very limited, if not negligible. It wasn't until 1975 that the doctrine of Nuremberg was amply taken note of.

Indeed, the codes from before 1975 omit the ethical treatment of experiments on humans or simply pay them rudimentary attention. In the codes of the time, one sometimes finds norms along the lines of this one from the Deontological Code published in 1950 by the Conseil Supérieur de l'Ordre des Médecins de la Belgique: "The doctor must avoid all unnecessary or reckless treatment and abstain from all medical acts which could be harmful. He may not provoke diseases or critical states except - for the sole reason of scientific observation - where formal consent has been given by the subject who has been duly informed about the risks involved". On the other side of the Atlantic, the Moral Medical Code (1954) of the Medical Federation of Columbia demands that "the doctor [shows] great respect for human subjects and therefore prudently [avoids] all thoughtless experimentation, ... and all acts which detrimentally affect the mentally sound person's independence of will or liberty. The doctor may not instigate the appearance of a disease or prolong it, not even in the name of scientific research".

However, one very often finds in Latin American codes the caveat that, under certain exceptionally grave circumstances, the doctor may proceed with experimental treatment when it seems to be the only way to save the patient's life. Here, both the patient's prior consent and the further recommendations from three other doctors are needed.

Before 1975, only Switzerland, Brazil, Costa Rica, Peru, and Venezuela had taken Helsinki I to heart. The Swiss Academy for Medical Sciences first published guidelines in its Directives for Experimental Research on Humans in December 1970; the Academy not only adopted the content of Helsinki I but even went further to include elements from the Nuremberg Code that Helsinki had left aside. Since then, the Directives have figured as an appendix to the Codes of Deontology of the Swiss Federation of Doctors and the Cantonal Societies of Doctors: they all basically state that scientific investigations on human beings are regulated by the corresponding directives of the Swiss Academy of Medical Sciences.

On 30 January 1953, the Medical Association of Brazil approved a Code of Ethics, officially recognized as Law No. 3268 on 30 September 1957. Article 57 of the law introduces for the first time in a professional code - albeit in a rather simplified fashion - the doctrine of free, informed consent for experiments on humans: "Even if consent has been given, experiments *in anima nobili* for speculative purposes are reprehensible. They may be tolerated for strictly therapeutic or diagnostic ends in the interest of the patient as long as they do not put the patient's life in danger or cause any serious harm. In such cases, one must obtain the patient's prior, expressed consent, and the mentally healthy patient must be fully informed of the possible consequences of the experiment".

On 12 March 1970, the Medical College of Peru inserted the complete text of Helsinki I into article 94 of its *Code of Ethics and Deontology*. The National Medical Union of Costa Rica set down guidelines for experiments on humans in three chapters of its *Code of Medical Deontology* on 18 August 1970. The chapters' titles are (1) Experiments posing risks for the subject, (2) Experiments with new medicaments, and (3) Research on humans for solving problems of knowledge outside the therapeutic domain. On 23 January 1971, the National Medical Union of Venezuela set down norms in its *Code of Medical Deontology* that are to a great extent quotations from Helsinki I.

Starting in 1975, such norms on human experiments began to gain momentum in Europe.[5] The Medical Code of Deontology, published the same year by the Conseil National de l'Ordre des Médecins de la Belgique, contains a clear and adequately complete treatment of the subject. The wording was clearly inspired by Helsinki II. The Order of Doctors of Italy set down rules for clinical experiments in 1978, dedicating an entire chapter of its *Nuovo Codice Deontologico* to the topic, while it took Spain until 1979 to come up with something similar. Also in 1979, a new *Code de Déontologie* was published in France, where mention is made of the material for the first time.

In Ireland, a code of ethical regulations was passed by the Medical Counsel in the form of the Medical Practitioners Act of 1978. In the first edition of the *Guide to Ethical Conduct and Behavior*, published in 1981, no mention is made of the ethics of human experiments. Not until the second edition (1984) is a paragraph on investigations on humans included and the text of Helsinki II added as an appendix. Both texts are kept in the third and fourth edition of 1989 and 1994.

Portugal's Order of Doctors dedicated a chapter of its *Code of Deontology* of 1985 to experiments on humans and included a large section of the doctrine of Helsinki II in it.

The case of Germany is surprising. Only after 1985 did the Deutsche Ärztekammer briefly and schematically mention in its *Berufsordnung* human experimentation and imposes the obligation to consult an ethics committee (IRB) as well as following the directives of the Declaration of Helsinki I and II (*Berufsordnung* 1985), Helsinki I, II and III (*Berufsordnung* 1988), and Helsinki I, II, III and IV (*Berufsordnung* 1993). The introduction of this norm was brought about by the necessity of including ethical criteria concerning experimentation on human embryos.[6]

The codes of medical associations of northern countries do not go into great detail concerning ethics in biomedical investigations. The author has been informed that after 1964 the Declaration of Helsinki constituted the commonly accepted ethical guidelines for Scandinavian medical associations and that ethics committees (IRB) have been active since then. The *Code of Medical Ethics of Iceland* (1992) states, for example, that: "The doctor must always take account in his investigations on human beings of the well-being of each of his patients or volunteers. The Declaration of Helsinki, with all its subsequent amendments, must be observed in all cases". The *Code of Medical Ethics of the Medical Association of Finland* (1988) and its *Manual of Medical Ethics* (1994) are based on Helsinki III and IV, presented from the point of view of a vigorous and generous development of patients' rights. In the manual, the Nuremberg Code holds a place of honor between the Hippocratic Oath and the United Nations' Universal Declaration of the Rights of Man.

Poland's *Code of Medical Ethics of the National Order of Doctors* (December 1991) dedicates Chapter II to scientific research and medical experimentation. Ample space is given to various nuances (10 articles), and the code conforms to the norms set down in Helsinki IV. The Code also includes norms for biomedical publications. In contrast, the *Medical Code of Ethics* from 1993 offers a comparatively simple set of guidelines.

The ways norms for human experiments are dealt with in Latin America are very irregular. On the one hand, they are still ignored by some countries today. For instance, up to today Argentina has stuck by its *Code of Ethics of the Medical Confederation* from 1964, which makes no mention of the ethics of medical experimentation on humans. Cuba's *Principles of Medical Ethics*, published in 1983, merely states that doctors must avoid doing harm to the healthy or the sick in the investigative work they carry out. The message of the *Nuremberg Code* has left no mark in the medical codes of ethics of some countries, such as Bolivia (1986), Columbia (1981), and Guatemala (1984 and 1993). These gaps in the deontological rules for the profession are frequently compensated for by relevant legislation.

The message of Nuremberg has nonetheless found conspicuous adherents in Latin America. Such is the case in Brazil, the first country to adopt the Code in its own *Code of Ethics of the Brazilian Medical Association* of 1953, hardly five and a half years after the ruling of the American military tribunal. The *Code of Ethics and Deontology of the Medical College of Peru*, approved in 1970, copied the complete text of Helsinki I in its article 94. As the Code of 1970 is still in effect (the renewing of Codes being generally slow in coming in Latin America), later versions of the Declaration have not yet been able to be added to the Peruvian Code.

In Costa Rica, the *Medical Code of Deontology* of 1970, produced by the Federation of Doctors, is surprising in that it anticipates the modern figure of ethical committees in the Declaration of Helsinki II: not only does it plainly adopt Helsinki I, but it also mandates the evaluation of the investigator's competence by an independent juridical organ and demands that each investigation involving mentally ill patients be first approved by a scientific committee formed for this purpose. In addition, it establishes guarantees for the protection of health and the compensation of harm caused to the subjects. The Code of 1981 establishes in Article 5 that "the doctor must observe ethical principles of the 'Declarations of Geneva and Helsinki adopted by the World Medical Association'". The text of these Declarations is added to the Code.

Chili also set down in its *Code of Ethics* (1986) the essentials of the conditions of Helsinki III, including (in the documents accompanying the Code) not only the Declaration, but also the complete text of the *Nuremberg Code*.

The Mediation of the Declaration of Helsinki in the Selective Incorporation of the Doctrine of the Nuremberg Code

Jay Katz is among the few authors who assert that the doctrine of the Nuremberg Code did not have the chance to establish continuity given the enormous difficulties involved in putting the code into practice. For Katz, the great ethical demand in the first clause meant that the Code would inevitably, if not immediately, be dethroned from its prominent position. He maintains that the Nuremberg Code was relegated to the history books at the moment of its conception.[7]

It is nonetheless universally accepted that, despite the regrettable lack of documentation on this topic, the Declaration of Helsinki was the impetus for the Nuremberg Code's entrance into codes of various national medical associations. There hardly is need for a detailed analysis to prove that such codes by national medical associations were indeed inspired by, if not copies or transcriptions of, parts or the whole of different versions of Helsinki and that Helsinki itself copied several points from the Nuremberg Code.[8]

What was Taken up Through Helsinki?

If we count up the codes that explicitly transcribe the ethical criteria of Nuremberg using the heuristic instrument mentioned earlier, we arrive at the results given in Table 3.

Table 3   Criteria from the Nuremberg Code (NC) adopted by medical codes of ethics that contain a deontological regulation of human experimentation

NC	B	SF	IRL	I	L	PL	P	E	CH	BR	RCH	CR	GCA	CO	PY	ROU	YV	Total
a	+	+	+	+	+	+	+	+	+	+	+	+	+	+	+	+	+	17
b		+	+		+	+	+	+	+			+			+			9
c	+	+		+		+	+	+	+			+	+		+		+	11
d	+	+		+		+	+	+	+					+			+	9
e	+					+	+	+	+							+		6
f						+	+	+	+								+	5
g									+									1
h	+	+				+	+	+	+			+			+	+	+	10
i		+		+	+				+	+		+			+		+	8
j	+							+	+	+	+	+	+		+	+	+	10
Total	6	6	2	4	3	7	7	8	10	3	2	6	3	2	6	4	7	86

This information gives us quite varying responses due to both the different countries listed and the content of the codes.

The Swiss Academy of Medical Sciences incorporated all the criteria in its Directives, while other countries (Ireland, Luxembourg, Brazil, Chili, Columbia, or Guatemala) only adopted two or three.

The criterion of the free consent of the subject met with universal acceptance. Other criteria were also by and large adopted: the condition of prior experimentation on animals (criterion c, 11 countries); the obligation to avoid or minimize the harm done to subjects (criteria d and j, 9 and 10 countries, respectively); the task of attaining a ratio of benefits to risks which favors the benefits (criterion b, 9 countries); and finally the demand that scientific investigators be quality-controlled (criterion h, 10 countries). Other criteria were only adopted here and there. Such is the case with criterion g.[9]

However, the numerous omissions were made up for by the numerous codes (Germany, Denmark, Spain, Finland, Ireland, Norway, Sweden, Switzerland, Chili, Colombia, Costa Rica, Peru, Uruguay) expressly establishing that successive versions of the Declaration of Helsinki are valid points of reference in evaluating the ethics of biomedical investigation in these countries. As for France, it established ethical guidelines for human experiments in laws to this effect. The same goes for Austria: the Chamber of Austrian Doctors has never passed a code of medical ethics. Rather, in Austria medical experimentation is regulated by the doctor's law, the law of drugs, and the law of health institutions. Nonetheless, the Austrian Chamber subscribes to the doctrine of the Nuremberg Code and to that of the Declaration of Helsinki.

What was Not Adopted from the Nuremberg Code?

Two clauses in the Nuremberg Code placing researchers and subjects under great moral scrutiny have, in my opinion, been unfortunately forgotten.

One of them, coming at the end of point one, places the ethical (not juridical, penal, or civil) responsibility in its personal, non-delegatible form squarely on the shoulders of all the members of a research team regardless of rank in assuring the ethical quality of consent: the subject's consent is thus not merely a legal or administrative formality that the researchers carry out perfunctorily but instead a serious moral decision whose authenticity must be guaranteed. Consenting or not consenting is thus not exclusively up to the subject but also involves an ethical ruling by the researcher.

The second Nuremberg clause that has been forgotten is the one formulated in point 9, which declares that the patient's participation is not something trivial that can be taken for granted. The subject, according to Nuremberg, is a morally responsible being who, after obtaining sufficient information and knowledge of the full implications of the experiment and a decision to participate, consents voluntarily. Of course, the patient reserves the right to end the experiment at any time. But at the same time, the subject does not lose the responsibility for all that in exercising that right, according to Nuremberg, when he "believes to have reached the threshold of mental or physical resistance beyond which he cannot go".

The successive versions of Helsinki have not taken up these two ethical demands, which also not longer appear in the codes. The first one disappeared without trace, having transformed itself into an occasional warning to the effect that the subject's consent "given of his own free will after receiving all the necessary information does not in any way diminish the project director's professional, civil, or penal responsibility".[10]

Reality has shown that this aspect of the first clause from Nuremberg has been abused everywhere. It goes without saying that Helsinki, unlike Nuremberg, opted for an minimalist conception of the experimenter's moral role. In order to provide a moral crutch for the moral weakness that is so frequently seen among experimenters, the WMA included in Helsinki II the obligation to submit the protocol of experiments on people to an independent committee set up for the very task of advising, thus wiping out the demand that the researcher personally guarantee the ethical authenticity of the subject's consent. From then on, the ethics committees (IRB) were in charge of guaranteeing that the subject's consent was free and well-informed. It could not have happened otherwise after the scandals denounced by Beecher[11] and Pappworth[12] showed that it was impossible to rely on the moral integrity of experimenters: according to Helsinki they are subject to administrative and external ethical control in an inexcusable way.

The second ethical demand has left a barely perceptible mark in the *Medical Code of Deontology of Venezuela* from 1971, which indicates in article 115, paragraph b) that every subject must be able to interrupt any experiment in progress at any time *when his personal situation demands it.*

Helsinki opted for a minimalist conception of the moral role of the subject: in order to obtain his consent more easily, he is given a permanently open door by which to leave the experiment when he sees fit without having to give any reasons. Thus, there is a consent à la Nuremberg and a consent à la Helsinki. For Helsinki, unlike Nuremberg, the consent given by the subject is not binding in any way: it is always a provisory decision, if not arbitrary and capricious. The subject's dedication to the project can be retracted at any moment: he is free to withdraw his consent whenever his heart desires. In my opinion, consent as defined in Nuremberg requires the addition of indispensable information about the consequences resulting from the subject's decision to withdraw from the experiment. This information makes the consent clearer, more voluntary and rational than the consent of the Helsinki type, which fosters a less responsible kind of behavior and may be behind all the clinical experiments rendered invalid - or weakened in import - by the many subjects who abandon ship.

To my knowledge, no one has recently studied the contrasts between these two types of consent. Beecher maintains in his critique of the Nuremberg Code that the consent demanded there is impossible,[13] but since then this most interesting question has not been taken up again.[14] In addition, the task of reconciling the subject's right to quit the experiment with his responsibility as a morally mature person to follow through with the experiment - except when circumstances justify an interruption - remains unresolved in the ethics of human experimentation.

It seems to me on this occasion that the problem merits reconsidering. Which just goes to show that the ethical heritage of Nuremberg has not been exhausted.

Notes

1   The surprising thing is that Nuremberg remained practically unknown (in Europe and Latin America) prior to Helsinki I. Many authors strongly believe that an influence was there from the start and wide-spread, neither of which has been demonstrated in my opinion. It has been maintained, without proof, that Nuremberg was behind the Geneva Declaration and the International Code of Medical Ethics, the fundamental documents of the WMA (see, for instance, S. Perley, S.S. Fluss, Z. Bankowsky, F. Simon, *The Nuremberg Code: An International Overview*. G.J. Annas, M.A. Grodin. *The Nazi Doctors and the Nuremberg Code. Human Rights and Human Experimentation*. New York; Oxford University Press. 1992: 149-173). Beecher claimed in 1959 that the ten points of the Nuremberg Code had become a sort of Credo of the West (H.K. Beecher. 'Experimentation in Man'. *JAMA* 1959; 169: 461-468), but this is a voluntaristic assertion for Europe and Latin America.

The truth is that only one of the Rules for Times of Armed Conflict adopted by the WMA in Havana in 1956 has any direct relation with Nuremberg: article 3 states, in the spirit of Nuremberg, that "experimentation on human beings is subject to the same laws in times of war as in times of peace; it is formally illegal on anyone who is not free, including both military and civilian prisoners or people in occupied countries".

It would be interesting to investigate, beyond institutional norms, what impact the Code had on actual practice. A glance through the most prominent medical journals of the period shows a general lack of interest in the Code. One striking example: the sentence against the Nazi doctors was published in *JAMA* in the form of a letter from the correspondent in Berlin containing a journalistic, non-technical version of the ruling and the Code (Foreign Letters. Berlin. From our Regular Correspondent. The Nuremberg Trial Against German Physicians. *JAMA* 1947; 135: 867-868).

2   The silence or ignorance surrounding the Nuremberg Code dissipated when the interest in medical ethics forced its way into public view in the 1970s. Articles on the Code are practically non-existent from 1947 to 1963 to judge from the bibliography in Ladimer and Newman (I. Ladimer, R.W. Newman, eds. *Clinical Investigation in Medicine: Legal, Ethical, and Moral Aspects. An Anthology and Bibliography*. Boston: Boston University Law-Medicine Research Institute, 1963: 493-516).

3   The exception is the second part of clause 5, authorizing the carrying out of experiments that can cause the death or disabling of the subject as long as the doctors carrying out the experiment are themselves the subjects.

4   The significance of the abandoning of these criteria, which I will discuss in a bit more detail at the end of this paper, merits an in-depth study of its own. Strangely enough, in transcribing the Code numerous authors omit the very text of, or commentaries on, the parts of the two clauses that demand both parties' involvement, that are themselves guarantees of the ethical quality of giving and retracting consent. See, for example, A. Fargot-Largeault. *L'homme bio-éthique. Pour une déontologie de la recherche sur le vivant*. Paris; Maloine, 1985: 154; et W. Schaupp. *Der ethische Gehalt der Helsinki Deklaration*. Frankfurt am Main; Peter Lang, 1994: 58.

5   It is surprising to see that between 1957 and 1977, contrary to what happened in the periods just before and after, the productive activity of professional codes remained practically paralyzed. This phenomenon has no parallel in Latin America.

6   Personal communication with Dr. Otmar Kloiber of the *Bundesärztekammer* in Cologne.

7   J. Katz. The Consent Principle of the Nuremberg Code: Its Significance Then and Now. In: G.J. Annas, M.A. Grodin. *The Nazi Doctors and the Nuremberg Code. Human Rights and Human Experimentation*. New York; Oxford University Press. 1992: 227-228.

8   For more on the reciprocity between Nuremberg and Helsinki, see S. Perley, S.S. Fluss, Z. Bankowsky, F. Simon, *The Nuremberg Code: An International Overview.* G.J. Annas, M.A. Grodin. *The Nazi Doctors and the Nuremberg Code. Human Rights and Human Experimentation.* New York; Oxford University Press. 1992: 157-160.

9   The number of codes ruling out the legality of experiments that can *a priori* cause the death or disabling of the patient were numerous. But here, only the codes that reflect the final part of clause 5 of the Code are counted. In an almost morbidly humorous vein, the Code allowed for one exception: the case in which the doctors carrying out the dangerous research could themselves serve as subjects. This criterion, which **ressent des ordalies,** was only taken up by the Swiss Academy of Medical Sciences in its *Directives for Experimental Research on Humans* of 1971, which reads in part: "It is not admissible that a research experiment be carried out when then project involves foreseeable risks of grave or irreversible nature or mortal danger, unless the subject is the very investigator in charge. No high risk study on oneself should generally not be carried out except in a group." This ethics for kamikazes of science **may have lasted:** its stay in the Directives was brief: it disappeared in the new version of 1981.

10   Academie Suisse des Sciences Médicales. Directives pour la recherche sur l'homme. Basel; Schwabe & Cie, 1971.

11   More interesting even than the original article (H.K. Beecher. 'Ethics and clinical research'. *NEJM* 1966; 274: 1354-1360) is without a doubt the article by Rothman, who gives a historical perspective of the matter (D.J. Rothman, 'Ethics and Human Experimentation. Henry Beecher Revisited'. *NEJM* 1987; 317: 1195-1199).

12   From the historical perspective, the original work is as interesting to read (M.H. Pappworth. *Human guinea pigs: experimentation in man.* London: Routledge, 1967) as the article by the self-same Pappworth commenting on the history of how the book came about and the reactions to its publication: M.H. Pappworth. '"Human guinea pigs" - a history'. *BMJ* 1990; 301: 1456-1460.

13   H.K. Beecher. *Research and the Individual. Human Studies.* Boston; Little, Brown and Co., 1970: 227-234 and 278-279.

14   G. Herranz. *The retraction by the research subject of his or her free and informed consent: an historical-ethical explanation.* International Bioethics Committee of UNESCO Proceedings, 1996 (in press).

12 The Nuremberg Code Turns Fifty

William J. Winslade and Todd L. Krause

Introduction

Ethics Codes regulating research involving human subjects may serve several purposes. Codes may articulate idealistic aspirations as well as express fundamental values, such as respect for persons or scientific integrity. Ethics Codes may also set standards for moral criticism of medical practices or policies that may violate the rights of human subjects. Finally, ethics codes may provide grounds for imposing civil or criminal liability on researchers who violate the rights of their human subjects. In these ways ethics codes seem to be potentially powerful means to prevent physicians or scientists from exploiting or abusing vulnerable persons such as children, the ill, prisoners, or soldiers.

Yet abuses occur. Nazi doctors, Japanese physicians, American scientists and physicians, and many other researchers around the world have been castigated for everything from torture thinly disguised as research, risky and harmful experiments on humans, and physically harmless observations of unwitting subjects that violate their dignity and privacy. In the name of science, medicine, or national security practices that would otherwise be crimes and moral offenses may be tolerated or even celebrated as sacrifices that individuals make for a greater good. The quest for knowledge and national security sometimes clash with the rights of individuals to be respected as autonomous persons and not to be harmed. Although ethics codes purport to establish a bulwark against abuse, critics often claim that ethics codes are too abstract to provide guidance, unenforced or even unenforceable, and not taken seriously or even appreciated by researchers.

It cannot be denied that abuses have occurred, but their frequency and seriousness is uncertain. Egregious cases may cause us to think that abuses are widespread or to conclude that few abuses occur apart from occasional outrageous incidents. Documentation of abuses of human subjects in the context of scientific or medical research is difficult to obtain because offenders naturally seek to conceal misconduct. Sometimes national security or governmental secrecy hides or buries abuses behind a bureaucratic barrier. When reports of abuse are investigated, documented, and exposed, ethics codes are among the tools for evaluating the nature, scope, and seriousness of violations of the rights of human subjects.

This chapter explores the influence of the Nuremberg Code in American jurisprudence and public policy. The Nuremberg Code is often referred to as the founding document of modern bioethics and health law. Despite this distinction, its place in American jurisprudence remains unclear. In the fifty years since its conception, the ideas expounded by the Code have been variously characterized as everything from a theoretical ideal to Constitutionally ensured. The unique heritage of the Nuremberg Code and its lasting influence on medical, ethical, scientific, and legal debate encourages a re-evaluation of its history and significance, on this, its anniversary. Part I of this chapter outlines the events that led to the Code's creation and examines the principles that comprise the Code. Part II gives a decade by decade account of the last fifty years of the Nuremberg Code's regulatory, legislative, and judicial life in America. Part III reflects upon the history of the Code and finishes with a discussion of its future.

The Birth of the Code

Nuremberg Trials

To understand the significance of the Nuremberg Code and its place in American science and ethical thought, it is necessary to look to its conception during the "Medical Trial" of the second Nuremberg Military Tribunal. The circumstances of the birth of the Code had a profound effect upon how it has been viewed ever since.

At the end of World War II the allies held two series of war crime trials. In the first series, held from 1945 to 1946, judges and prosecutors from the United States, France, Great Britain, and the Soviet Union jointly tried prominent Nazis such as Field Marshall Goering and Rudolf Hess for their war time activities. By the conclusion of the first series of trials the problems associated with conducting the trials in four different languages by judges from four different countries became apparent. In January of 1946, President Truman's proposal that the United States take sole responsibility for the second series of trials was accepted.[1]

The second series of Nuremberg trials involved the prosecution of Nazi officers and German citizens for further crimes during the war. This series of twelve trials involved the prosecution for a variety of crimes, including those related to human experimentation. The trials were held between October 1946 and April 1949. Defendants were tried by only American judges and prosecutors under a strange hybrid of American and German procedural rules. The military tribunal's jurisdictional authority derived from Law No. 10 of the Control Council of Germany.[2] The first of the trials, the *United States v. Karl Brandt*, commonly known as the "Medical Trial", began Dec. 9, 1946 and ended in August 1947.

The 24 defendants at the Medical Trial were charged with a variety of crimes. Most pertinent to the subject of human subject research were counts two and three of the indictment. Count three comprised crimes against humanity as defined under Article II of Control Council Law No.10. Count two listed the use of civilians, foreign nationals and prisoners of war as subjects in a series of grotesque experiments. The "experiments" enumerated in count two commonly caused suffering, injury or death of unwitting or unwilling subjects in experiments that included: 1) high altitude experiments, where they were locked in low pressure chambers and subjected to extremely low pressures; 2) freezing experiments, where they were bathed in tanks of freezing water or exposed to sub-zero temperatures outdoors until body parts froze or death ensued; 3) experiments where they were purposefully infected with malaria, epidemic jaundice, spotted fever, or other agents to study disease course or treatment; 4) experiments where they were exposed to lost (mustard) gas or phosphorous from incendiary bombs to study the wounds they inflicted and/or treatment options; 5) bone, muscle, and nerve regeneration and bone transplantation studies involving the excision of healthy tissue to study regeneration and treatment; 6) sea-water experiments, where subjects were forced to drink "treated" sea-water; 7) sterilization experiments, where subjects were forcefully sterilized by being exposed to x-rays, surgical procedures or various drugs to develop methods for mass sterilization of unwanted populations; 8) experiments with poisons to test their efficacy in killing human beings and to develop strategies and implement organized "euthanasia" programs; and 9) anatomical experiments where Jews were killed to study their anatomy and pathology and to enhance a University bone collection.[3] This list should not detract from the individual suffering of the thousands of people who were involuntary made the subjects in these "experiments". Even a glimpse look at the "selections from photographic evidence of the prosection" printed in the condensed version of the Trial's transcript brings to life, in graphic detail, the hideous nature of the acts committed by the defendants.[4]

As a result of the trial, seven of the 24 defendants were hanged, nine received sentences that ranged from 15 years to life, and the remaining eight were acquitted.[5] Although the Trial's verdict was front-page news in the *New York Times*, the defendants' execution was relegated to a backpage.[6] The verdict and decision were largely viewed as putting to rest a chapter of history that involved egregious breaches of morality by immoral agents under the direction of a dissolved government.[7]

Although the Nazi experiments generated moral outrage, the results of the experiments were subsequently published and used by the international scientific community. Japanese physicians who had engaged in similar experiments during the War were able to avoid prosection at the Tokyo War Crimes Trial by agreeing to hand over their findings to American scientists.[8] Some of the Nuremberg Trial's defendants were ultimately accepted into American science. Four of the defendants were later employed by the United States military.[9]

Trial Politics and the Code

Successful prosection of the defendants in the Medical Trial depended upon showing that the Nazi physicians deviated from accepted practices in their experimentation with humans. Indeed, much of their defense involved evidence of similar practices in other countries - most notably those in American science and medicine.

The lack of a defined ethical or regulatory code that governed the research practices of U.S. scientists caused some anxiety on the part of the American prosecutors. To help them in their efforts to understand the technical aspects of the case and the norms that governed international scientific practice, the prosecutors, at the direction of the American Medical Association (AMA), turned to Dr. Andrew Ivy.[10] Dr. Ivy was a well known physician and researcher who had been involved in experiments similar to the desalinization and high altitude experiments carried out by the Nazi defendants. After helping the prosecutors for several weeks, the AMA asked Ivy to submit a report on how the Nazi experiments had infringed medical ethics.[11] In September 1946, Dr. Andrew Ivy submitted the report to the AMA and the Nuremberg prosecution team. This report, claiming to represent standards "well established by custom, social usage, and the ethics of medical practice", formed the basis of a formal guideline on experimentation passed by the AMA in December of 1946, and established the foundation of the Nuremberg Code.[12] The prosecution at the Trial argued, somewhat ironically, that the Nazis had transgressed the AMA standards which were written in response to their transgressions. Although the AMA guidelines were published 19 days after the prosecution's opening arguments at the Trial,[13] Dr. Ivy only begrudgingly acknowledged this link in his testimony.

Although the report and Dr. Ivy's subsequent testimony were said to represent the "standards of practice in experimentation at the time", it is unclear that this was the case at the time or even now.[14] The lack of uniform adherence may have even extended, albeit unconsciously, even to Dr. Ivy. As pointed out earlier, part of the reason Dr. Ivy was selected for his role in the Nuremberg Trial was because of his experience with experiments similar to those carried out by the Nazi physicians. In some of these experiments, Dr. Ivy admitted using conscientious objectors as research subjects. Apparently Dr. Ivy was not bothered by the coercive environment under which the objectors gave consent to his experiments, although he acknowledged that the conscientious objectors had a choice of unpaid participation in the studies, manual labor, or imprisonment. Perhaps this did not bother him because as he indicated on cross-examination at the Nuremberg Trial, he had used conscientious objectors as research subjects because "[i]t was their duty".[15]

What did the Code Say?

The Nuremberg Code,[16] was laid out in the decision of the court in *United States. v. Karl Brandt et al.* Entitled "permissible experiments with humans", the code was divided into ten sections. The first, and most important, section of the Code dealt with the need for the informed consent of the research subject to the contemplated research. This section had four fundamental elements: 1) the subject must be legally competent to give consent, 2) consent must be given voluntarily without "any element of force, fraud, deceit, duress, over-reaching, or...coercion", 3) the subject must be informed of the nature, duration, purpose, method, risks, and possible side effects of the experiment, and 4) the subject must understand these elements (i.e. of 3) in such a way as to be able to make an enlightened decision about participation. The first section closes by noting a nondelegable duty of the investigator to ensure the quality of consent.

The next seven sections of the Code dealt with particular aspects of the proposed experiment. Sections two and three addressed the necessity of the proposed experiment. These sections required that the significance of the anticipated results of the experiment justify the use of human subjects. The fourth, fifth, seventh, and eighth sections required that the experimental protocol, being carried out by trained investigators, avoid physical or mental suffering or death of the subject. Interestingly, the fifth section makes an exception to this rule for physicians who serve as their own research subjects. The sixth section, perhaps a bit too vaguely, required that the risk to the subject not exceed the possible benefit of the information that the experiment was expected to provide.

The last two sections of the Code contemplated the termination of the experiment. The ninth section allowed the subject to withdraw consent to participate in the experiment at any time he saw fit. The Code's final section put a duty upon the researcher to terminate the experiment when she believed its continuation was likely to cause injury, disability, or death to the research subject.

Code in Application

1950s - The War Continues

New scientific optimism shaped the application of the Nuremberg Code in the 1950s. Dramatic discoveries brought two lines of scientific inquiry into prominence. Biomedical discoveries during, and shortly after, World War II made many lingering questions about human health seem finally addressable. Similarly, the development of atomic technology and the advent of the Cold War created new issues of military as well as medical importance. The attitude of the age and the intermingling of these forces was reflected in President Truman's address to the American Hospital Association in 1952: "Right now the Federal Government is supporting by research grants about a quarter of all the research done in medical schools. The Government is giving this aid without any control at all over the scientists or schools. That is the way it should be done and that is the way it must be done".[17] Truman went on to enthusiastically endorse the use of radioisotopes in medicine and the creation of an "atomic apothecary".

Indeed, during the 1950s scientific research greatly expanded. The ravages of World War II gave rise to technological advances and a new federal commitment to research and innovation. Recent discoveries of penicillin, the polio vaccine, and the structure of DNA seemed to point to unlimited possibilities in the fight against human suffering and disease. The optimism of the age was reflected by an unparalleled federal investment in peace-time scientific research. At the end of World War II, the National Institutes of Health (NIH) was completely restructured along the lines of the wartime Committee on Medical Research.[18] Support for the new research institutes was enormous - $700,000 were appropriated in 1945 for the war on disease; a decade later it had risen to $35 million.[19]

Continued support for the NIH was dependent upon discoveries that would address human disease and improve the health of Americans. This necessitated a commitment to clinical as well as basic research. In 1953 the NIH opened its Clinical Center to be able to put the new discoveries into action. The opening of the Clinical Center is significant as a symbol of the age's optimism[20] as well as the influence of the Nuremberg Code in American research. The Clinical Center put in place the first regulatory guidelines based upon the Nuremberg Code. Although not extensive, these guidelines required "voluntary agreement based on informed understanding" for all subjects and written consent for unusually hazardous studies. The written consent requirement was extended to all "normal" subjects in 1954.[21] These standards only applied to research carried out at the Clinical Center and did not extend to extramural research funded by the NIH or any agency.

While the NIH was busy waging war on disease, the U.S. armed forces were engaged in a Cold War and concerned with warfare in an atomic age. The dropping of two atomic bombs at the end of the World War raised new questions about how future wars would be fought and the effect of radiation on field troops.[22] These questions led to a pressing need for research on the effects of radiation. A burst of biological research began to try to characterize these effects.

In the same year that the Clinical Center opened, the Secretary of Defense adopted the Nuremberg Code for all atomic, biological and chemical warfare research by the military.[23] This is the earliest known adoption of the Nuremberg Code by any federal agency. However, enthusiasm for the boldness of this step is quickly tempered when one learns that the adoption was under an order of secrecy and it was only distributed to the heads of the three branches of the military. The letter was kept secret until 1975. Although the adoption led to little action by two branches of the armed forces, the Army Office of the Surgeon General issued the *Use of Human Volunteers in Medical Research: Principles, Policies, and Rules* the following year.[24] This unclassified document restated the Nuremberg principles for "medical research" involving humans and was distributed to some university investigators. Although labeled as "non-mandatory guidelines", there is evidence that some researchers adhered to its spirit.

Recent study of the Department of Defense's research policies have revealed that researchers were concerned about the Code being used to impose liability upon them personally.[25] In response to these concerns, Army lawyers advised the researchers that obtaining a waiver (i.e. consent) from the research subject would be the investigator's best protection.[26] These concerns were addressed more concretely in 1952 by Congressional action that indemnified investigators for any legal action that arose from their experimental subjects in Defense research.

These two statements, one covering the NIH Clinical Center and the other realistically effecting only the Army, were the only regulatory expressions of the Code in the 1950s. Perhaps one could understand a weak regulatory approach in the presence of vigorous judicial action. Alas, there are few cases reported from the 1950s of actions based on experiments. The few that did arise were within the realm of physician malpractice suits, rather than organized research.[27] Regulatory and judicial silence should not be interpreted to indicate the lack of any abuse. Indeed, suits brought in later years, many invoking the Nuremberg Code, were based upon abuses that occurred during these years.

American academic and professional communities were not awash with concern about the Code either. This indifference may have been due to not knowing about the Code or a feeling that it simply did not apply to American research. In the 15 years following the Trial, only few journals mentioned it[28] and the best known text on medical jurisprudence did not describe the Code until its 1956 edition.[29] The few comments that did surface from professional groups were not altogether approving. A 1959 meeting of the National Society for Medical Research,[30] while identifying the ten provisions of the Code as the "principal guideposts to the ethics of clinical research in the western world" indicated some unease with the stringency of the Codes' language.[31] The conference report made the Society's position clear; "[t]he protection of personal rights of individuals ... *can coexist* with the public necessity to use people - sick or well - as subjects for health research".[32] In the same year, Henry Beecher authored an article[33] that called the feasibility of some concepts of the Nuremberg Code into question. While praising the spirit of the Code, Beecher took issue with the lack practicality of its consent provision and the use of the Code as a model for rules governing American research.

1960s - Public Influence

The general acceptance of American research practices of the 1950s went through a radical awaking, if not transformation in the 1960s. Public outrage over the Thalidomide tragedy propelled the Nuremberg Code into national debate for the first time.

In 1961 stories began to emerge of severe physical deformities in the babies of European women treated during pregnancy with Thalidomide. Although Thalidomide had not been approved by the Food and Drug Administration (FDA), it was approved for use in Europe and was being tested in the United States. The deformities caused a public outcry for Congressional action. The *Drug Amendments Act*, passed in 1962, vitalized the concept of informed consent in American research. Indeed, it was the first federal law to require that a patient be informed that a drug was experimental and required the patient's consent for the administration of the drug.[34] Although consent was mandatory under the Act for the testing of drugs, it waived the consent requirement where obtaining consent was deemed "not feasible" or not in the best interests of the patient. The waiver in these cases was left to the discretion of the clinical investigator.

The Act required the FDA to regulate the clinical testing of drugs. The FDA created regulations, echoing many of the themes of the Nuremberg Code, that became effective in 1963. Among other things, they required information about the qualifications of the researcher, proposed duration of the study, proposed research protocol, and notification of the FDA in the case of "alarming" side-effects.[35] Despite these steps, the FDA did not elaborate on required consent provisions under the Act.[36]

As the Thalidomide tragedy began to be exposed, the American scientific community began to assess the new edifice it had created. In 1961 two studies of American research practices were published.[37] These studies indicated that very few research institutions had formal procedural guidelines for research and that institutions favoring review of research proposals were in the minority. Despite these deficiencies, a NIH funded study found that "normal subjects were fully informed".[38] In 1963 the NIH created the Livingston Committee to study the adequacy of consent. In a report published the following year the Committee concluded that no changes need to be made and that the creation of guidelines "would likely inhibit, delay, or distort...clinical research".[39]

The international community began to reformulate its concept of the Nuremberg Code at this time. In 1961 the World Medical Association published the precursor to the Declaration of Helsinki, the Draft Code of Ethics on Human Experimentation in Geneva.[40] The Declaration of Helsinki,[41] passed three years later, reshaped the Nuremberg Code in light of growing concerns about the future of biomedical research.[42] The Declaration divided the consent requirement according to the type of research. Research performed "combined with professional care" (i.e. clinical research) required the physician to obtain consent only if it was "possible" and "consistent with patient psychology". Requirements for non-clinical research were more stringent, requiring freely given informed consent in all cases. Subsequent revisions of the Declaration in 1975, 1983, and 1989 refined these ideas, but continued to give physicians greater freedom from consent requirements than the Nuremberg Code.[43] Henry Beecher, who had earlier voiced his suspicion about trying to apply the "legalistic" Code to American research, later praised the Declaration as a practical ethical guideline.[44] Although Americans were not involved in the development of the Declaration, it was applauded by American professional societies including the AMA.[45] The AMA adopted its own *Ethical Guidelines for Clinical Research* two years later in November of 1966.

As the problems of the Thalidomide tragedy had finally seemed to be resolved, new revelations of scientific abuse began to emerge. In 1966 Henry Beecher reemerged in the debate about the adequacy of controls on research. Although Beecher had voiced concerns in 1959 about attempts to apply the Code to American research, his new article ultimately lead to unprecedented controls on research. Beecher's article discussed twenty-two cases of ethical breaches in research published in recent medical journals.[46] One of these cases, the Brooklyn Jewish Chronic Disease Hospital study, involved the injection of live cancer cells into non-consenting patients. Another case, the Willowbrook study, involved investigators infecting retarded children with hepatitis virus under conditions of questionable consent. The Beecher article, and these cases in particular, were covered in the popular press[47] to such an extent that regulation of biomedical research became inevitable.

The same year, the Surgeon General issued a *Statement of Policy* that required institutions funded by the Public Health Service (PHS) to set up committees to review proposed research involving human subjects.[48] Although based upon ideas of the Nuremberg Code and the Declaration of Helsinki, the creation of a preliminary review mechanism went beyond the safeguards proposed in those documents. The spirit of the Code and Declaration were evident in the elements of the required review nonetheless. The committee's were to make three primary determinations: 1) the rights and welfare of the subjects; 2) the appropriateness of the method of securing informed consent; and 3) the risks and benefits of the proposed experiment.[49] Six months later the FDA published its own statement of rules to govern patient consent for investigational drugs. The FDA statement drew heavily from the Code and Declaration.[50] This borrowing was most evident in its definition of consent, which in many places copied the Nuremberg Code verbatim. This new definition got rid of the "not feasible" waiver for consent that was present in the *Drug Amendments Act* of 1962.

These dramatic events and regulatory controls were only a part of the influences that revived the Nuremberg Code in the 1960s. The civil rights movement, the Vietnam war, and their attendant issues of personal autonomy also lent to its revival. Respect for personal autonomy requires that "[p]ersons should be free to choose and act without controlling constraints imposed by others".[51] While it is difficult to disjoin the concept of respect for personal autonomy from informed consent philosophically, the legal union of the concepts is still struggling to take place. In this respect, judicial notice of the concept of autonomy is particularly significant. In 1965, a seven to two majority of the Supreme Court decided *Griswold v. Connecticut*.[52] The Court held that a state ban on the use, or the aiding of others in the use, of contraceptives was unconstitutional. The case was landmark in the law, reflecting a willingness of the Court to recognize the value of personal autonomy in the face of government regulation. This decision was a first important step to lead to a reinterpretation of the Code's meaning from a statement of physician liability to one of patient empowerment.

1970s - Study and Controls

The momentum of concerns raised about research practices spread into the 1970s. Although optimism about the potential of biomedical research to address persistent American health problems remained,[53] the drive to further refine rules governing research persisted. In 1971, the Department of Health, Education, and Welfare (DHEW) extended the Surgeon-General's 1966 directive into formal guidelines.[54] The guidelines spelled out for all DHEW supported investigators how its policies were to be followed and implemented.

Public anxiety about research practices over the Jewish Chronic Disease Hospital and Willowbrook studies was fueled by startlingly news of other exploitive experiments. Two shocking experiments were exposed in 1972. Although the experiments provoked concern about scientific merit, they also resonated with other volatile political issues such as civil rights, economic and social inequity and reproduction. News broke about the Tuskegee study as the civil and social rights movements were struggling to maintain the gains they had made in preceding years. In the Tuskegee study, hundreds of impoverished African-American men with treatable syphilis were deliberately left untreated for more than forty years to study the course of a disease that ultimately leads to dementia and death. This PHS experiment seemed to point to institutionalized indifference about the exploitation of research subjects, particularly when those subjects were poor minorities and raised questions about the adequacy of its six year old guidelines.

Public debate also centered on topics relating to reproduction. The Supreme Court handed down two significant decisions on reproductive autonomy in 1972 and 1973. *Eisenstadt v. Baird* expanded the scope of the *Griswold* ruling to allow for the distribution of contraceptives to unmarried persons.[55] The most controversial decision on autonomy came the following year in *Roe v. Wade*.[56] In *Roe*, the Court dramatically limited states' rights to control abortion by recognizing a "fundamental" right to privacy. Although decided by the Court in 1973, *Roe* was decided by a lower court in 1970 and had been argued in the Supreme Court in 1971 and reargued in

1972. In 1972 the *Washington Post* published an article on an experiment being carried out in Finland, but partially funded by the NIH, that involved the perfusion of the heads of aborted fetuses.

Despite expanding the recognition of autonomy, American courts remained largely silent on the application of the Nuremberg Code through the 1960s and 1970s. The dissent of one state case obliquely referred to the Nazi experiments in a 1969 dissent,[57] but never mentioned the Code or relied upon its principles. The only case to explicitly refer to the Code in the 1970s was decided by a lower state court. However, the decision in *Kaimowitz v. Michigan Dept. of Mental Health*,[58] reprinted the entire Code and used it as the basis of its analysis. Consistent with the Code's principles, the court held that the subject, a psychopath confined to a state hospital, could not give voluntary, competent, informed, or understanding consent.[59]

Shortly after the Tuskegee study was revealed, several bills were introduced in Congress to control human experimentation.[60] Although Senator Mondale had fought for the creation of a commission to study the topic since 1968,[61] Senator Edward Kennedy's bill ultimately prevailed. In 1974, Kennedy's bill became the *National Research Service Award Act*.[62] The Act endorsed new DHEW regulations and established the National Commission for the Protection of Human Subjects of Biomedical and Behavioral Research (National Commission). The new DHEW regulations required all institutions receiving DHEW funds to submit research proposals to institutional review boards (IRBs) before they were sent to the DHEW for funding review.[63] The National Commission was directed to identify "the basic ethical principles which should underlie the conduct of biomedical and behavioral research involving human subjects" and to develop guidelines for the Secretary of the DHEW.[64] Additionally, research using human fetuses was specifically banned until the National Commission produced a report on this subject. The National Commission's efforts led to a new set of regulations governing research within a year.[65] While the regulations reflected the spirit of the Nuremberg Code, they made several significant departures: 1) they placed ultimate responsibility to the research subject upon the institution rather than the investigator; 2) they allowed for consent from a representative of the subject; and 3) they did not require prior animal experiments, the inability to acquire the results by other means, avoidance of unnecessary suffering or prohibition of experiments likely to cause death or disability.[66] Although the regulations' consent provision quoted portions of the Code verbatim, it did not explicitly require subject understanding of the information given.[67] In light of the controversy about abortion, the greater stringency of the controls over fetal research was not surprising.[68]

The National Commission went on to publish 17 reports and appendix volumes before its statutory mandate expired in 1978.[69] The best remembered report of the Commission was the Belmont report , published in its final year. The Belmont report[70] identified three fundamental principles that should be applied in human experimentation: respect for persons, beneficence, and justice. Inherent in the "respect for persons" principle was a notion that had become increasingly evident over the National Commission's tenure - the vital importance of the subject's autonomy in the decision to consent.[71] As *Eisenstadt* and *Roe* foreshadowed, the legal concept of autonomy was beginning to take hold. The concept of patient autonomy was also born in these years. The case of *In re Karen Quinlan*[72] was a symbol of the struggle between a patient's rights and the interests of her physicians. In 1976 the New Jersey Supreme Court ruled that patient's rights took precedence in Karen Quinlan's case; deep in a coma, she was allowed to be removed from a respirator over the objections of her physicians that the court should not interfere with their medical decisions.[73] The issues raised in the *Quinlan* case were to effect the National Commission's successor in the 1980s in unexpected ways.

1980s - Deregulation

Although the President's Commission for the Study of Ethical Problems in Medicine and Biomedical and Behavioral Research (President's Commission) was authorized in 1978[74] at the close of the National Commission, it did not have its first meeting until 1980.[75] Part of the charge to the President's Commission was to get federal agencies to follow through on some of recommendations of its predecessor. An example of these efforts was a revision of the DHEW (now the DHHS) research regulations.[76] While the new regulations addressed some of the shortcomings of the 1975 regulations that have already been discussed, they made some significant new departures from the Nuremberg Code.[77] The new regulation defined "research" in such a way that it excluded novel therapies, research perceived to put the subject at little risk, and research devoid of physical contact, from its protections. In addition, the revised regulations allowed IRBs to waive the consent requirement if it found, among other things, that "[t]he research could not practicably be carried out without the waiver or alteration".[78] This is an obvious departure from the Nuremberg Code's imperative that "[t]he voluntary consent of the human subject is absolutely essential".

The President's Commission published 11 reports during a productive three year life. Its life was brought to an end by one of them. Their 1983 report, *Deciding to Forego Life-Sustaining Treatment*,[79] arguing for the withdrawal of feeding and hydration in certain cases, brought the ire of several conservative senators.[80] In response, Congressional action put an end to the President's Commission.[81] New, largely defanged, bioethics commissions were born of the 1985 *Health Research Extension Act*[82] passed over a veto by President Reagan.[83] These new commissions, the congressional Biomedical Ethics Board and Biomedical Ethics Advisory Committee, were utter failures, operating for about a year in the late 1980s.[84]

American courts began to struggle with the applicability of the Nuremberg Code in the 1980s.[85] The Code was cited in the dissent of a 1980 wrongful discharge action brought by a physician who said professional standards precluded her from doing certain proposed experiments.[86] The court's majority was reluctant to recognize the argument saying "[c]haos would result if a single doctor engaged in research were allowed to determine, according to his or her individual conscience, whether a project should continue."[87] The Code also made a rare appearance in a majority opinion in the case of *Whitlock v. Duke University.*[88] In that case, a tort action for inadequate disclosure to the subject of a University experiment was dismissed on summary judgment. The court noted that the informed consent of the subject met the requirements of the state's consent statute as well as the higher requirements of the Nuremberg Code.

The facts and holdings of two other cases referring to the Nuremberg Code were much more disturbing. Although the facts of both cases arose in 1950s, the court's decision's are an important indication of the status of the principles of the Nuremberg Code in contemporary American jurisprudence. Both cases arose from events that took place while the research subjects were in military service. In each case the subject did not provide informed consent for the experiment but lost the because soldiers "injured in the course of activity incident to service" are precluded from seeking damages from the government under the *Feres* doctrine.[89] In the summer of 1953 Stanley Jaffee, then a soldier, was ordered to stand unprotected in a field while a nuclear device was exploded a short distance away; he died in 1977 of cancer caused by his exposure to the radiation.[90] After pointing out that the Supreme Court had not ruled on such a case, the federal court of appeals held that Jaffee could not recover because of the *Feres* doctrine. The opinion stated that judicial review of military actions would compromise military efficiency.[91]

U.S. v. Stanley presented a similar issue to the Supreme Court in 1987.[92] Interestingly, *Stanley* is the only case in which the United States Supreme Court mentioned the Nuremberg Code. James Stanley sought recovery for injuries that resulted from his being secretly given lysergic acid diethylamide (LSD) in the course of an Army experiment. Stanley, an Army sergeant, had volunteered for the experiment thinking he was involved in testing protective clothing for use in the event of chemical warfare. In a five to four decision the Court dismissed the action citing a reluctance to intrude in military matters. Justices William Brennan and Sandra Day O'Connor were indignant in their dissents. Justice Brennan quoted the Nuremberg Code's consent provision and then seemed to raise the Code to constitutional status stating "experimentation with unconsenting soldiers, like any constitutional violation, may be enjoined if and when discovered."[93] Justice O'Connor stated "[n]o judicially crafted rule should insulate from liability the involuntary and unknowing human experimentation alleged to have occurred in this case"[94] and then quoted the Code's consent provision. When later reflecting upon the *Stanley* holding Brennan said "[w]asn't that an outrageous case? It was incredible! Some of us were so shocked by it when it came down that we were fearful it had started a trend. But, thank God, it hasn't shown its head again - not yet, anyway."[95]

1990s - Rediscovery

Though never far from the public consciousness, issues of reproductive and patient autonomy reemerged in the 1990s. In 1992, *Planned Parenthood of Southeastern Pennsylvania v. Casey* led the Supreme Court back into the center of the abortion issue.[96] Although the Court did not explicitly overrule *Roe*, it challenged the notion that abortion was a fundamental right and allowed states greater freedom in making laws that regulate abortion practices. An interesting aspect of the Court's decision is its upholding the state statute's "informed consent" provision. The provision provided that at least 24 hours before performing the abortion, medical personnel had to inform the patient of the procedure's risks, the probable age of the "unborn child" and the availability of materials describing the fetus and non-abortion alternatives. Although the provision is ostensibly included to protect the patient, its emphasis reveals a far greater concern for societal interest. In other words, this information is being forced on the patient in an effort to persuade her not to abort. The Court also addressed the concept of patient autonomy in hospital care. Two years before *Casey*, it had decided *Cruzan v. Missouri Department of Health*.[97] Nancy Cruzan had been in a persistent vegetative state for seven years following a car accident. Her parents sought to have the hospital discontinue Nancy's artificial hydration and nutrition to allow her to die. In a five to four decision, the Court said that although a competent person had a "...constitutionally protected liberty interest in refusing unwanted medical treatment", the state's interest in preserving life could outweigh this interest in the absence of "clear and convincing" evidence of the patient's preferences. These cases indicate a rather restrictive notion of personal autonomy in the face of government regulation.

In 1993 and 1994, reports began to surface of experiments conducted between 1944 and 1974 that had used human subjects in radiation research. Press coverage of the experiments began with an *Albuquerque Tribune* article in November 1993 that disclosed the names of individuals that had been injected with plutonium in an effort to understand the effects of radiation on the human body.[98] Subsequent reports spoke of federally funded experiments where radioactive materials were fed to retarded persons, cancer patients were subjected to "total-body irradiation", testicular irradiation of prisoners, and intentional environmental release of radiation on unsuspecting populations.[99] These reports generated an enormous public outcry. It is interesting that similar outrage was not expressed a decade earlier in response to the *Jaffee* case. Indeed, the case was followed by a similar one in 1984[100] and the release of a subcommittee report on the subject in 1986.[101] Nevertheless, the investigation of the 1990s was to prove more thorough.

President Clinton rapidly formed the Advisory Committee on Human Radiation Experiments and Energy Secretary Hazel O'Leary, who now headed the Department whose predecessor sponsored the experiments, promptly pledged to turn over her agency's files for the investigation. After extensive investigation and the publication of preliminary reports, the Advisory Committee published its final report on October 3, 1995. The report assessed the ethical, medical, and legal standards of research from 1944 to 1974, and made recommendations for subject notification and compensation for the research. President Clinton spoke of the creation of a National Bioethics Advisory Committee on the day that the final report was published. The Committee was appointed in mid-1996 and has just begun its work.

A federal court case arising out of these revelations has already been reported. In experiments carried out between 1960 and 1972, 87 patients, mostly impoverished African-Americans with terminal cancer, were exposed to radiation to study the effects of radiation on combat troops.[102] No consent forms were used for the first five years of the study and after that time the forms used did not disclose the risk to the patients or the purpose of the experiment.[103] The radiation exposure led to death, shortened life, and/or nausea, burns, and severe pain. The District Court found that the plaintiffs had a redressable cause of action against the defendant physicians and university. After the opinion reviewed the history and impact of the Nuremberg Code, it made the strongest judicial statement about the significance of the Code to date: "The Nuremberg Code is part of the law of humanity. It may be applied in both civil and criminal cases by the federal courts in the United States".[104] It remains to be seen whether this strong endorsement of the Nuremberg Code will be adopted by higher courts.

The civil suit of *In re Cincinnati Radiation Litigation* may not be the end of the matter. A coalition of groups representing radiation experiment survivors has also asked for criminal action against the scientists who lead the experiments.[105] They argue that criminal liability would arise, in part from the Nuremberg Code.

Conclusion

Lessons of the Past

The lesson that one takes away from the history Nuremberg Code in the United States is confused. Fifty years ago, seven of the twenty-four defendants in the *U.S. v. Brandt* were hanged for violating fundamental rules of medical ethics. Although it is difficult to argue that the sentences of the military tribunal were unduly harsh considering the defendant's actions, a question remains whether the Code truly reflected common medical practice of the time and whether it was ever meant to be applied outside of the circumstances under which it was generated.

The Nuremberg Code was part of the court's decision in *U.S. v. Brandt*. The purpose of the trial was not to formulate a code of ethics for experimentation with human subjects. The purpose of the trial was to prosecute and punish a series of horrendous tortures perpetrated in the name of science. The Code, as part of the decision, was used to impose liability by overcoming the defendant's claims of the lack of a uniform standard of experimental conduct. The Code and the events leading up to its adoption by the court in its decision, was presented not as an aspirational guide, but rather as a statement of fact regarding the present state of the rules guiding scientific research. In short, the Nuremberg Code was written to impose liability on scientists for their abuse of fellow human beings, not to guard the future rights of the research subjects.

The view of the Code primarily as a liability creating document dominated its application during the first decade of its existence. The Code was important to scientists during the 1950s because of its potential imposition of liability, not because of its significance to the rights of research subjects. Science, and its promises of societal health and prosperity, was now king. A whole new research infrastructure was being constructed. A series of discoveries, fundamental to the understanding of our world even to this day, were made. New, urgent, questions regarding atomic energy needed to be quickly answered. It was a time pressed with urgency for scientific inquiry that would benefit all Americans; it was a time to move forward.

It did not take long into the 1960s for the Code to be rediscovered and for what is perhaps the true spirit of the Code to be revealed. The Thalidomide tragedy has had a lasting effect on the way the scientific community is viewed by the American public. This graphic evidence of a science gone wrong led to questions about how science was conducted, and the price American society was willing to pay for it. Studies of research practices were published, government legislation and policy statements were made, and scholarly articles on the ethics of the use of human subjects in research began to appear. The Code, although not a secret before, was now at the center of the debate about the use of human subjects in experiments. It was in this environment that the first serious efforts were made to incorporate tenets of the Code into American scientific practice. It quickly became apparent that the Code would not be literally enforced; it was seen as burdensome on scientists and somewhat impractical. With several accommodations, elements of the Code were expressed in the Declaration of Helsinki and PHS and FDA policy statements.

While the 1960s marked an awakening of serious thought about American research practices, it also marked the beginning of the legal notion of personal autonomy. Unlike the preceding decade, the debate began to concentrate on the rights of the research subject rather than the liability of the scientist. Although the Nuremberg Code was not mentioned by American courts by name during the whole decade, this fundamental legal principle reshaped the significance of the Code in the decades that followed.

The revelations of the 1960s set the stage for the dramatic events of the 1970s. Growing national concerns with personal reproductive and civil rights were reflected in revelations about a number of scientific abuses exposed during this period. At the same time the Supreme Court was deciding pivotal cases in abortion rights and desegregation, evidence of NIH sponsored research with human fetuses and exploitive experiments involving African-Americans came to light. These events helped transform the already shaken public view of science from one of a noble, apolitical quest to one which not only reflected human frailties, but displayed political motives as well. It was in this environment that debate about the Code was almost entirely transformed into one of personal rights. Indeed, the *protection* of personal rights was the focus of what was the far reaching evaluation of human subject research by the National Commission.

The 1980s seemed to begin with a continued commitment to evaluate and protect the rights of research subjects. However, the brief life of the President's Commission was followed by a series of aborted efforts that fell prey to political infighting. The political struggles that plagued science during the 1980s were due, in part, to the recent recognition of the significance of personal autonomy. There were questions as to how far this recognition would extend. The ability of individuals to assert their rights was often seen in conflict with the moral and social values of the country as a whole. This tension is perhaps best illustrated by *U.S. v. Stanley* the only Supreme Court decision to discuss the Nuremberg Code. Without mentioning the Code, the majority of the Court, arguing on the grounds of military efficiency, set the rights of a research subject aside.

Thus far, the 1990s are marked by a rediscovery of the issues that gave rise to the Nuremberg Code. As a whole new generation learns of Tuskegee and the DOE radiation experiments, the same old question has been asked anew - how could we allow such things to happen? Perhaps we can draw comfort from the fact that most of the debate is over experiments done before serious national debate, policy statements, commissions, and legislation on the subject. Perhaps we cannot.

Are We There Yet?

The continuing irony about the Nuremberg Code is that we have never been able to get where we said we were 50 years ago. The irony is compounded, of course, when one contemplates whether we really ever wanted to get there. Despite 50 years of study, debate, and legal action, the substance of what makes the Code so important to American science and society has been largely forgotten. The Code was never meant to be practical. It was a device to facilitate the punishment of Nazi physicians. The Code was intractable, unyielding, and definite. It was written this way because it was written for "them" not "us". The problem of course is that the Code was our creation.

There can be no question that we have come nearer to meeting the standards of the Nuremberg Code in the last half century. However, problems remain to be adequately addressed. We consider here main themes rather than details of the present case law and regulations. The primary problems to be addressed in the Code's future are: 1) the union of investigator liability with personal autonomy and 2) the emergence of new thinking about the scope of human subject protections.

The Code's history has demonstrated that a fundamental shift of liability has occurred through regulatory law. The Nuremberg Code made the investigator ultimately responsible to the subject. Since 1966, American law has made the investigator's home institution responsible to the subject. As a result, the scientific superstructure created by the federal government has generated a class of highly-educated individuals who have the power to invade the lives of their research subjects, yet have no duty to them. The rules that a researcher will ultimately follow are those OKed by the IRB. IRBs, most of whose members are employed by the same institution as the investigator, are replete with conflicts of interest. Although they spend most of their time reviewing the proposal's consent forms,[106] they give little attention to implementation of the consent process or how the subjects are actually used in the experiment.[107] IRB review is essentially an administrative of documents - informed consent forms and research design - not oversight of how research is carried out. As a result, IRBs often end up either rubber-stamping the investigator's original proposal or requiring documentary revisions. Who is protecting the research subject? Investigators should have a recognized fiduciary duty to their research subjects.[108] Such duties have applied to the physician-patient relationship for some time. The lack of fiduciary duties in organized research may be due to the recent rapid growth of the American scientific community and deference to the scientific community on the part of lawmakers. The creation of such a duty will have little meaning if the subject's autonomy is not recognized and respected.

As this chapter has pointed out, fashions of interest in the subject of personal autonomy have come and gone, but commitment to the inherent value of more scientific knowledge has remained constant. At a fundamental level these efforts deny respect for the research subjects' autonomy in order to recognize a broader social agenda. The argument that our society should limit the rights of the individual for the sake of the scientific needs of society is ominously similar to those that took us to Nuremberg 50 years ago. Proponents of a middle-ground view would argue that we are a long way from Nuremberg - we have the benefit of years of debate, study and legislation to ensure the rights of research subjects. This may be true, but let us not forget that before the Nuremberg Code, the most comprehensive guideline guarding the rights of research subjects was in place during the Nazi reign.[109]

When one thinks of experiments requiring the Code's protection, images of the Nazi experiments, Tuskegee, Willowbrook, the Jewish Chronic Disease Hospital, *Jaffee, Stanley,* and *In re Cincinnati* come to mind. These cases are a grim reminder that the most vulnerable persons need the greatest protection from exploitation. Even well-intentioned investigators may be carried away by researchers' zeal rather than fiduciary duties to their patient subjects.

A recent change in FDA informed consent requirements clearly illustrates the dominance of scientific research over personal autonomy.[110] The new regulations waive the requirement for informed consent for research from certain human subjects who are in need of emergency therapy for a life-threatening condition. The waiver is limited to situations where research is needed because available treatments are unproven or unsatisfactory. For example, unconscious patients with severe brain injuries may benefit from new drugs or techniques for reducing brain swelling. The research must be conducted under an IRB approved protocol and after appropriate preliminary and animal studies. Other administrative rules also seek to assure responsible research. But the fundamental issue is that the waiver gives extraordinary discretion to physician investigators. They are permitted to enroll in research patients who are likely unknown to the physician. Patients who arrive in emergency rooms after vehicular accidents or gunshot wounds are often unconscious or, even if conscious, incompetent. Even physicians who try to protect their patients' best interests may be subtly influenced by the lure of research discoveries. Patients may be precipitously diagnosed as having a life-threatening condition. Existing therapies may be devalued in favor of research protocols. Efforts to obtain subsequent consent from family members may be subordinated to completing the research protocol. Research projects tend to acquire a momentum that may diminish the interests of individual patients. When their autonomy has already been sacrificed, it is critical that their welfare be vigorously and vigilantly protected. If exceptions to the voluntary consent of research subjects are to be made - even for their own benefit - it should not be left to researchers alone to protect patients' interests. At the very least such research should not only be prospectively reviewed by IRBs, but also continuously and independently monitored in its implementation. In the absence of such outside scrutiny, exceptions to the Nuremberg Code consent principle should be forbidden.

The debate in the research ethics community provoked by the FDA informed consent waiver rule brings out the continuing relevance and significance of the principles articulated in the Nuremberg Code. Whether or not one believes that exceptions to the consent requirement can even be justified in specific circumstances, the general importance of the Nuremberg Code is widely acknowledged. Our collective responsibility is to make sure that the Nuremberg Code is not only applauded in theory, but also respected in practice.

Notes

1   Reprinted in *United States v. Karl Brandt et al.*, "The Medical Case, Trials of War Criminals Before the Nuremberg Military Tribunals Under Control Council Law No. 10" at Vol I. ix. (Washington D.C.: U.S. Government Printing Office, 1949). [hereafter *U.S. v. Brandt*]

2   Annas G., Grodin M. (1992), *The Nazi Doctors and the Nuremberg Code* at 95. Oxford Univ. Press, New York.

3   *U.S. v. Brandt* supra note 1, at Vol. I, 11-16.

4   Ibid. at Vol. 1, 897-908. The prosection introduced an additional 570 written exhibits and 49 affidavits and called 32 witnesses.

5   Annas G., Grodin M., supra note 2, at 120.

6   Rothman D.J. (1991), *Strangers at the Bedside: A History of how Law and Bioethics Transformed Medical Decision Making* at 62, Basic Books.

7   *Final Report of the Advisory Committee on Human Radiation Experiments* (Washington D.C.: U.S. Government Printing Office No. 061-000-00-848-9 October 1995) at 150-155. [hereafter ACHRE]

8   Ibid. at 163n; see also Brackman A.C. (1989), *The Other Nuremberg: The Untold Story of the Tokyo War Crime Trials*. Collins, London; Williams P., Wallace D. (1989), *Unit 731: The Japanese Army's Secret of Secrets*. Hodder & Stoughton, London.

9   Mitscherlich A., Mielke F. (1992), 'Epilogue: Seven Were Hanged', in *The Nazi Doctors and The Nuremberg Code* at 106, 107 (George J. Annas & Michael Grodin (eds.); *that cited* Bower T. (1987), *The Paperclip Conspiracy: The Hunt for Nazi Scientists*. Little, Brown, Boston; and Hunt L. (1991), *Secret Agenda: The United States Government and the Project Paperclip, 1945-1990*, at 78-93, St. Martin's Press, New York.

10   ACHRE, *supra* note 7, at 132.

11   Ibid. at 133.

12   Ibid. at 133-136.

13   Grodin M., 'Historical Origins of the Nuremberg Code', in: *The Nazi Doctors and the Nuremberg Code* at 134, in: G.J. Annas, M. Grodin (eds) (1992).

14   Bassiouni M.C. et al. (1981), 'An Appraisal of Human Experimentation in International Law and Practice: The Need for International Regulation of Human Experimentation'. *Journal of Criminal Law. & Criminology* 72: 1597-1666.

15   *U.S. v. Brandt, supra* note 1, at Vol. 2, 113.

16   entitled "Permissible Medical Experiments," Ibid. at Vol. 2, 181-182.

17   *Public Papers of the Presidents of the United States: Harry S. Truman*, 1952-53, at 573. (Washington D.C.: U.S. Government Printing Office 1966).

18   Rothman, *supra* note 6, at 53.

19   *Id.*

20   Two years after the ground breaking for the Clinical Center in 1948 a prominent researcher remarked "[n]o clinical research has been undertaken in the fields of cancer, tuberculosis, or mental illness, since ... basic laboratory research has not advanced far enough to make possible clinical trials." Donald S. Fredrickson, 'Values and the Advance of Medical Research', in *Integrity in Health Care Institutions: Humane Environments For Teaching, Inquiry, And Healing* at 74 (R.E. Bulger & S.J. Reiser (eds) (1990).

21   ACHRE, *supra* note 7, at 113.

22   *See* Ibid. at Chapter 1.

23   *Reprinted* Ibid. at 105-107.

24   Ibid. at 109.

25   Ibid. at 99-101.

26   Ibid. at 100.

27   *Baldor v. Rogers*, 81 So.2d 658,659 (Fla. 1955); *Salgo v. Leland Stanford Jr. University Board of Trustees*, 317 P.2d 170 (Cal. App. 1957).

28   Rothman, *supra* note 6, at 62.

29   ACHRE, *supra* note 7 at 155.

30   The group was co-founded by one of the Codes' principal architects, Dr. Andrew Ivy.

31   ACHRE, *supra* note 7 at 155-156.

32   Rothman, *supra* note 6, at 67,68, italics added.

33   Beecher H. (1959), 'Experimentation in Man', *JAMA* 169: 118/470.

34   Faden R.R., Beauchamp T.L. (1986), *A History and Theory of Informed Consent* at 203, Oxford Univ. Press, New York.

35   Curran W.J., 'Governmental Regulation of the Use of Human Subjects in Medical Research: The Approach of Two Federal Agencies', in *Experimentation With Human Subjects* at 412-416 (Paul A. Freund ed. (1970).

36   Ibid. at 416-418.

37   ACHRE, *supra* note 7 at 138, 174.

38   *Id.*

39   Rothman, *supra* note 6, at 87.

40   Draft Code of Human Experimentation by WMA in Geneva 1961

41   Declaration of Helsinki adopted in 1962, *reprinted in* Annas & Grodin, *supra* note 2, at 331-333.

42   Faden R., Beauchamp T., *supra* note 34, at 203.

43   Katz J., 'The Consent Principle of the Nuremberg Code: Its Significance Then and Now', in: *The Nazi Doctors and the Nuremberg Code* at 231-234 (George J. Annas & Michael Grodin (eds) (1992).

44   Annas G., 'The Nuremberg Code in U.S. Courts: Ethics versus Expediency', in: *The Nazi Doctors and the Nuremberg Code* at 205 (George J. Annas & Michael Grodin eds., 1992).

45   Faden R., Beauchamp T., *supra* note 34, at 157.

46   Beecher H.K. (1966), 'Ethics and Clinical Research', *NEJM* 274: 1354.

47   ACHRE, *supra* note 7 at 177-178.

48   Faden R., Beauchamp T., *supra* note 34, at 208; Curran, *supra* note 35, at 437.

49   Appelbaum P.S. et al (1987), *Informed Consent: Legal Theory and Clinical Practice* at 217, Oxford Univ. Press., New York.

50   *See* Curran, *supra* note 35, at 419-430.

51   Faden R., Beauchamp T., *supra* note 34, at 8; For an excellent analysis of personal autonomy *see* Faden R., Beauchamp T., *supra* note 34, at 235-273.

52   *Griswold v. Connecticut*, 381 U.S. 479 (1965).

53   President Nixon declared war on cancer in 1971.

54   *Institutional Guide to DHEW Policy on Protection of Human Subjects* (U.S. Guidelines on Human Experimentation).

55   *Eisenstadt v. Baird*, 405 U.S. 438 (1972).

56 *Roe v. Wade*, 410 U.S. 113 (1973).

57 *Strunk v. Strunk*, 445 S.W.2d 145 (Ken. Ct. App. 1969).

58 *Kaimowitz v. Michigan Dept. of Mental Health*, 42 U.S.L.W. 2063 (Mich. Cir. Ct. July 10, 1973).

59 Annas, *supra* note 44, at 207.

60 ACHRE, *supra* note 7 at 180.

61 *See* Rothman, *supra* note 6, at 168-189.

62 Pub. L. No. 93-348, 88 Stat. 342 (1974)

63 39 Fed. Reg. 18914-18920 (1974).

64 Glantz L.H. (1992), 'The Influence of the Nuremberg Code on U.S. Statutes and Regulations', in: *The Nazi Doctors and the Nuremberg Code* at 187 (George J. Annas & Michael Grodin (eds).

65 45 CFR §46 (1975).

66 *See* Glantz, *supra* note 64, at 187-190.

67 *See* 45 CFR §46.103(c) (1975).

68 Glantz, *supra* note 64.

69 Faden R., Beauchamp T., *supra* note 34, at 215.

70 National Commission for the Protection of Human Subjects of Biomedical and Behavioral Research, *The Belmont Report: Ethical Principles and Guidelines for the Protection of Human Subjects of Research*, DHEW Publication No. (OS) 78-0012 (April 18, 1978). [hereafter Belmont report]

71 ACHRE, *supra* note 7 at 181.

72 *In re Quinlan*, 355 A.2d 647 (N.J.1976).

73 *See* Rothman, *supra* note 6, at 222-246.

74 Public Law 95-622 (1978).

75 Faden R., Beauchamp T., *supra* note 34, at 221.

76 45 CFR §46.

77 Glantz, *supra* note 64, at 190-191.

78 45 CFR §46.117(d)(2) (1983).

79 President's Commission for the Study of Ethical Problems in Medicine and Biomedical and Behavioral Research, *Deciding to Forego Life-Sustaining Treatment* (Washington D.C.: Government Printing Office, 1983).

80 Cook-Degan R. (1994), *The Gene Wars: Science, Politics, and the Human Genome* at 259, 260, W.W.Norton & Co., New York.

81 Ibid.

82 Public Law 98-158 (1985).

83 Ibid.

84 *For a personal account see* Cook-Degan, *supra* note 80, at 260-262.

85 *See* Annas, *supra* note 44, at 201-222.

86 *Pierce v. Ortho Pharmaceutical Corp*, 417 A.2d 505 (N.J. 1980).

87 Ibid. at 514.

88 *Whitlock v. Duke University*, 637 F.Supp. 1463 (M.D.N.C. 1986).

89 Annas, *supra* note 44, at 208-215.

90 *Jaffee v. United States*, 663 F.2d 1226 (3rd Cir. 1981).

91 The court stated: If claims for injuries sustained by members of the armed forces in the execution of military orders were subjected to the scrutiny of courts of justice, then the civil courts would be required to examine and pass upon the propriety of military decisions. The security and common defense of the country would quickly disintegrate under such meddling. Ibid. at 1229.

92 *United States v. Stanley*, 483 U.S. 669 (1987).

93 Ibid. at 687, 690.

94 Ibid. at 709-710.

95 Hentoff, Nat, 'The Justice breaks his silence: for the first time since his retirement, Supreme Court Justice William Brennan delivers the closing argument on his colleagues, the constitution and what this country faces', *Playboy*, July 1991, at 120.

96 *Planned Parenthood of Southeastern Pennsylvania v. Casey*, 112 S.Ct. 2791 (1992).

97 *Cruzan v. Missouri Department of Health*, 497 U.S. 261 (1990).

98 ACHRE, *supra* note 7 at 2.

99 Ibid. 2-4.

100 In that case, former Navajo uranium miners brought suit against the government for injuries related to their exposure to uranium. The PHS conducted an epidemiological study on the miners from 1949 to 1960, but did not warn the miners about potential health risks. The court dismissed the suit, saying that the PHS study was "consistent with the medical ethical and legal standards of the 1940s and 1950s....The PHS physicians were not experimenting on human beings...[t]hey were gathering data..." *Begay v. United States*, 591 F.Supp. 991, 997-998 (D. Ariz. 1984).

101 *See* Annas, *supra* note 44, at 221n.

102 *In re Cincinnati Radiation Litig.*, 874 F. Supp. 796 (S.D. Ohio 1995).

103 Ibid. at 803-804.

104 Ibid. at 821.

105 *Cold war experiment patients want researchers tried*, Reuters, Ltd., Oct. 12, 1995.

106 Arguably because this is the only part of the proposal that they can understand.

107 Appelbaum P.S. et al. (1982), 'The Therapeutic Misconception: Informed Consent in Psychiatric Research', *Int. J. Law Psychiatry* 5: 319; Gray B.H. et al. (1978), 'Research Involving Human Subjects', *Science* 201: 1094.

108 *See* Delgado R., Leskovac H. (1986), 'Informed Consent in Human Experimentation: Bridging the Gap between Ethical Thought and Current Practice', *U.C.L.A. L. Rev.* 34: 67.

109 The 1931 Reichs Circular, reprinted by Grodin Michael A., 'Historical Origins of the Nuremberg Code', in *The Nazi Doctors and the Nuremberg Code* at 132-133 (George J. Annas & Michael Grodin (eds) (1992).

110 45 CFR §46, Rule 61 FR 51531.

13 Ethical "Norms" and the Law: Legitimacy of "Experts" and Democratic Legitimacy

Bertrand Mathieu

Introduction

The existence of ethical "norms" suggests that there may be rules governing human conduct within a social context other than those derived from the law. Such norms are not the concern of positive law. In other words, they are not issued by a body, i.e., the constitutive authority, an international organization, the legislator, an administrative authority, or the judiciary, whose purpose it is to produce legal imperatives, the violation of which is subject to punishment.

Certainly, morals and religion are, as much as the law, capable of elaborating principles of human, individual, or collective conduct. Their connection with the law is, however, the result of their mutually accepted relationship of independence and interference. "In the secular state, the law tends to bring about a synthesis of political and moral chemistries. The law cannot be confused with morals, nor can it sever itself from them".[1] In any event, morals are formed without the intervention of the state; they are binding in society only when they have been transmuted by way of the law and embodied within a legal precept. To be sure, one may contest a civil law that is contrary to a moral principle but it is by no means permissible to shirk a law (except if doing so in the name of a moral demand that overrides any civil authorization), nor is the violation of a moral principle a punishable act.

The relationship between ethics and law is different. To begin with, ethics sets itself off from morals, which compete with it; on the other hand, the relationship between ethics and the law is less definable.

Briefly stated, morals express a universal demand for individual rules of conduct held to be valid on a universal basis, while ethics are supposed to regulate social problems and set up standards of conduct for new issues

163

and unknown situations that arise, requiring quick solutions. The essential difference between morals and ethics is in the way they evolve and the philosophy that inspires them. Morals are normative, deriving standards of behavior from fundamental rules, i.e. principles in keeping with a superior law such as natural law. They tend, insofar as required by the social order, to be embodied in legal regulations. Ethics, on the other hand, strives to find solutions based on references which are to be restored, to a great degree, by relying extensively on the individual judgments of "experts" or "savants."[2] Whereas morals intend to dictate rules, ethics intends to describe the status of mores, inviting political authorities to draw up statutes on the basis of the evolution of such mores. Ethics has a less intimate rapport with the law because of its distrust of it. Yet, ethics is more closely dependent on public intervention than are morals. Ethics is the word of the "experts" who must, however, be empowered by public authority. As "counselors to the prince", these "sages" replace the clergy of former times. However, it is up to the government in the end to give ethical "norms" their democratically based legitimation, without which they could not become legal standards.

In medicine, as in other fields (though medicine has done pioneer work before ethics ever was), ethical norms of conduct have been elaborated on the fringes of positive law such that the legal aspects play a more significant role than they do in morals: we are referring here to deontological rules. Like ethics, deontological rules constitute applied morals to a certain extent. They differ from one another, however, in several significant respects. To begin with, it is the personal obligation of the physician to adhere to deontological guidelines, while ethics is not limited to therapeutic activity alone but rather is also interested in scientific activities (research) and social issues (i.e., *in vitro* fertilization and other medically assisted reproductive procedures).[3] Furthermore, unlike deontology, ethics is not subject to legal sanctions. Last of all, ethics is not limited to the members of one profession, as is the case with deontology.

Nevertheless, within the context of this discussion, deontology interests us as much as ethics does, since both deal with fundamentally the same matter. In other words, how can "norms" of conduct that have been formulated outside any democratic institution be translated into positive law? And what if the formulation of these laws is left up to private organizations? Or should the secular arm of government carry out this function?

This problem is not only encountered in medicine and medical research. In the French legal system, other private organizations are endowed with functions and prerogatives that are in the public interest (for instance, sport federations). In addition, the development of independent administrative agencies (for example, in audiovisual communications) with regulatory powers is a sign of the crisis in which traditional legislation is involved. In this regard, however, particular circumstances affect the field of biomedical ethics. On the one hand, ethics committees have been set up outside the field of professional deontology; on the other hand, the legal status of these ethics committees has not been clearly stipulated, as if it were difficult to decide on an adequate manner for establishing rules in this field.

Among the existing committees, several have the task of formulating general ethical norms; others are entrusted with regulating a certain practice. Some have been created to address a particular issue and are dissolved after completing their mission (*ad hoc* committees), while others are permanent. Some are involved with research protocols, while others deal with clinical decisions. Some have been created by public authorities, others by private organizations.[4] Their legal status as well as the legal basis for their intervention are further differences. Yet, in reality, these differences are not as marked as they may seem. Contemplating the ethical implications of a certain practice can just as easily become deontological and influence a physician's conduct. For instance, considerations concerning research cannot simply ignore medical practice. Nevertheless, we can distinguish between two types of committees that interest us most here in terms of legitimacy: those that formulate principles and those that regulate certain practices.[5] The former type will be our main concern here. Indeed, intervention by a body entrusted with regulating certain procedures questions the so-called "unique dialogue between the doctor and the patient" rather than the conditions for formulating the rules. A body entrusted with regulating a procedure sees to it that a decision or act affecting the individual conforms to the entire body of applicable regulations. In addition, it acts as a means of assisting the individual in the decision-making process. However, aside from the relative nature of the difference as outlined above, the committees that are entrusted with regulating practices may stipulate practices which the law itself cannot ignore.

Finally, the phenomenon of ethics committees affects international law just as much as national law. A certain number of international organizations - such as the Council of Europe, the European Community,[6] or UNESCO[7] - have their own ethics committees. Even if their methods differ, in practice all are dealing with a similar question as to the origin of the laws, i.e., how can bodies that have been authorized by international law to formulate legal acts confer upon committees the task of stipulating ethical norms and of creating instruments of international law.[8]

The present study, beginning with the situation in France, will be restricted to considering how law-making in the biomedical field is affected by ethical "norms" formulated by agencies which, in a given situation, have been given a special status at the Government level.

The Government confers the task of resolving ethical problems to committees that have been set up outside the traditional professional organizations (I). The ethical "norms" formulated by these committees have a different kind of legitimacy than the one on which legal regulations are based, i.e. legitimacy through "experts" (II). However, these ethical norms have an innate weakness in terms of legal aspects, hence implying and necessitating the intervention of a sovereign state based on democratic sovereignty (III).

Professional Organizations and "Committification": Governmental Authorization

Traditionally, professional organizations intervene in the formulation of medical law. They are established by governmental authorities and empowered by them to lay down or prepare provisions of a regulatory nature. As a result, a professional group is responsible for creating a legal system that is officially endorsed by the government. As doctors' work began to spill over into fields other than therapy, ethics committees appeared alongside these professional organizations for doctors. In the beginning, the government did not intervene with the work of these ethics committees. This "spontaneous generation" of committees gave rise to a phenomenon that has been inelegantly termed *"comitologie"* (approx. equivalent to "committification", a boom in ethics committees; translator's note) The fact that a neologism had to be created for this phenomenon shows its uniqueness. However, in a later phase, public agencies took up the idea and created committees of their own that were authorized to find solutions to ethical problems and worked within a legal framework that determined the way it functioned and its powers.

Ethics without Government

This contribution is not intended to be a historical study of the phenomenon of ethics committees. Nevertheless, it is fitting to illustrate some of the milestones in that have ensued in the relationship between ethics and law. On the international level, two key texts marked the birth - or dawn - of ethical thought: the Nuremberg Code of 1947 and the Declaration of Helsinki of 1964. The latter was amended in Tokyo in 1975, in Venice in 1983, in Hong Kong in 1989 and ultimately in Somerset West, South Africa, in 1996; it stipulates that study protocols for experiments involving human subjects must first be submitted to the careful scrutiny of an independent committee designated especially for this purpose. This landmark text was produced by the World Medical Association, a private scientific organization. Other norms of international biomedical ethics have also been defined by non-governmental organizations (NGOs).[9] Thus, the relationship between ethics and law is quite unusual: private organizations, acting without powers from public officials to do so, define norms later to be used as a basis for both lawmakers, on a national level, and for authorities at the supranational level.

At the national level, the origin of ethics committees is just as interesting. Around 1980, local committees were formed within hospital systems in France. The creation of these committees went hand in hand with both the birth of ethics as the moral reflection on consequences of scientific undertakings.[10] In broader terms, any group of individuals entrusted with the task of making a decision on an ethical matter or deliberating together to solve a bioethical problem can be called an ethics committee.[11]

The recommendations formulated by these ethics committees have no legal significance whatsoever. This is also the case for the guidelines stipulated by the Center for the Study and Preservation of Sperm (*Centre d'études et de conservation du sperme*). On the other hand, the local committees have no legal status: they were not called into being by any legal document, except for the committees of the Parisian social welfare assistance, which owe their existence to a circular from the general director of this agency.

Yet, one of the main features of these committees is "that they are called on to issue general or specific ethical directives on conduct that is contrary to the law",[12] especially when medical activities or research proposals are involved when their chief aims are other than therapeutic. The idea behind these committees could be formulated somewhat dramatically as follows: The developments in science and medical technology inevitably lead to practices that could be dangerous. For this reason, ethical norms must exist to keep these practices in check and to put them into a certain moral framework. The reasoning behind this is not false and certainly has its advantages. Yet it conveys an unusual thought about the relationship between science and the law, namely that science has precedence over the law and that a legal ban is only valid in keeping with a scientific or ethical opinion. Thus, informal committees contribute to the emergence of elaborate practices at the periphery of deontology that are at times in opposition to the legal ruling. This type of self-regulation within the scientific and medical community is moving toward its own normative system bordering on general law.

None of the regulatory or legislative texts that were introduced later on in order to create ethics committees has provided for the dissolution of these local committees. Even though these committees are not legally recognized, nothing prevents them from continuing to function. Legislators or regulatory agencies certainly could have given them a status. A number of suggestions had been made to this effect,[13] but this way has not been chosen. The constitutional right to freedom of association that applies to those committees that are official associations and the right to freedom of research as recognized by the *Conseil constitutionnel*[14] prohibit any ban of ethics committees that are not recognized or authorized by governmental agencies. And yet, these ethics committees only play a role in terms of legal doctrines. Although these committees may contribute to advancements in law and may induce doctors and scientists to focus more of their attention on the practices of their professions, their analyses cannot in any case legitimize conduct that violates the law nor can they incorporate their opinions or recommendations by way of a process of legal decision-making.

Organizations Authorized by the Government

Two types of such organizations are known to exist. One type comprises professional bodies. The French government grants this type of organization regulatory competence and entrusts it with the task of formulating a deontological code. The other type comprises ethics committees (review boards) which owe their existence to laws and legal provisions yet have often an ill-defined legal status.

Professional bodies Here we shall only be concerned with medical bodies, although others, in particular the professional organization of pharmacists, are just as authorized to formulate deontological guidelines. The French Medical Association (*Ordre des Médecins*) was created by a law that dates back to October 7, 1940 and was amended after the Liberation. Article L 382 of the *Code de la santé publique* (French public health code) must "see to it that the French Medical Association keep watch over the principles of moral integrity and devotion towards one's patients so indispensable to the practice of medicine and that all of its members observe their professional obligations and comply with the rules of the code of deontology".[15]

Hence, the French Medical Association is a private law corporation legally authorized to exercise a regulatory function under the control of the administrative judge.

This regulatory function can be exercised in several ways. For instance, in a decree dated July 22, 1977, the *Conseil d'État*[16] (Council of State) granted regulatory power to the *Conseil national de l'ordre des médecins* (National Medical Council) in order to ensure that it be able to carry out the tasks conferred upon it by law. But this power is limited. In fact, the French Medical Association (*Ordre*) does not hold any generally implied regulatory powers in the field of deontology.[17] By the same token, no deontological code may encroach upon a domain that is constitutionally designated for the law.[18] This regulatory power can be more clearly visualized by the fact that it is possible to issue model contracts, some of which contain binding clauses providing for the possibility of redress before an administrative court for immoderate exercise of said power.[19] The *conseils de l'ordre* of the various French Departments can also institute measures against doctors that may entail an administrative court action. Hence, any agreement involving the practice of medicine must be reported to the *Ordre*, which can then give instructions to those concerned.[20] In addition, the *Ordre* is also vested with the power to exercise disciplinary authority over doctors, a power subject to the control of the *Conseil d'État*, the supreme court of appeal. Exercising this disciplinary power leads to the establishment of legally binding rules of conduct.

The principle role of the French Medical Association with regard to the rules of professional conduct is to prepare a deontological code. The *Ordre* plays an important role in determining the deontological rules in that it prepares and revises the code; however, for it to become applicable, the code must be sanctioned by the government. In fact, this professional code begins to look like a decree issued by the *Conseil d'État*. This means that the executive power deems the code as set up by the medical profession effective after the *Conseil d'État* has stated its opinion with regard to the contents. The rules stipulated in this deontological code thus become statutory rules. Some have a simple regulatory function, while others are of a legislative nature, whereas the code limits itself to adopting certain provisions from legal texts. This is the case, for example, with regard to a doctor's freedom to prescribe medication and with regard to professional secrecy as stated in Article L 162-2 of the French public health code (*Code de la santé publique*) in the section on legal regulations. Finally, some provisions may even be granted constitutional status, such as the freedom to choose one's doctor. Although the constitutional council (*Conseil constitutionnel*) has not as yet discussed this possibility, it has not ruled out an amendment of this nature either.[21] The connection between the rules of professional conduct and the law is thus perfectly defined: a committee of medical professionals is set up by the legislative power which authorizes it to define deontological principles that have the status of rules in terms of positive law. This status is attained either by express and limited authorization from the legislative power or by ratification by the executive power.

Such deontological rules are applicable, however, only to a limited degree. On the one hand, they only apply to doctors and cannot be referred to with regard to third parties. On the other hand, an agreement that is not in keeping with the deontological rules does not necessarily become nil and void before the civil court judge.[22] Contrarily, under certain conditions, third parties may apply these rules against a doctor.[23]

Even though, as opposed to ethical "norms", deontological rules can also be legal rules, the rules of professional conduct may be influenced by and may originate from ethical principles. Such a development can be seen in the professional code for doctors that was issued by decree on September 6, 1995.[24] For example, the new code includes a rule elaborated by the *Comité national d'éthique* and adopted by the administrative arm of justice, according to which the respect for human beings must also be maintained after death (Art. 2).

Ethics committees While the professional medical organization exerts regulatory and disciplinary power over doctors, regulatory or legislative texts have created ethics committees entrusted with the task of acting in an advisory capacity on certain research projects or for certain clinical practices. There is a wide variety of such ethics committees. Two such committees merit a more detailed discussion, namely the *Comité consultatif national d'éthique* (CCNE) and the *Comités consultatifs de protection des personnes dans la recherche biomédicale* (CCPPRB).

The committees created by public authorities by way of legislation or regulations are particularly numerous and offer a variety of legal status. Some of these committees are legal bodies and public institutions. Others, such as the *Agence du médicament* and the *Agence française du sang,* are vested with regulatory powers, the latter also being endowed with an ethical mission. The law of January 4, 1993, which spawned this agency, provides in particular that "the entire process involving transfusions be carried out in strict compliance with ethical principles". The *Commission nationale de médecine et de biologie de la reproduction et du diagnostic prénatal*, established by law 94-654 on July 29, 1994 and organized by decree on May 6, 1995, is especially supposed to take a stand on biological research projects on embryos. Thus, such a committee does *de facto* have true decision-making powers. The *Conseil constitutionnel* agreed to have this power relegated to the *Commission* without the legislature filing to recognize its competence.[25] Such bodies constitute advisory agencies and can, as the case may be, take on the form of independent administrative committees without any legal status.

As mentioned above, among the organizations referred to as ethics committees, two types will be subject to closer examination here. First, protection of human subjects in biomedical research will be discussed. These committees were created by the law of December 20, 1988.[26] There is one committee per region and each one must be approved by the Minister of Health. Members are nominated by the prefect of each region according to "a list of proposals compiled by organizations and authorities whose task it is to do so under conditions stipulated by decree". The members state their position regarding the conditions under which biomedical research may be conducted on human subjects, taking into account the protection of test subjects, the relevance of the project and the appropriateness of the objectives and means used. These committees have legal status. The protocol of each research project must be submitted to them. While a decision in favor of a project is not binding for the minister, a decision opposing a project means that such a project must be discontinued for a period of two months as of the date of receipt in the ministry. In theory, these committees are not commissioned to formulate ethical rules, but merely to regulate practices. Nevertheless, their recommendations are part of a legal decision-making process. However, these committees are not confined to technically and/or scientifically controlling the submitted protocols nor do they limit their control to the respect of regulatory or legislative legal rules; nor do they really help in making medical decisions;[27] but they are able to draft ethical reference standards. For this reason, such boards can be considered ethical committees.

The *Comité consultatif national d'éthique* belongs to the second, more distinct category. Created by the decree of February 21, 1983, this committee was given a legal foundation with law number 94-654 of July 29, 1994. This law states that "the Committee is designed to give advice on ethical problems raised by the progress of knowledge gained in the fields of biology, medicine, and health and to publish recommendations on this subject". It may be consulted to this end by public authorities (members of the government and the presidents of parliamentary assemblies) or research institutes. The *Comité consultatif national d'éthique* is composed of five personalities from the principle schools of philosophy and religious denominations and chosen by the President of the Republic, nineteen experts designated by the presidents of the parliamentary assemblies, the ministers and heads of supreme courts and administrative courts, and fifteen members from the research sector who are appointed by academic or research organizations. The President and the President of Honor are nominated by the President of the Republic.

Legally, this committee is sometimes defined as an independent administrative authority. In fact, this name is inappropriate. To be sure, the CCNE is independent, but it is not an authority. Rather, the Committee only makes advisory statements (or recommendations) without legal authority and without any formal appearance in any legal decision-making process. In fact, the CCNE is an institution *sui generis*. This specific status of the committee, this indefinite status with respect to existing legal categories, precisely expresses the particularity of its mission. Paradoxically, the organization set up to issue statements on ethics at the highest level is not involved in the legal process. But its actual influence on law-making is inversely proportional to its formal role in drafting legal rules.

In the following we will venture to characterize the competing legitimacy on which ethics and the law are based by taking a look at the role filled by the *Comité consultatif national d'éthique*, and incidentally also by the Committees for the Protection of People, and we will attempt to trace some paths in which these competing roles have affected ethics and law.

The following description takes a look at the legitimating foundations of ethics and law, describing the role of the *Comités de protection des personnes* and, above all, the Comité consultatif national d'éthique.

The "Guidelines" of Ethics or Legitimacy through the "Experts"

The making of an ethical "norm" observes principles that bring out its specificity. Ethics can only be expressed under certain conditions. In fact, the ethical norm is only legitimate when drafted by "experts" - who are recognized as such - according to a procedure that is based on a consensus. This concept is not neutral; instead, it aims at defining a value system that is free both of the constraints of pre-existing moral standards and of the majority vote decision process inherent to the field of politics (1). Usually deprived of any legal value, the ethical "norm" thus created is incapable of developing a legal character of its own (2).

The Procedure at the Core of Ethics

Ethical reasoning observes its own set of rules. These rules have, by the way, been defined by the ethics committees themselves and are a result of the phenomenon of "committification" described above. Thus, the system produces not only its own norms, but also its own legitimacy. Basically, these rules depend, on the one hand, on the structure of the ethics committees and, on the other hand, on the pursuit of consensus as the only legitimate decision-making process.

Fundamental rules regarding the structure of ethics committees The three commonly acknowledged fundamental principles for legitimating an ethics committee are independence, multidisciplinarity, and pluralism.

The committee autonomy is based on a fundamental text that has no legal basis, namely the Declaration of Helsinki of 1964. The autonomy of the Committees for the Protection of People, that were established by the law of 1988 (Article L 209-11 of the French Public Health Code), is expressly affirmed in this constituent document. Thus, these committees are supposed to carry out their mission in full autonomy. Public support can be retracted if they do not meet the requirements for autonomy. This autonomy is not expressly stated in the texts regarding the *Comité consultatif national d'éthique*. This is perhaps because said autonomy is taken for granted and it is of less benefit to protect it than that of the organizations responsible for judging research protocols as these organizations must be autonomous, especially with respect to project sponsors and investigators. Autonomy in terms of political power is not threatened as such by the political arrangement for nominating members. Rather, on the one hand, the French constitutional court judge, for example, is nominated by political authorities, and his autonomy is not questioned; on the other hand, it would be difficult to find a more legitimate form of nomination for these positions, especially since these committees should also be autonomous in terms of medical and scientific "power". This type of autonomy is conceivably the one that is the most difficult to accomplish. The logic of the "knowledgeable one", who is both wise and competent, presupposes that every committee member will give precedence to the ways of wisdom over the sweet talk of science. If the caliber and the success of the *Comité national d'éthique français* may raise hopes that this often is the case, it would be nonetheless unrealistic to be too optimistic at this early stage: Only the multidisciplinarity of the committees can guarantee their autonomy.

Multidisciplinarity is thus the second major principle underlying the organization of ethics committees. Yet often this multidisciplinarity is just an illusion and in reality most ethics committees, especially those in Europe, abound with representatives from the medical community and the biomedical sciences.[28] In France, more than 60% of the members of the CCNE are from the medical and scientific worlds and less than 10% are from the legal community.[29] Article L 209-11 of the French Public Health Code states that members of the CCPPRB must reflect the full spectrum of competence in the biomedical field regarding ethical, social, psychological, or legal issues. Yet, the decree of September 27, 1990 does not provide for more than one jurist. Even though it is perfectly justified to have a predominance of practitioners and scientists in committees assigned to assessing research projects or clinical practices from a technical point of view, this disproportion is less tolerable when it comes to determining reference standards. The distrust, specifically toward jurists, may reflect a rejection of the traditional normative system, and a desire to cut off science and medicine from the view of others. In defining ethics, scientific logic most certainly surpasses legal logic. However, despite its shortcomings, multidisciplinarity is most likely the most prolific principle underlying these ethics committees.

The third principle, pluralism, governs the structure of both the CCNE, in which five members of the philosophical and religious mainstream must be represented, and the CCPPRB, to which, after consulting with the representatives of different schools of thought, four individuals are appointed. Here we see in a sense how certain currents of thought as sources of morality, in the traditional sense of the term, play a role within the framework of defining ethical "norms". This pluralism is absolutely necessary in response to the notion that ethics emanates from many sources. However, these representatives from the major streams of thought do not have a very comfortable position within ethics committees. Since they, by definition, are there to defend a doctrine, they must make concessions in order to draft norms established by a consensus.

These principles are crucial for the existence of ethics committees and constitute as such their seal of approval by the authorities whom they will later advise. In turn, nothing prohibits, for example, certain schools of thought from formulating their own rules of ethics based on recommendations from committees that are not governed by pluralism.

It should be noted, lastly, that in France, unlike countries such as Denmark, the general public is not represented in these committees of ethics. The presence of the "common element" within ethics committees could be a ploy: how should these individuals be chosen and appointed, in what context, and by whom? People living in a democracy must speak out. Those who speak out, however, cannot be chosen at random. Yet it is the very task of ethics committees to inform and educate the public.

The principle of consensus The decision-making process at the ethics committee level is a response to certain requests that are not directly seated in the field of law yet are at the very heart of the notion of ethics. Contrary to morals or law, ethics is not decided upon by authority; instead, it is the product of a consensus.

This process is common to all ethics committees, especially in Europe. It is designed to determine, outside any rigidly fixed normative system, what is ethically acceptable and what isn't. The opinions expressed by the "experts" are compared with each other and discussed so as to reach an ethical consensus produced by expert knowledge and circumspection.[30] The legitimacy of a recommendation by these experts can be assessed as a function of the degree of consensus reached. Such a recommendation is "the fruit of patient, meditative work with a view to reaching a precarious and fragile equilibrium between conflicting values and interests".[31]

With regard to this point, the approach in bioethics constitutes a challenge to the democratic principle of majority rule.[32] In a democracy, discussion and reaching a consensus may contribute to the drafting of rules.

However, majority opinion will always affect a decision, even in the absence of a consensus. From its beginnings, bioethics has exhibited a genuine distrust of the traditional democratic system. The Nuremberg Code was the attempt to make fundamental principles prevail over a perverted system under which a democracy had collapsed in the process of even nurturing it to some extent.

The notion of supraconstitutionality, which is highly contestable from the democratic standpoint,[33] is based on a similar concept. The constitutional court judge presides over the people. An assembly of "sages" delimits the people's sphere of intervention according to principles that it considers inviolable. German constitutional law is especially explicit on this subject. In addition, the existence of independent administrative authorities are proof of this need for an out-of-court, regulatory power whose decisions are accepted as the outcome of a consensus.[34]

Yet, the constitutional court is still a legal authority whose rulings are based on preexisting reference norms. And, some of the independent administrative authorities mentioned have a delegated regulatory power which is limited and subject to compliance with superior laws and to control by the administrative arm of justice. The situation is altogether different for ethics committees. The ethics committee freely produces its own norms according to its own legitimation, independently of the democratic process.

The approach of the ethics committees is typical for this new decision-making process which does, however, pose certain risks. First, the availability of sufficient information may enable us to assess a problem correctly, but it does not provide any set of values with which to solve it.[35] Second, it must not be overlooked that some of the expert's reports presented as the consolidated opinion of the foremost "sages" of a community are none other than the lowest common denominator of their respective opinions.[36]

This system professes to be a competitor of the democratic one to the effect that its legitimacy for establishing reference values is superior to that of the democratic system. Here, we are again confronted with the old debate about natural law and positive law.[37] However, the issue in question is not quite the same one. While natural law is based on a coherent, preexisting normative system, bioethical norms have established a system of reference under the hallmark of negotiation, diversity, and a consensus of opinion. Ethical norms do not have legal authority with the force of law, nor do they have the permanence of moral imperatives. On the contrary, ethical norms are relative, constantly changing and subject to discussion. The situation-dependent nature of ethical rules is exacerbated by the fact that questioning a principle by a certain practice tends to further the evolution of the principle and not to transform the practice.[38] The relativism of the ethical norm relies in part on the preconceived notion that science has about man. Ethics, therefore, has the chore of subjecting this notion to closer scrutiny and imposing limits upon it.

However, this pessimistic and critical view of bioethics must be brought into the proper perspective. To begin with, in a society in which everything is relative and there is little compliance with authority or where reference systems have deteriorated, the ethical approach still remains the lesser evil provided that it seeks to safeguard the values upon which said society is based. On the other hand, bioethics professes to lay the foundation for a set of values. Herein lies the actual reason for its existence. Though the manner in which these bioethical norms are elaborated as well as their great variability may be subject to debate, their existence is still invaluable as they can be used in conflicts with scientists without their legitimacy being challenged. This system of values gives absolute priority to the human being and the respect of his dignity. However, such incontestable principles, rightly deemed as being absolute, are subject to major misinterpretations and are relativized depending on how they are used. The human being is not defined as such; challenging certain rules derived from the principle of dignity can in turn attack this very principle.[39] Responsibility in this situation does not, however, rest entirely on the shoulders of the ethics committees: the law has not proven to have been more effective in this area, either.[40]

The Shortcomings of the Ethical "Norm"

Being born of a different logic and a different legitimacy than a legal norm, the ethical "norm" is capable of influencing the law. Below we will see that the intervention of democratically legitimated organizations is usually necessary for transforming the ethical "norm" into a law. In the majority of cases, the ethical "norm" cannot attain the force of law on its own. This is because ethical principles or expert opinions are weak in terms of normative status and have only a limited validity. Moreover, the legal responsibility of the ethics committees has not been clearly defined.

Weak normative status and limited validity The ethics elaborated by the committees, though understood in terms of recommendations or suggestions, is not normative in nature. The expert opinions concerning research projects or clinical practices enter the decision-making process and culminate in an individual decision;[41] however, neither the jurisprudence that may be formulated on the basis of these expert opinions nor the recommendations of the CCNE are normative. Both only have a moral authoritativeness. Thus, the violation of a deontological provision that had not been approved by the authorities in the first place will not lead to disciplinary action.[42] This holds all the more for the expert opinions or statements made by an ethics committee. Since they cannot be contested, they are not subject to litigation. Though not legally binding in terms of legal norms, these recommendations nonetheless do have a definite influence on the conduct of scientists and practitioners. A misconstrued understanding of their legal bearing or uncertainties ensuing from their at times vaguely formulated contents may cause some legal uncertainty. Thus, an ethics expertise that runs contrary to a law or even a legal regulation in no way relieves anyone of their civil or penal liability. However, the wording of some expert opinions makes them seem like legal rulings, especially when they have been formulated in the imperative mode or a peremptory tone.[43]

While the validity of deontological codes is limited to the professional *per se*, ethics codes stipulate rules concerning scientists and medical practitioners, in general, again without the force of law. Subjects who claim to be the victims of malpractice or of medical experimentation cannot, as with deontological rules, implement these ethics principles against doctors. On the other hand, ethics principles are not compelling for those receiving care or participating in research projects. This is why informed consent of the individual is so important.[44]

The unsettled question of the liability of ethics committees Ethics committees are endowed with a weighty moral responsibility.[45] However, the question whether they are subject to civil and even penal responsibilities has not been precisely clarified. It is likely to undergo major developments. We will only take a brief look at it here.

An ethics committee can be called to account only to the extent that it has a legal status. Thus, the liability of the committees set up in public hospitals only covers the hospital departments, which are legal entities of their own. Otherwise, it would only be possible to fall back on the liability of one of its members. But this would mean the elimination of a number of obstacles (e.g., the question of causality regarding the damages suffered by the conduct of one of the committee members). On the other hand, in my opinion, the liability of an ethics committee can certainly be established if said committee is a legal entity and if its expert opinions are subject to dispute.[46] Such is the case with regard to the CCPPRB, especially when a negative statement delays a research project.[47] In this context, the jurisprudence of the *Conseil d'État* has opened new perspectives toward determining responsibility in France's "contaminated blood" affair. The *Conseil d'État*[48] believes that the Government can be held liable on the grounds of negligence in supervising blood banks while the Government concurrently could start a lawsuit against the blood banks.

The Validation of Ethical Guidelines by the Law or Democratic Legitimacy

Normative competence at the government level is determined by the constitution. No organization can proclaim universally applicable rules without being directly or indirectly authorized by the constitution to do so. In keeping with the Constitution, the people are vested with sovereign power and may exercise it directly or indirectly via representatives.[49] More precisely, Article 3 of the Declaration of Human Rights and the Rights of Citizens of 1789 proclaims that "the principle of all sovereignty resides essentially in the nation; no association, no individual may exercise authority that does not expressly emanate therefrom".

Ethics directly involves fundamental liberties and rights; it does so on the basis of constitutional norms. It also concerns fundamental civil rights, especially those rights regarding the status of the individual which, pursuant to Article 34 C, fall under the domain of the legislators. Regulatory competence is, theoretically speaking, a by-product pertaining to provisions of a technical nature.[50] After all, the courts are responsible for interpreting the law[51] and, in so doing, are expected to fill any "legal voids".[52,53]

Thus, in principle ethics committees do not have any normative competence. The intervention of organizations, that are constitutionally entrusted with ruling on the law, is indispensable for conferring legal status upon an ethical "norm". Thus, this form of democratic legitimacy is at the basis of the ethical rule. Although legitimacy through the "experts" may lend weight to the ethical "norm," only democratic legitimacy can transform such a "norm" into a legal norm. The intervention of organizations authorized to rule on laws is not a pure formality by virtue of which the ethical "norm" automatically turns into a legal norm.

The linkage of an ethical "norm" and of positive law can operate in several ways. First, and within a context without legal status, the expert opinions written by ethics committees may influence the authorities commissioned to formulate legal texts. The authorities may also entrust, along formal legal lines, ethics committees or professional organizations with contributing to the formulation of legal texts. Finally, these professional organizations and ethics committees can, under certain conditions and within certain confines, be entrusted with the power to enact legal texts. In this case, even though this conferral of power can be justified by legitimation by the "experts", the binding quality of the thus enacted ruling is, after all, based on democratic legitimation.

This interaction between ethics and the law affects all of positive law. It makes itself known in one or the other form mentioned schematically, both in jurisprudence and in provisions and laws.

Ethical "Norms" and the Judiciary: An Influential Power

The influence of ethical "norms" on jurisprudence can be measured indirectly by whether a judge rules in favor of a solution advocated by an ethics committee or not. Such ethical "norms" exert a more direct influence when a judge formalizes an ethical "norm" so that it becomes a standard or general legal principle.

The influence that an expert's opinion by an ethics committee has on jurisprudence seems to be particularly significant. This question was emphasized in the parliamentary debates that took place before the 1988 bill was passed.[54] Ethical and deontological stipulations can also be of assistance in guiding judges in their decisions on matters of medical responsibility. Hearing ethics committees members may also further influence. As the former CCNE president, Professor Jean Bernard, stated: "The judges often consulted us, and we, as it were, clarified questions pertaining to jurisprudence through our work".[55] Thus, in an unprecedented plenary session the French Supreme Court of Appeal (*Cour de Cassation*) heard the President of the *Comité national d'éthique* as an *amicus curiae* on the so-called "surrogate mother" affair.[56] Yet, the judge sometimes does keep his decision-making autonomy in the face of the expert opinions of the ethics committees. This was, for example, the case when a judge gave preference to the opinion of a local ethics committee, that had no legal status, over the CCNE's opinion concerning the implantation of embryos following the death of the mother.[57] In a case involving non-implanted embryos, a constitutional judge did not adhere to the opinion maintained by the CCNE that human embryos are potential individuals.[58]

The ethical "norm" can become a rule of positive law in terms of jurisprudence when a judge uses it as a standard or general principle of law. Such was the case when the *Conseil d'État*[59] upheld that the respect for human beings even continues after death and that this constituted such a principle. Recognition of this principle was clearly inspired by the CCNE.[60]

Incorporating the Ethics Expertise in the Decision-making Process

Legally, the expert opinions of the ethics committees can enter the law by way of the process of enacting regulatory legal norms. Thus, some expert opinions of ethics committees constitute an integral element of the advisory process. Some ethical or deontological provisions can be ratified by the regulatory authority, thereby acquiring regulatory significance. Finally, under certain conditions, the Constitution allows for certain organizations to be granted regulatory power, such could be the case with ethics committees.

While committees like the CCNE, whose role is to provide expert opinions and general recommendations, do not enter into the administrative decision-making process, this is not the case for a certain number of committees set up to regulate medical and scientific practices and which are legally established by competent authorities. These commissions may be granted the power to formulate supporting, compulsory or optional expert opinions. In principle, the expert opinion is not open to legal action; it does not constitute an administrative decision, nor is it subject to appeal. However, in some cases, an appeal may be lodged against an administrative decision that has been made in accordance with an expert opinion.[61] Moreover, if an expert opinion restricts the decision-making power of the administrative authority or produces its own effects, the expert opinion may itself be deemed an administrative decision.[62] Such could be the case with the opinion of the CCPPRB, which prohibits the use of a research protocol for a certain time,[63] or the expert opinion of the national commission of medicine and biology and prenatal diagnostics[64] concerning research on human embryos. In any case that principally concerns decisions which the Constitution solely reserves for the laws, the legislator has the competence to oblige the regulatory agencies to carry out an advisory procedure.[65]

It is possible to imagine, though the case in point does not occur in positive law, other complexities involving ethical "norms" and regulatory decisions. Thus, just as the deontological code, drawn up and revised by the *Conseil national de l'ordre des médecins*, is ratified by the regulatory authorities in the form of decrees, it is conceivable, provided that the provisions in question stem from the regulatory domain, that if the CCNE, for example, were to draft an ethics charter, said charter could become legally binding by way of ratification through the regulatory authorities under common law. The Government could, as with the deontological code, be committed to the contents of the proposed project but would have the possibility of refusing to endorse it.

It is also imaginable that regulatory power bestowed on an organization like the CCNE. In fact, the *Conseil d'Etat* feels that "the constitutional provisions do not prevent the legislator from conferring the task of establishing the norms for implementing a law to a public authority other than the Prime Minister, provided that this would only involve measures of a limited scope, both in terms of their applicability and content".[66] This legal authorization may especially involve independent administrative authorities,[67] or, by way of conventions,[68] the social partners (doctors or social security administrations). The specific features of an ethics committee are apparently no obstacle to such a legislative authorization.

Ethical "Norms" and the Law

It may be reasonable to assume that the basic principles of biomedical ethics are embodied in the Constitution.[69] However, most countries (except Switzerland) have at best relied on their legislators to establish these principles. France has quite a comprehensive set of laws of this type. The legislator has intervened in a number of issues raised by the CCNE. This committee's influence on the content of laws is not negligible. However, there is an influence of ethics on law, more contestable perhaps and which consists in the legislator being guided by methods specific to ethics when drafting laws. The outcome is not always satisfying.

The influence of the ethical "norm" on the contents of the law As President Braibant put it, "one of the purposes of a law can be to consolidate and generalize already extant principles that, for example, have been laid down by the CCNE".[70] The influence of ethical norms on the law can be seen in that the committees call upon the legislators as well as in the fact that legislators orient themselves around the expert statements of the ethics committees. Thus, the CCNE began to draw the attention of the legislative body, starting with its first expert's report in 1983.[71] In its recommendation of July 18, 1990 pertaining to the organization of gamete banks, the same committee stated that "the result can only be reached by the indispensable and compelling support of legislative provisions".

Although the legislator admits being motivated for the most part by the statements of ethics committees, some members of parliament are voicing their objections to the fact that the laws are being made outside the legislative setting.[72] As Professor J. F. Mattéi put it, "the legislation that we are about to pass rests, in many respects and *a posteriori*, on the recommendations and expert's opinions handed down to us over the past ten years by the *Comité consultatif national d'éthique*".[73]

It would be going too far, however, to see in the law a mere replica of the expert opinions of ethics committees. For instance, the laws of July 1994, also known as "bioethics laws", were drafted some ten years after the first CCNE expert's reports and were the subject of a parliamentary debate that lasted ten years under two different parliamentary majorities. These laws were preceded by five excellent reports[74] stemming either from the parliament or ordered by the executive body yet in no way constituting a synthesis of the expert's reports of the ethics committees. The legislative body, on the other hand, disregarded some of the CCNE's expert's reports. As a result, the law of December 20, 1988 departs from the CCNE's expert reports concerning tests of new treatment methods for humans and regarding local ethics committees.[75] Also, in 1994 the legislators disregarded the solution advocated by the CCNE with regard to the implantation of embryos after the death of the biological father.[76]

The law "contaminated" by ethical "norms" Even if it were to be assumed that in the debates prior to enacting a law, the discussion, the free exchange of ideas, and the pursuit of a consensus would dominate over the decision of an authority that must choose from among several solutions while being committed to a fixed reference system, the role of the law is a far different one. As President of the National Assembly P. Seguin put it, "Laws must be enacted that provide solutions to bioethical issues and these solutions must be as precise as possible for, according to the famous words of Portalis, 'The law permits, commands, and prohibits' [La loi permet, ordonne, interdit]".[77] Even if the author of these lines may agree with this analysis, he does not seem to believe that it fully mirrors reality. The law is also affected by the general crisis of authority.[78] This is not the place to reflect on the reasons why coercive rules are less easily accepted today than before. In any event, counsel tends to take the place of orders, negotiations replace authority, and arguments supplant constraint. The freedom of the individual has not necessarily gained from all of this, yet society's grip on the individual's private and family life, on private conduct, does seem to have grown.[79]

The law thus becomes a text that can be discarded in accordance with the will of developments brought about through scientific knowledge. This is the result of a precarious compromise. Aside from the fact that legal security is not really taken account of here, principles solemnly asserted as absolute are relativized in practice. Some of these principles are, incidentally, shaky in their scope and tenure. For instance, this is the case for the principle of the dignity of the human being.[80] The constitutional judge himself admits this frailty of the legal norm and adapts his control accordingly. For bioethical laws, he believes that control is assured in keeping with the state of research and technology and that the rulings are not definitive.[81] This statement recognizes that the law adapts itself constantly to the status of science and technology even when it ought to serve as a frame by enacting certain principles.

Conclusion

More than any other phenomenon, ethics committees reveal that there is a problem involving legitimacy. The ethics model becomes the dominant model of social regulation. It has almost become a banality to say that the representative system, a corollary of contemporary democracy, is in a crisis. This crisis of legitimacy arises in a context where the problems, especially those linked to the future of man and our understanding of the human being, necessitate, now more than ever, a reference system of values. The crucial question is, thus, to determine who, i.e., which organization, is capable of defining these values. In the field of morals, both churches and political ideologies have lost their monopoly as authorities. A new system of the oligarchic type now aims at defining a new type of legitimacy based on using consensus as a method and human rights as a reference system. The reference system, though uncertain and evolving, has the merit of existing. It is a system, perhaps transitory, in which political legitimacy, itself crumbling, is necessary in order to guarantee those rules coming from elsewhere. The fact remains that the assimilation of ethical legitimacy into a renewed form of democratic legitimacy is still a myth.

Notes

1   P Jestaz, *Pouvoir juridique et pouvoir moral*, RTD civ., 1988, p. 625 ff.

2   Cf. G. Mémeteau, *les régles éthiques*, R.I.D.C., Journ. interal. drt. comp., Vol. 14, 1992, p. 343.

3   Cf. M.H. Douchez, *la déontologie médicale*, in: Hecquard-Théron, *Déontologie et droit*, Presses I.E.P. de Toulouse, 1994.

4   With regard to these classifications, cf. G. Mémeteau, *les régles éthiques*, idem.

5   Cf. C. Byck, G. Mémeteau, *le droit des comités d'éthique*, ed. Lacassagne et Eska, 1996.

6   Cf. esp. A. Rogers, D. Durand de Bousingen, *une bioéthique pour l'Europe*, Editions du Conseil de l'Europe, 1995.

7   The international committee of bioethics which is preparing a project for a Declaration on the Protection of the Human Genome.

8   Nonetheless, if these international conventions are subject to ratification by each country, said ratification provides a legal foundation for these decisions in terms of internal law.

9   Cf. the exhaustive list of international texts of ethics drawn up by the WHO. My thanks to Mr. Sev Fluss, WHO Geneva, for this information.

10   Cf. N. Lenoir's report, *Aux frontières de la vie*, Doc. Franç. p. 307.

11   Cf. G. Mémeteau, idem.

12   Cf. C. Byck, G. Mémeteau, *le droit des comités d'éthique*, idem, p. 189.

13   Cf. ibid., p. 190 ff.

14   Cf. *décis*. 71-4 DC, RIDC-I-24 and *décis*. 94-345 DC, B. Mathieu and M. Verpeaux, resp.; *Chron. juris. constit., Les Petites Affiches*, 1994, No. 125, p. 7.

15   With regard to this question, cf. *Déontologie médicale*, in: *Dictionnaire permanent bioéthique et biotechnologies, éd. législatives*.

16   Barry, R. 368.

17   CE *Ass. syndicale des médecins*, February 14, 1969.

18   Cf. C. Maugüe, *conclus; sur CE collectif nal*. Kine-France, December 20, 1995, AJDA, 1996-139.

19   Cf., for example, CE May 13, 1987, D 1989, SC, p. 65; footnote, Chelle and Prétôt.

20   CE October 25, 1974, Valton, DA 1974, No. 414.

21   *décis* 89-369 DC, R.I.D.C., I-392

22   Cf., for example, *cass civ*, May 4, 1982, D. 1993, IR, p. 378 and *cass civ*; 1, November 5, 1991, *bull civ* I, 297

23   Cf. CA Paris, March 13, 1996, S.A ed. Plon c. Consorts Mitterand. The Court feels that the petitioners have an interest in acting to stop a clearly illicit disturbance resulting from a breach of professional confidentiality, the latter being embodied in the law and solemnly professed by every doctor by reading aloud the Hippocratic Oath upon entering the profession.

24   *décret* 95-1000 on the medical code of deontology, J.O., September 8, 1995, p. 13305, with regard to this text, cf. L. Boulouis, *le nouveau code de déontologie des médecins*, R.T.D.S.S., 1995, p. 725.

25   *décis*. 94-343-344 DC, cf. B. Mathieu, R.F.D.A., 1994, p.

26   With regard to these committees, cf. Y. Gaudemet, *les CCPPRM*, J.C.P., 1993, ed. G, I-3653 and A. Langlois, J.I.B., 1995, No. 1, p. 61.

27   Cf. N. Lenoir's report, *aux frontières de la vie*, idem.

28   Cf. Conseil de l'Europe, *les instances nationales d'éthique*, Editions du Conseil de l'Europe, 1993.

29   Cf. the list of the 41 members of the CCNE, J.I.B., 1994, Vol. 5, No. 2-127.

30   Cf. S. Hubac and E. Pisier , in: *les A.A.I*, sd C.A. Colliard and G. Timsit.

31   C. Byck and G Mémeteau, idem, p.33.

32   Cf., in this context, N. Lenoir's relevant remarks, in: Diogène, 1995.

33   Cf. B. Mathieu, *la supra constitutionnalité existe-t-elle? Les Petites Affiches*, p.

34   Cf. H. Maisl, in: C.A. Colliard and G. Timsit, *les Authorités administratives indépendantes*, idem.

35   Cf. R.Thomas, *Bioéthique et démocratie*, J.I.B., 1994-511.

36   Cf., in this context G.Mémenteau, *recherches irrévérencieuses sur l'autorité juridique des avis des comités d'éthique*, R.R.J., 1989-159.

37   Cf., with regard to this subject, A.Sériaux, *le droit naturel*, Q.S.J. , P.U.F., 199.

38   Cf. C. Ambroselli, *le Comité d'éthique*, Q.S.J., P.U.F., 199.

39   Cf. our study, *la dignité de la personne humaine, quel droit, quel titulaire?*, D. *Chron.*, 1996 (in press).

40   Cf. infra III-3.

41   Cf. infra III-2.

42   Cf. Cass 10, January 1995, cf. C. Rozet, *la déontologie notariale, Les Petites Affiches*, 1996, No. 46, p. 25.

43   C. Byck and G. Mémeteau, idem.

44   Cf. D. Thouvenin, *éthique et droit en matière?*, D. 1985, C., p. 21.

45   In speaking of this responsibility, President Mitterand stated in his address to the CCNE on December 2, 1983 that it is shared by the State and the researchers.

46   With regard to this notion, see infra III-2.

47   In this case, responsibility would have to be exercised in keeping with the jurisdiction of the judiciary pursuant to Article L209-22 of the Public Health Code.

48   CE April 9, 1993, D. 1993, J. 312, *conclus. Légal.*

49   Article 3 of the Constitution.

50   Cf. CE July 21, 1989, R. 163. Nevertheless, due care must be exercised as, in this context, the techniques are difficult to distinguish from the principles that they may question.

51   Thus, according to the *Conseil constitutionnel* (*décis.* 77-83 DC), the *Cour de cassation* (French Supreme Court of Appeal) is commissioned with the task of providing a conclusive interpretation of the law. Cf. B. Mathieu, *droit constitutionnel civil, juris. class. adm. fasc.* 1449, No. 24 ff.

52   Cf. A.Sériaux, *question controversée: la théorie du non droit*, R.R.J., 1995-1-13.

53   Article 4 of the [French] Civil Code states that "the judge who refuses to make a ruling under the pretext of the elusiveness, the obscurity, or the insufficiency of the law, may be found guilty of a denial of justice."

54   Cf. Senator Sérusclat, *débats Sénat*, J.O., October 13, 1988, p. 543.

55   Cf. N. Lenoir's report, idem, Vol. 2.

56   Ruling of May 31, 1991, *conclus.* Y. Chartier; footnote D. Thouvenin, D. 1991, J. 417.

57   T.G.I. Angers, December 10, 1992, obs. by X. Labbée, D 1994, S.C., p.30.

58   *Décis.* 94-343-344 DC; footnotes B. Mathieu, idem.

59   CE Milhaud, July 2, 1993, R. 194, *conclus.* Kessler.

60   Session of November 7, 1988, quoted by the government's representative in his conclusions about the judgment.

61   Regarding this notion of preparatory measures, cf. R. Chapus, *droit du contentieux administratif*, Montchrestien No. 514

62   Cf. CE January 31, 1991 Rovoola cf. R Chapus, *droit administratif général*, T.1, No. 1128.

63   Cf. in this context Y. Gaudement, *les CCPPRB*, J.CP. 1993 ed. G, 3653.

64   Cf. Art. L 184-3 of the Public Health Code, cf., similarly, the judgment of May 6, 1995.

65   Cf. *décis.* CC 73-76 DC and, with regard to the National Commission of Medicine and Biology and Prenatal Diagnostics, *décis.* 94-343-344 DC, idem.

66   *Décis.* 89-260 DC, R.J.C. I.-.

67   Cf. , for example, decis. 91-304 DC R.J.C. I.-.

68   Cf. *décis.* 89-269 DC, footnote B. Genevois, R.F.D.A., 1990, p 405.

69   Cf. in this context our study, *la difficile appréhension de la bioéthique par le droit constitutionnel, Les Petites Affiches*, 1993, No. 70, p. 4.
70   *Pour une grande loi, Pouvoirs*, 1991, No. 56, p. 109.
71   *Rapport* 1984, *La Documentation Française*, 1985.
72   Cf. in this context F. Sérusclat.
73   Cf. *débats*, A.N., J.O 26 November 1992.
74   Listed according to author: *rapport* G. Braibant in 1988, *rapport* N.Lenoir in 1990, *rapports parlementaires* F. Sérusclat and B. Bioulac in 1992 and *rapport* J.F. Mattei in 1994.
75   Expert opinion of October 9, 1984 and November 7, 1988.
76   Cf. expert opinion 40, J.I.B., 1995, No. 1, 61, also cf. J.Massip, *obs. sous Cass. civ.* 1, January 9, 1996, *Les Petites Affiches*, 1996, No. 41, p. 11.
77   Speech before the 3rd session of the I.B.C. (International Bioethics Committee) of UNESCO, December 1995.
78   With regard to this question, cf. C. Ambroselli, *le Comité d'éthique*, idem, p. 21 and esp. the quotations of H. Arendt.
79   Cf. B.Mathieu, *La loi*, Dalloz, 1996, esp. p. 98 ff.
80   With regard to this principle cf. esp. B. Mathieu, *La dignité de la personne humaine, quel droit?, quel titulaire*, recueil Dalloz, *chron.*, 1996 (in press).
81   *Décis.* 93-343-344 DC idem.

14 The Interrelationship between Ethical Codes and the Law: "Legitimacy" Seen from the British Point of View

Paul Honigman

What is meant by "Legitimacy". The author has decided, like Humpty Dumpty[1] to make the word mean what he chooses it to mean. In the context of the overall theme "Reflections on Nuremberg and the Role of Ethical Codes in Law and Medicine" and the context of the subtitle "The interrelationship between codes and the Law" it is assumed that the purpose of a paper on "Legitimacy" is to consider the extent to which medical ethics, that is to say good and bad ethical practice in medicine, can and should be given the full force and effect of the law of the state, or of a larger grouping such as Europe or of a worldwide international grouping such as the United Nations.

It is self evident that the detailed approach to medical ethics will vary from country to country, with important regional variations. Politics, economic circumstances and social mores are bound to affect doctors who are not immune to societies in which they reside and practice. Nevertheless, medicine, like illness, is not contained by national frontiers. Problems of medical ethics in one country are likely to be common to the world community of medical practitioners. Therefore, in the short space available, it is proposed to concentrate on the law relating to medical ethics in the United Kingdom which happens to be the authors principal sphere of work.

For medical ethics to be effective, they must be incorporated either directly or indirectly in the law of the land, at least in a democratic society. "Indirectly" means that the state may delegate to a subsidiary body the responsibility for ensuring that ethical standards are maintained and enforced. Medical ethics which are divorced from the law of the land are likely to be merely academic and lacking in effectiveness. This does not mean that there can never be occasions when in moral and idealistic terms it is the duty of the medical practitioner to uphold abstract principles of medical ethics even if the law of the land dictates otherwise. The whole purpose of the Freiburg Project is to commemorate work which was started at Nuremberg almost 50 years ago. However, it is submitted that in general terms "the Law" and medical ethics should go hand in hand.

What is meant by "the Law" in this context? Broadly speaking it means that the law of the land impinges on medical ethics in a least three different ways, namely the criminal law, the civil law and the license to practice medicine as a profession. First, it is obvious that a doctor who behaves unethically may thereby be committing criminal offenses, for example a doctor who indecently assaults a patient or steals a patient's money in the course of a medical consultation. However, medical ethics and the criminal law can change. Until 1967 in the United Kingdom, it was for almost all purposes a criminal offense for a doctor to carry out a termination of pregnancy and any doctor who did so was likely to find himself not only imprisoned by the state for performing an illegal abortion, but also erased from the Medical Register. After the passing of the Abortion Act 1967[2] it became possible to terminate pregnancy, strictly speaking under various controls but in effect virtually upon demand and this also became ethically acceptable except for those doctors who for reasons of religion and conscience do not wish to engage in the practice of abortion.

Again, so far as civil law is concerned, a doctor behaves unethically if he fails to carry out a thorough examination of a patient and thereby misses critical medical conditions which cause damage to the patient's health. Such a doctor is likely to be sued for damages in the civil courts of the land by the patient or the patient's family, and the doctor is also likely to be find himself in trouble with his medical licensing body.

Third, the law impinges on medical ethics in the realm of the license to practice. Certainly so far as the United Kingdom is concerned, and also probably in many other countries, the doctor who offends against the established medical ethical code of the country concerned is likely to lose his license to practice, or to have that license severely curtailed. Without the license to practice the extent to which a doctor can practice medicine without breaking the law is likely to be severely limited if not completely nullified.

This brings me conveniently to the role of the General Medical Council in the United Kingdom (in this paper called "the GMC"). The GMC has been the governing body regulating the medical profession in the United Kingdom since 1858 when it was decided by Parliament that the medical profession should be a self regulating profession. The governing statute is now the Medical Act 1983.[3] This is not the time or place to describe in detail the workings of the GMC but one of its principal functions is to consider whether a person who is a registered medical practitioner and therefore licensed to practice should have his or her registration curtailed in some way. It is interesting, that until 1978, once a doctor had been registered with the General Medical Council his name could only be removed from the Register, other than by death, if either the doctor had committed a serious criminal offense which was regarded as having some relevance to medical practice or if the doctor had committed serious professional misconduct. Only in 1978 did Parliament give power to the GMC to suspend or impose conditions on the registration of a doctor whose fitness to practice was seriously impaired on health grounds and only by the *Medical (Professional Performance) Act* 1995[4] has Parliament given the GMC power to introduce similar procedure for doctors whose professional performance is seriously deficient. In other words for most of its existence since 1858 the GMC's jurisdiction to prevent a doctor from practicing has been on the grounds of a serious beach of medical ethics.

It can be seen, therefore, that serious professional misconduct is the practical and legal basis for the enforcement of medical ethics under English law. In Germany this enforcement role is carried out by the Landesärztekammer and in France the license to practice is generally granted by the Prefecture of Police on a departmental basis rather than by the profession centrally as a self regulating profession. The GMC gives guidance to the profession both in the form of booklets describing the duties of a doctor and good medical practice[5] and in the form of literature and precedents backed by decided court cases describing the kind of misbehavior which may be regarded as serious professional misconduct.

So what is meant by this crucial expression "serious professional misconduct" ("SPM") or "infamous conduct in a professional respect" as it used to be known? The problem is that there is no satisfactory definition. Indeed, insofar as definition implies codification, and insofar as codification implies an element of rigidity it may be felt that legal definition is less important than a broadly acceptable concept which commands acceptance and respect in the context of the time. To quote an old adage it is impossible to define an elephant, but most people will recognize an elephant when they see one!

There have been many attempts to define SPM in the English courts. In *Allinson v The General Medical Council of Medical Education and Registration*[6] the Court of Appeal adopted the following definition: "If it is shown that a medical man, in the pursuit of his profession, has done something with regard to it which would be reasonably regarded as disgraceful or dishonorable by his professional brethren of good repute and competency, then it is open to the General Medical Council to sax that he has been guilty of infamous conduct in a professional respect".

In *Rex v General Medical Council*[7] Lord Justice Scrutton stated that "Infamous conduct in a professional respect means no more than serious misconduct judged according to the rules, written or unwritten governing the profession".

In *Doughty v The General Medical Council*[8] Lord Mackay of Clashfern delivering the judgment of the Board said: "...in their Lordships' view, what is now required is that the Council should establish conduct connected with his profession in which the dentist concerned has fallen short by omission or commission of the standards of conduct expected among dentists and that such falling short as is established should be serious".

It does not require close analysis of these decisions to recognize that what constitutes SPM is highly subjective; it means that SPM is behavior which is regarded as professionally reprehensible by a group of doctors and lay people sitting in judgment on a particular day and considering the facts of a particular case. However it may be felt that guidelines which provide a balance between on the one hand consistency of approach and on the other hand flexibility to adapt to changing circumstances may be the only way to maintain and enforce ethical standards which command a broad measure of acceptance.

It should be borne in mind that the importance of the enforcement of ethical standards in medicine (and particularly medical research) does not lie in the provision of interesting theoretical dilemmas to be resolved by academics. In the last resort such ethical standards are meaningless unless they exist to protect the public at large, and in particular those sections of the public who by reason of age, mental and physical incapacity, political persecution or many other factors are unable to protect themselves.

In this context it may be felt that the consideration of SPM should be approached from the other end. In other words the relevant question may be "Does the behavior /misbehavior of this doctor require that his license to practice should be withdrawn or restricted in order to protect the public?" If so, then it is serious professional misconduct. If not, then sanctions restricting the license to practice are not required.

Strictly speaking, it is not unlawful, in theory, for a person who is not a registered medical practitioner to work as a doctor in the United Kingdom, but in practice the medical work which an unregistered person may do is so severely restricted as to make it impossible. He or she may not describe themselves as being a physician or surgeon, may not work in the National Health Service which is still the employer of well over 90% of medical practitioners, may not prescribe controlled drugs or sign death certificates. Thus to be erased or suspended from the medical register for breach of medical ethics is a heavy penalty for any doctor.

Bearing in mind the historical background of the Freiburg Project, it may be appropriate to say a few words about ethical committees. Broadly speaking it is now very difficult if not impossible, for any meaningful research in the field of medicine and pharmacology to be carried out, and indeed funded in the United Kingdom unless a clear protocol for that research has been approved by an ethical committee. That is obviously a desirable safeguard in the public interest. In practice, it is surprising, however, to note the many different ways in which ethical committees are created. Some are appointed at a national level, others at a local level, for example by the teaching hospital under whose auspices the proposed research will take place. However, there are some private ethical committees which exist simply because a group of people have chosen to form themselves into such a committee. It may be felt that the use of such self created groups is open to abuse, and thus that their "Legitimacy" should either be under strict public control, or discontinued altogether.

Next, it is desirable to give some consideration as to how voluntary codes originate, how fields of medical ethics are identified and how the authors dealing with new fields of ethics are chosen.

Voluntary codes have originated, at any rate in the twentieth century, because medical practitioners operating in new fields of medical specialty see a need to define what is or is not ethically acceptable. This can happen both at the national and international level since medicine as previously suggested knows no frontiers. The following is an example from a case dealt with by the GMC in 1989 an 1990. About 20 years earlier surgeons had begun to perfect the techniques for successful kidney transplants. Until then the ethics of transplantation were largely irrelevant because the technology did not exist. Once kidney transplantation became possible questions arose as to the circumstances in which it would be ethical to transplant kidneys from a donor to a recipient. This was a matter which exercised both the British and no doubt other national transplantation societies and the International Transplantation Society a special interest group of surgeons and nephrologists who are specialists in that field. In 1989 a nephrologist and two surgeons who had been involved in the transplantation of kidneys between unrelated donors where large sums of money were changing hands, were brought before the GMC which had to consider whether this behavior was or was not serious professional misconduct. In reaching their decision as the governing body of the medical profession, the GMC took evidence from the British transplantation society as well as other bodies. All three medical practitioners were found guilty of serious professional misconduct and one of them was erased from the Medical Register. One can see, therefore, that what started as a voluntary code of conduct by interested specialists in a particular field acquired the legitimacy of the form of law because that code of conduct was adopted by the GMC which is vested by the law of the United Kingdom in regulating the medical profession.

Medicine is a profession with very rapid technological advances of which one of the most recent is in the field of the mapping of the human genome and genetic engineering. This has led to many groups becoming involved in trying to establish voluntary codes of good ethical conduct relating to advances in the genetic field. For example at the end of 1996 the Council of Europe gave approval to its own *Convention on Human Rights and Biomedicine*. It is anticipated that in 1997 the International Bar Association will submit to the United Nations the text of a draft treaty for the regulation of the human genome.

How are fields of ethics identified? It may be felt they are identified by special interest groups, such as the transplantations societies, who realize that new technologies generate new ethical dilemmas which have to be addressed. If the specialists themselves are unable or unwilling to address those issues and problems then sooner or later public opinion will become involved and that may lead to political action. For example at the height of the kidney transplantation furor a short statute was rushed through Parliament known as the *Human Organ Transplant Act* of 1989[9] which prohibited commercial dealings in human organs.

Who decides who will become involved in the preparation of voluntary codes of medical ethics? I believe that to a large extent people are self chosen. They express an interest or they see a need or they see the problems of new technology which cannot necessarily be covered by ethical codes which were sufficient for medicine in the past. The Hippocratic Oath simply cannot cope with the medical problems of the 20th and 21st Century and therefore persons come together to grapple with new dilemmas of medical ethics. The self chosen then bring in other specialists such as lawyers and representatives of patient organizations who are able to contribute their own specialist expertise to the ethical debate, on the basis that medical ethics are much too important to be left simply to doctors. For example HUGO, the Human Genome Organization, has held a series of workshops, funded by the European Community, to discuss the ethical implications of its own research.

It is, of course, possible for the state to initiate its own discussions on issues of medical ethics. In the United States this might be by way of special committees of Congress. In the United Kingdom, the Government might set up a Royal Commission, or Parliament might set up a so called Select Committee. However, it may be felt that progress is achieved when the specialist practitioners themselves see the need to debate new codes of conduct as new dilemmas emerge. It may be felt that it is right and proper that members of a caring profession should be the principal map makers when charting new territories of medical ethics.

[NB The references are principally to Statutes of the United Kingdom, or to United Kingdom Law Reports.]

Notes

1   "Alice Through The Looking Glass" by the Reverend Arthur Dodgson, more commonly known as Lewis Carroll.
2   The Abortion Act 1967, Chapter 87.
3   The Medical Act 1983, Chapter 54.
4   The Medical (Professional Performance) Act 1995, Chapter 51.
5   "Duties Of A Doctor - Guidance From The General Medical Council" published by the GMC and obtainable from 178 Great Portland Street, London W1N6JE.
6   1891 1 Queen's Bench Reports, Page 750.
7   1931 King's Bench Reports, Page 562 at Page 569.
8   Privy Council Appeal No 15 of 1987.
9   Human Organ Transplants Act 1989, Chapter 31.

15 The Genome Project: Legal and Ethical Thoughts for Coping with Problems to Come

Joel Levi and Markus Plantholz

One can hardly put the general conflict of interests in modern medicine in more poignant terms than this American judge, whose job it was to rule on the legality of a planned kidney transplant from a mentally retarded child to the child's loving father. Modern medical methods and the genome project in particular - once the human genome has been completely decoded - are already opening up new opportunities and, hence, new dimensions.

On the other hand, there is hope that in the future illnesses will be able to be identified even before the first symptoms are apparent, that risks for future generations will be made out, and that such illnesses will be able to be treated or prevented at such an early stage. But the new possibilities also nourish the old dream of a perfect and constantly healthy individual. Skeptics are likewise worried that people will be selected out according to their health, their ability to survive, or even their personality traits. We are not concerned here with the potential influence genetics could have on personalities. Rather, our attention is focused on the new dimensions and problems that are currently cropping up in the vehement conflict of interests mentioned above. A look at history - especially in this century - will shed much light on the issue for both medicine and law. The historical development will show to what extent fundamental ethical rules have been reconcilable with technological advances.

The first section will deal with the history of eugenics, especially in the Third Reich. This will be followed by a discussion of the consequences that were drawn from this history in the years after the war. Special emphasis will be given to the development of general legal guidelines as seen from the present. Finally, the applicability of these legal guidelines to present-day genetic research will be investigated, especially concerning the question of whether they are capable of protecting humanity from another situation analogous to the events in the Third Reich. The juridical view of history will also raise the central question of "informed consent" - the willing participation of a patient who understands the issues sufficiently.

Development of Eugenics up to 1945

Foundations up to 1933

This history of eugenics will concentrate on the events between 1933 and 1945. This period begins on 14 July 1933 with the law for the prevention of deliveries of infants with hereditary diseases and ends with the extermination of 6,000,000 Jews and 500,000 "Gypsies". However, contrary to what is sometimes assumed, the theoretical basis and its reworking as an ideology predate this period by far.[1]

The beginnings of eugenics are to be found in the ideology of the 19th century, in a science that was absolute and applicable to all fields of life. Darwin's theory of evolution and natural selection is the focal point.[2]

At the end of the 19th century, biologist Ernst Haeckel reduced this theory to the selection principle, though he did not give up the belief in the hereditary transmission of newly developed traits.[3] Haeckel radicalized the idea of natural selection but also was concerned that under certain conditions the "unfit" might prevail. He thus advocated a forced natural selection, otherwise known as *Rassenhygiene*. The category "unfit" included outsiders (the *asozial*), those who were unfit to make any useful contribution to society. Here are the beginnings of the efforts to replace welfare with considerations of the usefulness of the individual for the collective.[4]

In 1895, Adam Jost proclaimed that there are cases in which individuals as well as society have the right to end people's lives when their lives are no longer desired.[5] He had very rigid arguments to support his claim: what is good for society cannot be bad for individuals. Thus, killing was not only seen as a good deed for society, but also for the individual. Cynically reminding us of the suffering of family members and the costs for society, Haeckel also demanded somewhat later that "crippled, deaf-dumb, and mentally retarded" newborns be killed. Lastly, the finishing touches on the term *Rassenhygiene* were given by Alfred Ploetz. In demanding that the lesser part of humanity be weeded out, i.e. that the protection of the ill and weak be done away with in the name of the survival of the fittest, he softened the term "race" and added social worth to purely hereditary selection.[6] Procreation was only to be allowed among couples of great worth, while weak newborns were to be killed, "say, with a dose of morphine".[7]

This idea was kept alive even after the First World War by a lawyer held in high standing even today, Karl Binding, along with psychiatrist Alfred Hoche, who together denied certain types of people the capability of having a will. At any rate, they also argued, the individual must bow to the will of society when the two are in conflict.[8]

In 1924, Gustav Boeters, a physician, brought forward a bill that he had presented to the government of Saxony in the form of a memorandum in 1923.[9] This bill proposed the sterilization of epileptics, imbeciles, and those born blind and deaf-dumb. Even at that time, the bill was an exception as it acted completely without the consent of the person concerned to the point of providing for force if they resisted. This bill was to serve as a precedence in 1933. Eduard Kohlrausch's comment shortly before the Third Reich can serve as an example of the extent to which economic-utilitarian considerations had already become predominant: "If we only compare the savings to the costs, we can see that the former would greatly outweigh the latter! In many cases, the otherwise necessary and costly internment following operations could be done without. And in most cases, doing without one's descendants who would almost always be in need of care would bring such enormous financial benefits to the *Volk* that the costs could be given back to the welfare budget without further ado".[10]

The years leading up to 1933 were thus drenched in a theoretical conflict of interests. Achievements such as the welfare state were to be dismantled and replaced by a new value equation between, on the one hand, the financial burden and the usefulness of the individual for society and, on the other, the life and integrity of the individual. With the exception of the examples above, however, the principle of consent remained untouched.

Development from 1933 to 1945

In order to realize these ideas, the *Strafgesetzbuch* (penal code) had to be amended. The amendments had already been approved by the *Strafrechts-ausschuß* (committee for criminal law) in 1932. While sterilization for eugenic purposes was still part of section 224, section 226a made it clear that such an act with the victim's consent was only to be seen as a crime against good manners.[11]

Thus, the way had been paved for the "law for the prevention of deliveries of infants with hereditary diseases" of 14 July 1933. Section 1 of this law stated that people were to be made sterile through surgical intervention "when medical science states that the descendants will in all probability be afflicted with severe physical or mental hereditary defects." The law stated that hereditary diseases were "congenital mental deficiencies, schizophrenia, circular (manic-depressive) madness, Huntington's disease, hereditary blindness, hereditary deafness, severe hereditary physical deformation, or severe alcoholism." From the legal standpoint, section 2 laudably and explicitly stipulates that sterilization can only be carried out by supplication and official court order; however, according to section 3 not only the patient, but also a court doctor or, in the case of the institutionalized, the director of the institution could file for a permit. Moreover, section 12 states that force can be applied. The demand for the patient's consent was thus completely undermined by giving doctors the right to petition the court for permission at their discretion; their opinion alone sufficed.[12]

The step from sterilization to "euthanasia" was small.[13] It was simply a matter of bringing the "stamping out of life unworthy of living", of so-called "people along for the ride" (*Ballastexistenzen*) and the "less worthy", to its logical conclusion. In 1940 and 1941, some 7,000 patients were killed in gas chambers at the psychiatric clinics in Grafeneck, Branden-burg, Hartheim, Pirna, Bernberg, and Hadamar. The basis for these killings had been given by Hitler in October 1939 in a command misleadingly dated back to 1 September 1939 in which he gave doctors the "power to decide according to their best judgment and critical analysis when the in-curably ill should be granted a mercy killing".[14] The killing began with a systematic census of the patients at the clinics. Questionnaires were sent out in which the patients were categorized according to whether they were "1) curable, 2) capable of improvement through therapy, 3) incurable but capable of being productive within the clinic, 4) capable of being produc-tive in normal labor, 5) incurable and incapable of being productive (in sense 3)". These questionnaires were then sent to three of the fifty-odd members of a psychiatric recommendation committee. Ten of them were university professors. They were paid a few *Pfennige* for each patient. An "X" was a death sentence; a check meant life. If the doctors disagreed, the decision was settled by a head doctor. Because of this procedure, the doc-tors were soon nicknamed the Xers. The intensity with which questions of life and death were dealt with can best be seen from the number of ques-tionnaires filled out in six months by the director of the clinic at Eglfing-Haar, Dr. Pfannmüller: he managed to fill out 5,475 along with his regular duties as director of the institute.[15] The patients were murdered in a gas chamber camouflaged as a laundry room. The psychiatrists themselves re-leased the carbon monoxide into the room. Due partly to the protests of family members, the residents of the clinics, and churches, the killings were temporarily halted. There is little indication that the psychiatrists protested.[16] The gist of this policy was summed up by a eugenics specialist in the winter of 1940: "From life unworthy of living to treatable and curable *Volksgenossen* [people's comrades]. From biological refuse to biological high quality".[17] Thus, "useless eaters" were undesired.[18] After the protests from the population, the period of "wild euthanasia" began. The killings were no longer carried out in gas chambers; rather, the pa-tients were left to starve to death, or they were given an overdose of bar-biturates and opiates.[19] By these means, some further 150,000 patients were murdered.

After years of terror against the Jews, the Nuremberg laws were passed on 15 September 1935 - according to the Nazis, they were "constitutional amendments" - which in combination with countless other regulations made the Jews second-class citizens. The Law of Citizens of the Reich (*Reichsbürgergesetz*) divided the population up into "members of the state" and "citizens of the Reich". Jewish citizens were thus deprived of their rights, as only the *Reichsbürger* had "all of the political rights guar-anteed by the state".

Basing their decisions on supposedly scientific findings, the Nazis then defined what a Jew was in section 5 of one of the regulations: "A Jew is someone who has at least three racially pure Jewish grandparents..., but also whoever is a mixed-breed product of two pure Jewish grandparents":

a) whoever was a member of a Jewish religious community at the time this law was passed or at any time hence,
b) whoever at the time of the passing of this law was married to a Jew or has married one since,
c) whoever is the product of a Jewish marriage in the sense of section 1 that was consummated after the law for the protection of German blood and German dignity was passed in 1935,
d) whoever is the product of extramarital coitus with a Jew in the sense of section 1 and was born after 31 July 1936. *Reichsbürgergesetz*, Section 5.

Whoever had belonged to a Jewish religious community (!) could be counted as a Jewish grandparent. Mixed marriages and extramarital sex between Jews and "German citizens or those of similar blood" were punishable by law. These laws also show clearly that the theoretical underpinning that was based on a hateful view of mankind even before 1933 was ripped out of its context and exploited by the Nazis for their increasingly extensive annihilation frenzies.

In July 1941, the Reinhard Campaign began with the beginning of the construction of three concentration camps: Belzec, Sobibor, and Treblinka. In these three camps alone, some 2.5 million Jews were murdered. Because the usual facilities for murder did not suffice, the Nazis searched for additional ways to kill. They finally came across the idea of using the personnel and facilities of the euthanasia program. Thus, the first director of Treblinka was Dr. Eberl, who had been the director of the killing facilities in Brandenburg and Bernburg until then. He was relieved of his position when he proved incapable of disposing of all the corpses quickly enough. His successors, Franz and Stangl, had also learned their trade in the field of euthanasia. Wirth had developed the carbon monoxide method. He was the first to try out this procedure in Brandenburg, and he later worked at Hartheim and Grafeneck. His method was not only used in Belzec but was also the basis for the use of cyclon B in the gas chambers at Auschwitz and elsewhere.

At the Wannsee Conference on 20 January 1942, the proposal to solve the "Jewish question" with mass sterilization was discussed. It was found to be impracticable; killing was easier. The scientists, doctors, and physicians were primarily responsible for not only keeping the killing machine going, but also refining it to perfection.

The doctors' participation in the selection of prisoners for the gas chambers should also be noted. They made decision on the value of the life of the individuals and their usefulness for the *Volk*. They were the ones standing at the forefront - but not only there - and deciding who was to be murdered and who was to be spared; and, of course, they made these decisions according to their supposed scientific knowledge.

When speaking of the crimes of science during the Third Reich, one should emphasize the killing of so many helpless people. On the one hand, these killings served the ends of the Nazis - whether they were scientists or not - in wiping out the "others". On the other hand, the conditions of the Third Reich gave scientists loyal to the regime the opportunity to carry out experiments regardless of their disastrous effects, to publish, and to climb the professional ladder in ways unimaginable before.

Reappraisal after 1945

After the capitulation of the German Reich on 8 May 1945, the extent of the atrocities committed by doctors gradually came to light and had lasting detrimental effects on the trust patients and doctors need for one another. In the following year, preparations began for the trials against those responsible. Between 9 December 1946 and 20 August 1947, the so-called trials against Nazi doctors took place at the first American military court in Nuremberg. Twenty-three doctors and scientists stood trial; 13 were found guilty.

Which consequences were drawn and which changes were made in ethical norms in the wake of these trials?

The principle reaction to these events was undoubtedly the Nuremberg Code, which states the fundamental laws regulating doctors' conduct with patients and subjects of medical experiments. Aside from some partial changes dealing with rules for certain experimental interventions, this Code is still basically valid. In this context, the first section of the Code is of special interest. The first sentence states in the manner of a preamble that the patient's **voluntary consent** is required. Sentence two then stipulates that voluntary consent can only be obtained when the patient understands the facts and when no force, deception, threats, etc. are used; the patient has to be free to decide. A further requirement for voluntary consent is an understanding of the risks and type of intervention planned. Thus, the well-known need for the doctor to inform the patient came to be, a point I shall come back to shortly.

Sections 2-6 of the Code establish a sort of principle of relations. The experimental treatment employed must be necessary, and the success of the procedure should not be attainable through conventional methods. The formulation of the Code is thus far quite reserved but nevertheless represents significant progress in light of what preceded it. Section 4 states common-sensically that unnecessary suffering is to be avoided, while sections 5 and 6 rule out experimental methods that are a priori too risky on the basis of a means-ends calculation. The other sections describe certain cautionary procedures to be carried out during the experiment.

The lessons drawn from the Third Reich have also influenced the constitutions of several countries. The German constitution states in article one, section one that the dignity of human beings is inviolable. In addition, the founding of the World Medical Association (WMA) was appropriately commemorated with the formulation of a modern version of the Hippocratic Oath that was intended to bring back some of the lost credibility to the profession. Furthermore, the WMA was fundamental in the Declarations of Helsinki (1964) and Tokyo (1975). On the other hand, its ethical demands concerning human subjects of medical experiments in genetic transferals, *in vitro* fertilization, and embryo research are not binding as the organization has no power to enforce these guidelines. The German *Ärztekammer* gave them the force of laws by adopting them into their statutes. These guidelines have also been adopted by some countries, such as Israel. At any rate, their effect is strong and their validity generally recognized.

It is, however, strikingly obvious that German scientists, and among them doctors and anthropologists, have yet to formulate a critical analysis of these events. Even the documentation of the Nuremberg trials published by Alexander Mitscherlich and Fred Mielke[20] fails to critically document the personal involvement of each person. Initially, the reaction was to calm everyone down, and the arguments of confidentiality, collegiality, and the necessary sense of trust between doctor and patient were used to justify silence or speechlessness. Only after around 1970 was the reassessment of history taken more seriously.

The Patient's Consent

Some Thoughts on the Principle of Informed Consent

As we have seen, eugenics had earth-shaking consequences in its beginning stages as well as during the Third Reich, by which time it had been established and legitimated as a scientific discipline. In saying that, we do not mean to speak of this as the much-taunted historical accident. It goes without saying that, unlike an earthquake, the events of 1933 were well planned. After the war, the principle of consent - never formally done away with, but clearly deprived of its efficacy - was not revived in the Nuremberg Code for nothing. Patients were to be able once again to decide individually and freely whether the planned intervention into their bodily and spiritual integrity should be carried out. In many countries today, the demand for informed consent is either constitutionally guaranteed or part of some legal codex that cannot be amended by a simple act of law.

The latter is true for Israel. For instance, in article 2 of the *Law of Human Freedom and Dignity* from 25 March 1992, there is a phrase about the protection of life, the human body, and human honor which much resembles article 2, section 2 of Germany's constitution. Neither can be changed by the legislative. Considerations of informed consent and the prevention of other laws which would undermine this consent are the result of an anticipated weighing off of, among other things, the rights of integrity, personality, and self-determination as rights of the highest order against the rights of third parties or society at large, which are usually seen as less important in light of the historical events discussed above. Without special protection of these highly personal rights, general human rights would be meaningless. Both are therefore indissolubly linked.[21]

As rule of thumb for every doctor, informed consent requires that the patient be informed about the type, necessity, consequences and extent of the operation before being asked to consent. The information the patient must receive is directly related to the diagnosis and the proposed treatment and is thus a mandatory requirement for valid consent. Without this information, any treatment by the doctor is illegal.

The relation between mandatory information and treatment is often emphasized in legal texts,[22] whereas doctors sometimes still hold that the health of the patient is most important in calculating the risks and benefits, especially where contraindications are concerned. [23] Such attitudes are dangerous as they disregard the patient's right to self-determination. Aside from a few rare cases, namely when there is a contraindication or other justified concerns about the potential lethality of the prognosis, the doctor remains bound both ethically and legally to the calculation of pros and cons described above. This is true above all when, as in the case of a contraindication, the interests of third parties or society are contrary to those of the patient.[24]

In many countries, finally, the passing on of patient data is dependent on the consent of the patients. Germany is not the only country where this special protection is guaranteed by the constitution within the context of human dignity and general personal rights.

Consequently, in some countries medical intervention is punishable by law as a form of bodily harm, despite some disgruntlement among physicians, when the patient's informed consent was not obtained, even when the operation was otherwise carried out according to all regulations.

The Possibilities of Modern Medicine

Genetic analysis will some day give doctors access to multitudes of formerly inaccessible information about patients. Genetic analyses can be carried out clinically on a patient or simply on certain organs, cells, proteins, chromosomes, or even the DNA itself. By means of these various techniques and methods, certain illnesses or anomalies in the chromosome structure can be detected and genetic blueprints can be drawn up.[25]

Especially interesting in this context is the fact that this information is new. Legal and ethical problems result above all from the genetic analyses that predictions will be based on. Illnesses will be diagnosed before the first symptoms have appeared, and dispositions will be able to be determined and risks for future generations predicted. In the field of science, many are warning not to mystify genetics in light of all these advances. Luis Archer points out that the human genome is only one of many factors, such as social and environmental variables, that determine a person's state of health.[26]

At the same time, the problems of the future are already taking shape: genetic analyses will reveal the susceptibility of a colleague to disease as well as give insurance salesmen indications of risk and expecting mothers signs of the potential illnesses of their children. In all of these examples, the genome analysis portends a conflict of interests that is already at hand but will take on new dimensions in the future.

Just imagine the following scenario: an employer makes DNA-analyses part of job applications or demands that such documents be presented as part of an application; or an insurance salesman refuses to complete a contract without a DNA analysis. Such situations are by no means unknown today in lesser forms, but they will include much more information in the future and will allow predictions about the future to be made with a remarkable degree of certainty.

The development of gene research has only increased the danger of what has come to be called the "man of glass". Knowledge of what has happened in history is essential here; the danger that science will further the suppression of self-determination in the name of progress is greater than ever.

In closing, we would like to cite a passage written by an Israeli physician, Benjamin Moses: "The role of society is to convince everyone who wants to live that this end is best met through medicine. Everyone has the right to take advantage of medical services. The use of modern medical services requires of individuals that they sacrifice themselves, that they give themselves up to new therapeutic methods that are uncertain. The basis of this is the idea that experiments on people are the basis for medical progress and that there are no alternatives. Traditional ethical principles on this topic do not serve this purpose any longer. Therefore, they must be changed and replaced without any bias or discrimination. The social control over experiments is being taken over by commissions that have the status of those empowered by society".[27]

Due to their intellectual prowess, Moses argues, a panel of experts should make decisions for the people: a demand that would make scientific goals the measure of all things in a totalitarian manner and open the doors to abuse. We have already witnessed science in the service of a racist regime placing itself over the individual once. It must not be repeated.

Will the principle of informed consent as we know it today pass the test of future developments?

Notes

1   The term "eugenics" was coined by scholars associated with Darwin, especially in Francis Galton's *Inquiries into the Human Faculty*, London 1883, p 24f. The initial purpose of eugenics was to "regulate the birth rate of the unfit.... The second goal was to improve the race by furthering the fit by means of earlier marriages and the more healthy upbringing of children" (quoted in G. Baader, *Rassenhygiene und Eugenik - Vorbedingungen für die Vernichtungsstrategie gegen sogenannte "Minderwertige" im Nationalsozialismus*; Bleker/ Jachertz (1993), *Medizin im "Dritten Reich,"* 2nd ed., p. 36 ff.).

2   Darwin C. (1859), *On the Origin of Species by Means of Normal Selection*, London.

3   Haeckel (1924), *Natürliche Schöpfungsgeschichte* 1. Teil, Leipzig, Berlin, pp. 176-180.

4   Cf. Simon J. (1993), 'Die Erbgerichtsbarkeit im OLG-Bezirk Hamm', *Juristische Zeitgeschichte* Vol. 1., Justizministerium NRW, p. 131 (132).

5   Jost (1895), *Das Recht auf den Tod*, Göttingen.

6   Ploetz (1895), *Die Tüchtigkeit unserer Rasse und der Schutz der Schwachen*, Berlin, p. 116 and 145.

7   Ibid.

8   Binding/Hoche (1920), *Die Freigabe zur Vernichtung lebensunwerten Lebens* [sic], *ihr Maß und ihre Form*, Leipzig. See especially p. 29 and 31, where the authors describe as "unworthy to live" (*lebensunwert*) "those who are unretrievably lost due to illness or injury, those who in full comprehension of their condition are possessed by the urgent wish for relief..., as well as the incurably imbecilic or, say, those who are like the paralyzed in the last stage of their suffering. They have neither the will to live nor to die".

9   Geheimes Staatsarchiv Berlin-Dahlme, Per. 84a, Nr. 868, in Simon, p. 134.

10   Kohlrausch (1932), *Sterilization und Strafrecht*, 8fStr, 52, p. 404.

11   The requirement for consent had already been in use but was created by the courts, not the legislature. Eugenic sterilization without consent had not, however, been legal (cf. Simon, p. 135f.).

12   The cynicism of the law becomes clear in the passage about "brotherly love for the coming generations" where it is also argued that "asocial descendents will be a burden for the collective". The weighing off of interests (in favor of society) is clear here.

13   For details, see Müller-Hill B., *Tödliche Wissenschaft, Die Aussonderung von Juden, Zigeunern und Geisteskranken 1933-1945*.

14   See Bastian T. (1995), *Furchtbare Ärzte. Medizinische Verbrechen im Dritten Reich*, p. 50.

15   See Bastian.

16   There is, however, evidence that it was possible to refuse to fill out the questionnaires without fearing retribution. See the approach of Professor Gottfried Ewald in Bastian, p. 50.

17   Quoted in Schmidt G. (1995), *Selektion in der Heilanstalt*, Frankfurt/Main, p. 100.

18   The term itself probably was coined by Hitler himself; Viktor Brack mentioned the term during the Nuremberg Trials in 1946.

19   Bastian, p. 38ff.

20   Mitscherlich A. (1947), *Das Diktat der Menschenverachtung: e. Dokumentation/* Alexander Mitscherlich; Fred Mielke, Heidelberg Schneider,.

21   This is further made clear by the insistence of the *Bundesverfassungsgericht* [German Constitutional Court] that the protection of personal rights in Article 2 be seen in connection with article 1 on human dignity.

22   Cf. for Germany BGH, Verse R 1954, p. 98.

23   See Laufs A. (1984), *Arztrecht*, 3rd edition. Rn. 111ff., 126.

24   The construct of "presumed consent" as proposed in German law does not represent a real exception, as it is based on the fundamental principles of "management without commission" (*Geschäftsführung ohne Auftrag*) and is only designed to prevent the doctor from carrying out operations without the patient's consent when the will of the patient is known or recognized to be contrary to such actions.

25   Archer L. (1996), *Looking for New Codes in the Field of Predictive Medicine*, Lisbon, p. 1-3.

26   Ibid, p. 41f.

27   Moses B.(1986), *Modern Medicine - Decision-Making in Uncertainty*, Tel Aviv, p. 1.

The Paradigm Shift in Medical Ethics: Patients' Rights, Education, Institutions

16 The Paradigm Shift in Health Care and the Patient-Physician Relationship from an American Perspective

Ronald A. Carson

Health Care and Human Values

Throughout human history, the practice of healing has been part science, part art, part social service, part spiritual quest. And yet, during the past fifty years, American medical education focused almost exclusively on training students to master the explosively expanding biomedical sciences and increasingly powerful technologies. As a result, our health-sciences universities produced physicians sophisticated in the diagnosis and treatment of disease, but largely untutored in the meaning of illness for individuals and the purposes of medicine in society.

About thirty years ago, a conversation was struck up between medicine and the humanities. Medicine was becoming morally unsettled in those days. As the decade of the seventies dawned, questions arising at the intersection of health care and human values became pressing. An awareness was growing of the need for public mechanisms to govern medical research involving human subjects (1, 2). A mounting public unease was palpable regarding the use of new technologies that often seemed to prolong life at the expense of dignity in dying. Surgical and pharmacological advances in the transplantation of vital organs were accompanied by challenges to widely accepted notions of how to recognize and properly acknowledge death.

In response to the post-World War II increase in publicly funded medical research, the emergence of a vast hospital industry, and the enthusiasm for specialty and sub-specialty training, medical educators worried about the withering of the virtues of personal care and engaged practitioners of the humanities in a dialogue about the legitimate scope and purposes of medicine in modern society. Academic physicians concerned about these matters turned to the humanities in search of conversation partners because the humanities are fundamentally disciplines of moral inquiry.

In any endeavor, power without critical insight and self-awareness tends to be dangerous. Yet, insight and self-awareness are not second nature; they must be learned both directly and by example. In the context of medical education and practice, they present special challenges: doctors must maintain a certain distance from suffering in order to alleviate it. They must summon the confidence to act quickly and decisively in situations where the life or death of fellow human beings rests on their skill and judgment. They must be capable of relating to people from all walks of life. They must often make extraordinary physical and emotional demands on themselves that put them out of touch with their own well-being, making it even harder for them to understand the vulnerabilities of others.

In the face of all this, encouraging introspection and imagination, and teaching moral reasoning cannot be left to chance and convenience, to the traditional curricula of medical schools or the good intentions that lead so many to take up the study of medicine. Biomedical science provides physicians and researchers with the knowledge and tools of their professions but not with the broader understanding to wield these wisely in a world that technology, economics, and cultural diversity are daily making more socially and morally complex. The humanities can help provide that understanding, especially when they take medicine as their subject and medical people as their conversation partners.

History illuminates the evolution of the health-care professions and the roles they have played in societies through the ages. Literature permits a vicarious encounter with the emotional and relational complexities of human suffering and healing. Art history reveals how various cultures have viewed the body-its beauty, its infirmities, and its demise, while it helps us look more closely and clearly at what we see. Philosophy subjects to critical scrutiny the methodologies of science and the way we conceptualize medical issues. Jurisprudence opens a window onto how society can protect the rights of individuals and give procedural guidance to professionals. Religious studies illuminate the relationship between spiritual ideas and traditions of health care. Ethics delineates the professional values and the community and individual values that touch on every aspect of healing. And social and political philosophy make use of these insights to forge public policy.

Fruitful as these disciplines are when they examine health care singly, they have even more profound potential when they engage in dialogue with each other as well as with the healing arts and the biomedical sciences. The interdisciplinary bridges built by these dialogues provide paths to fresh perspectives on perplexities as timeless as the meaning of suffering and the nature of life and death and as current as equitable distribution of health-care resources, the uses of genetic research, and the moral quandaries surrounding abortion and euthanasia.

As the post-World War II era extended through the economically prosperous 1950s and into the socially turbulent 1960s, the American people became exorbitantly optimistic about medicine. It would be only a mild overstatement to say that the broad public came to believe that doctors could cure just about every ailment - if not now, then surely soon. It was an era of wonder drugs and the magic of high technology interventions to delay the spread or slow the progress of diseases such as cancer. Patients who would previously have died of respiratory failure could be sustained by artificial means. The training of doctors was becoming highly specialized; new specialties were proliferating.

As exhilarating as it admittedly was, all of this activity did not amount to an unalloyed advance in the conquest of disease. For example, once it became possible to maintain respiratory function in the absence of brain stem function, new moral questions arose about when and under what conditions to attach someone to a respirator and about when and in what circumstances to withdraw the respirator. As moralist Paul Ramsey put it in a seminal book of the time entitled *The Patient as Person,* the new question was how to resist the mechanical ventilator - "a devilishly efficient instrument".

Questions such as these fundamentally human questions, prompted by medicine's progress-began to open up medical ethics, which heretofore had been *doctors'* ethics, to public debate. Increasingly, patients expressed the desire to be included in decisions regarding their own medical care (3). Three notable events of the 1960s and 1970s are suggestive of the then growing need for special attention to the *human* dimensions of medical research and medical care.

In 1965 the United States Congress passed progressive social legislation establishing Medicare, a program that is as close as the United States has come to providing universal access to health care-in this case, for that segment of the population made up of older Americans. This massive federal program, added to the enormous public commitment of funds to support medical research and education through various grants and subsidies of the National Institutes of Health and other federal and state agencies, ensured that the public sector would be integrally involved in shaping medicine's future. These developments also paved the way for ethics commissions at the federal and state levels.

A different sort of event occurred in 1968, namely the promulgation of the so-called Harvard Brain Death Criteria, aimed at defining irreversible coma. Such an attempt at an explicit uniform "definition of death" which had previously been a matter of clinician discretion and judgment was prompted by advances in the surgical transplantation of vital organs, a practice rife with ethical concerns.

Finally, in 1976, the Supreme Court of the State of New Jersey ruled in the Karen Ann Quinlan case - the first of several high-profile court cases having to do with end-of-life decisions regarding the appropriate treatment of patients incapable of speaking for themselves - that decisions to stop life-support measures cannot be made by family members in the absence of appropriate public review.

These three otherwise unrelated examples are suggestive of the ferment characteristic of the decades during which American medicine was becoming morally troubled. The story of post-World War II American medicine is, in the main, a story of machinery and money, and of rapid bureaucratic and technological development. It is a story of "big" science (government-sponsored and, more recently, corporate-sponsored, science) and one of "rescue" medicine, the attempt to stave off death one individual at a time with massive expenditures of time, effort, skill and matériel. Hospitals have grown in size and number and in sophistication of staff in order to house and support the rescue efforts.

Americans have generally welcomed these developments but they are becoming increasingly ambivalent about some of what medicine has to offer. To put it plainly, if perhaps a little oversimply, we Americans fear death and want to enlist medicine in fending it off, but we tend also to want to avoid unnecessary suffering, including suffering brought on by medicine's sometimes painful remedies. It is in this context that the medical humanities are engaged in reflections on the changing relations between patients and doctors-not only at the end of life, but perhaps epitomized there-aimed at answering such questions as: what ought society realistically to expect from medicine? And, how should doctors be educated for the kinds of relationships we as individuals want?

In order to understand why the humanities are well-suited to this task, one other matter should be noted. The notion of science uncritically adopted by American medicine in its heyday and still dominant today is a much narrower conception than that prevalent in most other societies. It is a positivistic conception in that it imagines itself to be limited to the study of non-normative phenomena. A typical contrast case is the broader German understanding of science in which there are *Naturwissenschaften*, *Sozialwissenschaften*, and *Geisteswissenschaften* - natural, social and human sciences. Sciences, on this view, are understood to be systems of knowledge acquired by sustained study. Not so in America, where the displacement of the humanities by "science" (narrowly conceived) had until recently become so thoroughgoing that the moral aspects of medicine seemed to have no place at all-a situation which, in an enterprise as deeply involved as medicine is with social, cultural and personal life, could not be sustained. As medicine became morally problematic the humanities became necessary again, not as self-contained academic disciplines but as modes of inquiry adept at various interpretive practices. Plainly put, the humanities have become central to thinking through the moral muddles of late twentieth-century American medicine because mainline scientific and professional medicine has retreated into a formal, technical rationality ill-suited to taking the moral aspects of its practice into account. It lacks a language for addressing human questions.

What characteristics of the humanities prepare their practitioners to engage in a fruitful dialogue with medical people about these issues? First, as I have already mentioned, the humanities are interpretive in orientation.

They aim not so much at explanation as at critical understanding. In this sense, they are a culture's means of making sense of itself to itself and to others. Second, except where they become overly preoccupied with themselves, the humanities deal with matters which are interesting and accessible to everyone, or at least to everyone who is sufficiently protected from the worst of life's vagaries-hunger and poverty and the like-to be able to reflect a little on what it all adds up to. Put another way, although there are specialists in the humanities, one doesn't have to possess specialized knowledge to be interested in the subject matter of the humanities, namely human experience in all its variety. Third, this subject matter, these varieties of human experience-for our purposes, experiences of sickness and suffering, health and well-being-are inextricably woven through with human meanings and values which require not only understanding but critical evaluation as well. The humanities are an important repository of a culture's methods and approaches and texts that deal with complex questions of value. The humanities are adept at testing and contesting interpretations and at debating the advisability of one or another course of action.

Over the past thirty years, the humanities have engaged American medicine in a dialogue aimed at exploring its philosophical grounding and historical context and at clarifying the values and probing the assumptions of its practices. On a wider public stage, this dialogue aims at cultivating tolerance for the intractable ambiguities of health and health care, and at encouraging both an appreciation for experience that eludes quantification and a disposition toward self-examination on the part of doctors and patients alike (4, 5). Although this dialogue is wide-ranging, consideration of three of its central subjects-patients' rights, medical ethics education, and institutional change-will suggest its character.

Patient's Rights

In general, we understand a right to be a just claim, that is, a claim on something to which one is entitled by law or moral custom or tradition. The language of *individual* rights central to Anglo-American political philosophy was influentially articulated in the seventeenth century by John Locke. Locke's social contract theory turned on the idea of trust. The social contract was understood to be constituted between individuals who yielded certain rights to their government in return for the government's pledge to act on behalf and in the best interests of those individuals in certain agreed upon matters. A contract view presupposes the notion of voluntary agreement. Relations established by contract are authorized, not by divine or sovereign decree, or by experts, scientific or otherwise, in possession of arcane knowledge and its derivative power, but by consent.

Voluntary informed consent, as formulated with regard to research subjects in the first article of the Nuremberg Code, is the central idea in the critique of medical paternalism that accompanied the growing recognition of *patients'* rights beginning in the 1960s when the American civil rights movement made great strides on behalf of black Americans. Competent patients, it was argued, are free agents and as such have: 1) a right to know the truth about their condition and about treatment options, 2) a right to refuse treatment, 3) a right to have confidences kept, and 4) a right to access to a fair share of society's health-care resources. Physicians and other health-care personnel are obligated, in turn, to ensure that those rights are secured by: 1) informing patients about their diagnosis, prognosis, and treatment options and 2) seeking their permission for medical manipulations and interventions. Thus were the rights and corresponding duties of patients and physicians contractually specified.

As medical ethics became increasingly *professionalized,* a social contract view of the doctor-patient relationship came to prevail (6, 7). This view continues to be a useful antidote to the hegemony of medical and scientific aristocracies of moral expertise. Evidence for the *codification* of rights-based principles is to be found in such documents as the reports of the President's Commission for the Study of Ethical Problems in Medicine and Biomedical and Behavioral Research, various patients' bills of rights, the extensive literature on informed consent, and bioethics textbooks.

Rights language is assertorical and procedural. In the parlance of biomedical ethics, it asserts that patients have a right to be treated respectfully and beneficently as self-determining individuals. It sets out the terms of agreements, especially those having to do with the *limits* of responsibility and liability. The language of patient rights embodies the notion that consent is a necessary condition of relations among free persons in doctor-patient relations as elsewhere in civil society. Sustained attention to consent as the cornerstone of contractual relations will continue to be necessary to meet the challenges posed by new scientific knowledge and medical technology. This is especially so in the domain of human subjects research, but is also the case in clinical practice. However, although similarities exist, doctor-patient relations cannot be subsumed without remainder under the model of the researcher-subject relationship, not least because contractual relations are minimalist in orientation (that is, they err in the direction of *negative* liberty) and tend to be inflexible in dealing with the contingencies with which patient care is replete. (It is easier to abide by the principle of nonmaleficence than it is to discern what, in an individual instance, beneficence requires.)

The widespread acknowledgment of consent as a non-negotiable feature of responsible medical practice has eventuated in an increasingly egalitarian doctor-patient relationship (8). Patients expect not only to have their rights recognized, but also look to be treated as full partners in a relationship of *moral equals.* The codification of patient rights is an important exercise for medicine as a *profession.* Codes announce a profession's best intentions and publicly declare the standards by which the profession will conduct its affairs. But actually relating to patients as moral equals day-by-day is the responsibility of *individual* physicians - patient after patient - and is in large measure a function of the way physicians are educated and of the organizational structures in which they practice.

Medical Ethics Education

Education in medical ethics has burgeoned in the past twenty-five years. Most United States medical schools provide some instruction in ethics as a regular component of the curriculum. Commonly, these courses focus broadly on the many morally relevant aspects of relationships between patients and health-care professionals-truth-telling, confidentiality, attitudes toward suffering, end-of-life care, financial considerations, caring for the destitute, and the like. Codes and guidelines of professional medical societies play a modest role in such teaching.

Among the various models for teaching medical ethics, two predominate: an applied ethics approach and an interpretive, pragmatic approach. On the applied ethics model, students are familiarized with the defining features of certain moral principles believed to be centrally significant to medical practice. They are expected subsequently to appropriately apply the principles in patient care settings. Instruction typically consists of lectures and reading assignments augmented by case materials that illustrate an action-guide approach. This analytic philosophical approach mimics the basic science/clinical science arrangement of most American medical school curricula. The teaching is for the most part didactic and is sometimes supplemented by preceptorial instruction in clinical settings. The chief advantage of this approach is that it provides students with a portable conceptual framework for dealing with moral problems in medicine. On the other hand, the quandary ethics framework it provides is best suited for decision-making in moments of crisis and in conflict situations which, though not uncommon in the emergency and intensive-care settings of institutional practice, are unrepresentative of medical practice generally (9).

The second of the two models of medical ethics teaching is predicated on the assumption that moral reasoning in medical practice, like clinical reasoning generally, is less abstract and deductive than it is descriptive and inductive. It is a form of practical reasoning about concrete moral concerns. Teaching practical reasoning using an interpretive-pragmatic approach sets out from the observation that most of what ails us is chronic in nature and is not going to kill us, at least not soon. We may need help in determining our options and in understanding what is best for us under circumstances altered by illness or injury. This requires of the doctor that he or she be a knowledgeable conversation partner but seldom a decision-maker, and virtually never unilaterally so. And to the extent that illness *is* an intimation of mortality, what ails us may well give us pause and cause us to reconsider the meaning and direction of our lives in its light.

Being sick may be confounding, confusing, unnerving, unsettling, discomfiting, or dismaying, but seldom does sickness come bearing clear moral *choices.* What is required is a probing of the experience with a view to trying to make livable sense of it and its likely implications. For this, the help patients need is from someone who is: 1) versed in varieties of illness experience, 2) capable of critically reflecting on the received wisdom embodied in societal mores and morally sound practice patterns, and 3) skilled at assessing what is plausible and reasonable under the concrete circumstances of a particular patient's current condition. Acquainting students with a rich range of lived experience, cultivating in them habits of critical reflection, and sharpening their interpretive skills requires pedagogic approaches derived from the humanities, that is, from the careful reading of historical and literary, as well as philosophical and religious, texts (10).

Institutional Change

Many institutional responses to changes in the relationship of patients and health care professionals have occurred in the United States since the mid-1960s. Two federal commissions were convened. The National Commission for the Protection of Human Subjects of Biomedical and Behavioral Research was charged to develop guidelines for conducting ethically sound human subjects research and issued reports on experimentation with human fetuses and pregnant women, children, prisoners, and institutionalized mentally ill or retarded persons. These guidelines provided the basis for federal regulations. A subsequent President's Commission published reports on making health-care decisions, securing access to health care, screening and counseling for genetic conditions, genetic engineering, compensation for injured research subjects, whistle blowing in biomedical research, defining death, and deciding to forgo life-sustaining treatment. The latter two reports were widely influential in shaping hospital policies. A National Bioethics Advisory Commission has recently been established.

A number of commissions have also been active at the state level. Task forces in Michigan, Minnesota, New Jersey, New York, and Oregon have developed policy recommendations on issues ranging from physician-assisted suicide to fairness in the allocation and distribution of health care resources. Professional medical societies have established ethical practice standards and articulated what, for example, the American Board of Internal Medicine calls "essential humanistic qualities required in certified internists ... integrity, respect, and compassion" (11). The American Medical Association publishes *Fundamental Elements of the Physician-Patient Relationship;* its Council on Ethical and Judicial Affairs issues *current opinions* as part of its regularly updated *Code of Medical Ethics* (12). The U.S. Catholic Conference promulgates *Ethical and Religious Directives for Catholic Health Facilities* and the American Hospital Association has a *Patients' Bill of Rights.* The Joint Commission on the Accreditation of Healthcare Organizations requires hospitals to provide evidence that they conduct their relations with patients and the public in an ethically defensible manner. Ethics committees are a common feature of most large hospitals, and ethics consultation services are proliferating.

Hospital ethics committees, though by no means flawless in concept and easily co-opted in practice by the organizations they serve, constitute the single most pervasive institutional change in recent years. There is great variation in the way such committees function, but all of them make ethical issues an explicit concern in hospital care and governance. Many committees serve primarily a pedagogic function, educating hospital personnel regarding basic ethical considerations in patient care. Some also assist in the development and revision of ethically sound hospital policies. A few are involved in clinical case review. Hospital ethics committees symbolize a commitment to openness and inclusiveness in decision-making in place of the relatively closed and exclusive practice patterns of earlier eras of medical paternalism. Their very existence signals society's acknowledgment that medical ethics is not limited to professional ethics but is a function of an ongoing broad-gauged public dialogue about moral values. How these positive developments are likely to be affected by the corporatization of a growing segment of the American health care enterprise is a concern to many.

Conclusion

All in all, the recognition of patients' rights, and the special consideration of ethical issues in health professional education and health care institutions, have heightened public awareness and deepened the seriousness of attention given to the quality of patient care. Whether this is an adequate response to changes in the relationship of patients and health care professionals remains an open question.

As to the question of the general utility of codes of conduct for shaping behavior, what seems increasingly clear is that the relation of ethical principles to morally responsible practices is internal and reciprocal. That is, only to the degree that the principles enshrined in codes of conduct both accurately *reflect* moral practice *and* function as touchstones to *transform* practice, is it reasonable to expect codes to provide serviceable standards and useful guidance. Conversely, and perhaps even more important, it is only to the extent that codified norms are embodied in the everyday work of individual practitioners that we may speak of morally responsible medicine. The work of embodiment is not principally accomplished by exhortation but by thoughtfully and deliberately shaping both the minds and sensibilities of practitioners-in-training and the organizational structures of health-care institutions.

References

1　Reiser, S.J. (1994), "Misconduct and the Development of Ethics in the Biological Sciences", *Cambridge Quarterly of Healthcare Ethics* 3: 499-505.

2　Rothman, D.J. (1991), *Strangers at the Bedside: A History of How Law and Bioethics Transformed Medical Decision Making*, New York: Basic Books.

3　Callahan, D. (1993), "Why America Accepted Bioethics", *Hastings Center Report* 23 (6): 8-9, November-December.

4　Coles, R. (1979), "Medical Ethics and Living a Life", *New England Journal of Medicine* 301 (8): 444-446.

5　Jonsen, A.R. (1983), "The Therapeutic Relationship: Is Moral Conduct a Necessary Condition?" in *The Clinical Encounter*, Earl E. Shelp, ed., Dordrecht: D. Reidel, pp. 267-287.

6　Churchill, L.R. (1977), "The Professionalization of Ethics: Some Implications for Accountability in Medicine", *Soundings: An Interdisciplinary Journal* LX (1): 40-53.

7　Fox, Renee C. (1989), "The Sociology of Bioethics", in *The Sociology of Medicine*, Englewood Cliffs, N.J.: Prentice Hall, pp. 224-276.

8　Veatch, R.M. (1991), "Contemporary Bioethics and the Demise of Modern Medicine", in *The Patient-Physician Relation: The Patient as Partner*, Bloomington, IN: Indiana University Press.

9　Pellegrino, E. D. (1993), "The Metamorphosis of Medical Ethics: A 30-Year Retrospective", *Journal of the American Medical Association* 269 (9): 1158-1162, March 3.

10　Carson, R.A. (1995), "Interpretation", in *Encyclopedia of Bioethics,* revised edition, Warren Thomas Reich, ed., New York: Simon & Schuster Macmillan, pp. 1283-1288.

11　American Board of Internal Medicine (1983), "Evaluation of Humanistic Qualities in the Internist", *Annals of Internal Medicine* 99 (5): 720-724, November.

12　Council on Ethical and Judicial Affairs (1995), *Code of Medical Ethics: Current Opinions with Annotations,* American Medical Association.

17 Means and Ways for the Protection of Patients in France

Jean Michaud

Specific Institutions

Science, especially biology and medicine, are no longer matters for specialists only. This does not mean that everyone will be able to understand the details of progress that is made as the complexity of the information increases more and more. But some of this progress could have such a profound influence on the evolution of society and the fate of its members that we should not simply deliver everyone up to these effects without considering what this entails.

The objective of researchers, aside from their fundamental passion for knowledge, is the common good, the betterment of the human condition. But what is good - and what better? The answers from the various vast domains of science are not uniform. They may even be contradictory depending on the philosophy, the ethics, of those who are answering.

Will the evolution of techniques for artificial insemination lead up to the complete dismissal, except in exceptional cases, of natural insemination? Will prenatal diagnostics mean that only fetuses without any imperfections will ever see the light of day? Will we be able to modify genetic traits, not to mention genetic diseases?

No doubt, the solutions are a matter of law. In France, three texts were published on this subject in July 1994. But these texts were a long time in coming, and one of them is already scheduled to be revised in the near future.

In this respect, such considerations are being carried out in France and elsewhere within committees of ethics. These institutions have been set up in the course of the last few years. They are characterized by their pluralism, the interdisciplinarity, and their utter lack of decision-making power. After airing the points of view of researchers, physicians, lawyers, sociologists, and philosophers, their sole task is to sum up the opinions on the new problems posed by science, especially concerning their implications for society. The questions raised above illustrate the type of issues these committees deal with. Though the opinions are not binding in any sense,

215

they do serve as reference points for governments and researchers. Thus, they can be the basis for an ongoing dialogue between those involved in the evolution of science and are widely seen as serving democracy by formulating such texts.

Such is the role of the *Comité Consultatif National d'Éthique Français*. It mediates between the committees of ethics in hospitals, which are largely not officially recognized outside the hospital, and the committees concerned exclusively with one particular aspect of health care.

Biomedical ethics goes beyond national borders. The problems, at least at the European level, are comparable between nations. For this reason, the *Comité Directeur de Bioéthique* of the Council of Europe included the following phrase in the preamble of the convention that it adopted in June 1996: "in light of the importance of promoting public debate on the questions raised in applied biology and medicine as well as on the responses that will be brought forward ". The idea is taken up again in article 28 of the text. In an effort to bring their experiences together, the European committees of ethics have met three times in Madrid, Stockholm, and Budapest. It is possible that the growing public awareness of these new scientific problems, whose very solutions will determine the future, will enable us to create effective obstacles against any actions that, under the pretext of progress, would threaten the rights of man by means of the establishment of these original institutions such as ethics committees.

The Recognition of Patients' Rights

Patients have the same rights as all people. But unlike healthy people, the ill are more vulnerable to dangers they cannot ward off. They thus deserve special protection by, though not from, the people caring for them. Indeed, physicians can only treat and diagnose the ill based on the principles of integrity and the inviolability of the human body. These principles are laid out in articles 16-1 and 16-3 of the French Civil Code of law 94653 of July 29, 1994. In addition, article I of the *project de convention* passed by the *Comité Directeur de Bioéthique* of the Council of Europe in July 1996 also mentions the rights of the integrity of the body. But article 16-3 of the French Civil Code gives doctors special dispensation to these principles in the name of the patient's right to receive treatment. This right to be treated regardless of the integrity and inviolability of the human body depends on the patient's consent as set out in articles I6-3 of the Civil Code and 5 of the convention cited above.

The laws which demand the freedom of this consent also allow for special arrangements for those unable to give such consent: minors and adults who are incapacitated. But this freedom presupposes sufficient knowledge about the treatment to be undergone as well as its possible consequences - hence the term "informed consent".

But there are limits to the patients rights. Patients cannot ask for treatment that will not lead to a cure. In French law, the doctor is obliged to provide the best care attentively and in line with the latest findings. His obligation is of means, not results. Medicine is not a science. In certain domains, the demand for consent is enforced by ever-increasing formalities. In tests, for example, the consent must be written. In medically assisted pro-creation, the consent is necessary to obtain official permission from the authorities in order to receive an embryo.

Finally, for some methods that could have grave consequences, there are protective measures limiting the powers of the doctor in favor of the patient. Organ transplants, artificial insemination, and diagnostic prenatal care cannot be carried out outside of certain establishments or specially designed sites. The tendency is thus towards more rights for the patients, which is itself a sign of the - irreversible? - will to never again view human beings as mere laboratory material.

Training in Medical Ethics

Physicians follow professional regulations that make up their deontological code whose earliest form is the Hippocratic Oath. An understanding of these texts is as much a part of their training as the purely technical aspects. By the same token, every member of the medical profession is obliged to respect certain rules of conduct in dealing with patients. One could speak of medical morals. Some scientific events that took place in the second half of the 20th century have necessitated further regulations. The progress that has been made goes far beyond what preceded this century, requiring us to question our conscience anew.

Artificial insemination will allow us to cultivate the human embryo in the laboratory, to isolate it outside the maternal organism, to preserve it frozen for long periods of time. It is easy to see how one could be tempted to make such embryos part of scientific experiments. Diagnostic prenatal treatment allows us to detect *in utero* defects or abnormalities in the fetus, which also opens up a whole new field of research. Research on the human genome is significantly increasing man's knowledge of man.

These are only some examples that show the extent of recent progress - and its implications. The evolution of medically assisted procreation could produce a state of affairs in which parents put off birth until it is convenient; diagnostic prenatal care could lead to the elimination of embryos and fetuses that have some malformation or disease - or that simply do not display the "preferred" traits; and genome research could further the crazy scramble to find out everything about human beings.

The goal of what is still called bioethics - we could speak of medical ethics - has to be to make distinctions between the good and the bad in scientific progress. Not everything that is new is necessarily good. New findings can only be beneficial for society when they are applied with an understanding of what is at stake. Physicians and others in the medical profession are at present ill-qualified to make such rulings. Therefore, it is important that their training should have ethical characteristics considered as influential as any other parts of their university curriculum. But ethics goes beyond the realm of therapeutics and biology. It is both interdisciplinary and pluralist, being fundamentally part of philosophy, law, and sociology, among others and, with respect to the answers needed, of the different strands of ideas. Hence the need for institutional training in the field of law as well as of the humanities.

After all, this concerns every citizen. The fate of everyone - and their family - is at stake. When patients consent to participate in a modern operation, they must understand more than ever what it will entail exactly. What better place to do this than in committees of ethics where they can be informed as well as inform. But education of this sort does not mean preaching the one truth. Rather than dictating a moral truth, such organisations should sensitize people to new problems that society must rule on. How can we make such decisions without understanding the problems?

It is possible that this education in ethics and the research that will go along with the teaching will, by training them to question their conscience, help to arm citizens of whatever camp against the dangers to which they have hardly been exposed yet.

References

Baudouin, J.L. and Labrusse C. (1987) *Produire l'Homme de quel droit?* Riou / P.U.F.

Aux débuts de la Vie - ouvrage collectif / éd. La Découverte, 1990.

L'Ethique et la Vie - France Queré /éd. O. Jacob, 1991

Ruffié J. and Jacob, O. (1993) *Naissance de la médecine prédictive.*

Les Avis du Comité National d'Ethique - 1983-1993. Centre de Doc. INSERM.

'L'Ethique, seul rempart véritable contre la paranoia étatique' - *Th. Feral / Rev. Psychiatrie Française,* Avril 1996, pp. 73-88.

18 The Paradigm Shift in Health Care and the Patient-Health Professional Relationship

J. Stuart Horner

During the last fifty years ethical approaches in the United Kingdom have been influenced by a recognition of patients' rights and the move from paternalism to patient autonomy. Medical education has played a rather minor role in this paradigm shift, but a variety of institutions have played key roles in the process. In order to understand these developments, it is desirable to place them in an historical and cultural context. Medical ethics in the United Kingdom had been influenced for at least a century, and probably for considerably longer, by three major factors:

- the organization of the health care system;
- prevailing ideas in philosophy and the law; and
- medical technology.

Historical Background

In the United Kingdom the health care system has been largely influenced by developments taking place in hospital. There has always been an inherent tension between those practicing medicine in institutional settings and others providing healing services outside such institutions. These tensions can be traced back at least five hundred years in the United Kingdom. Initially the tension was between apothecaries and traditional healers on the one hand and the university trained physicians on the other. These tensions were brought into dramatic focus during the civil war in the sixteenth century. Over the last one hundred and fifty years the tension has been between general practitioners and the community health team on the one hand and hospital based staff on the other.

Nevertheless, it is with the hospital that this review is primarily concerned, since these are the *institutions* which have most influenced attitudes to patients and the control of ethical teaching. Two hospital systems originally developed side by side:

- voluntary hospitals; and
- state financed hospitals.

Voluntary Hospitals

These hospitals in turn were created in one of two ways. Firstly, by the church, although the destruction of the monasteries by King Henry VIII seriously disrupted this process. Secondly, and more recently, by the philanthropy of individuals such as Thomas Guy (Guy's Hospital) or a group of local philanthropists working together, who created the major teaching hospitals in most of our cities.

In these voluntary hospitals consultant medical staff mostly gave their services free of charge, deriving their incomes from private practice, based on reputations established within the voluntary hospitals. The junior medical staff, who normally provided on site medical care at the hospitals, were either in training under one of the consultants, or paid relatively poorly as a salaried doctor by the institution itself. Inevitably, within the hospitals, this created a system where the doctor had all the knowledge and all the power. Patients were naturally grateful to receive such expert care, either at a cost they could afford, or even free of charge. Many of these voluntary hospitals established a subscription service, which allowed an individual to contribute relatively little whilst in health, in return for free treatment when disease occurred.[1] All of these patients were grateful for this 'medical charity'. Unfortunately it produced a system of medical paternalism in which the doctors' conclusions and decisions were accepted without question by patients normally afraid even to inquire about their diagnosis.

State Funded Hospitals

These began early in the nineteenth century when local boards of guardians (a group of local worthy men appointed for their 'good works') found it necessary to provide medical care to the paupers incarcerated in the workhouses which they maintained. At the beginning of the present century those who were not paupers could also receive treatment in these hospitals.

In 1929 local government took over responsibility for these state funded hospitals from the local boards of guardians and for twenty years some of them invested heavily in medical service programs. Others did not and provision was geographically patchy. Thus the main task of the National

Health Service, which took over both groups of hospitals in 1948, was to create a common system of care throughout the country and spectacular success has been achieved during the period under review, despite a series of revolutionary changes in the way that the hospitals have been managed in recent years.

Given their *Poor Law* origins, however, these hospitals too created an approach in which the patient was the supplicant and the salaried medical staff (whilst usually earning less in overall terms than those in the voluntary hospitals) could nevertheless be identified by patients as holding all the keys to their treatment.

This historical background has been set out since it explains why paternalism has been so deeply ingrained in the United Kingdom. Indeed it is alive and well in many hospital institutions where consultants still maintain a hierarchical structure and the needs of patients receive relatively less attention, with scant regard for patient autonomy. Very few patients are offered a range of treatment options and some even today scarcely know their diagnosis or why they are receiving the particular treatment which the doctor has determined.

It can nevertheless be set in an even wider historical context. Albert Jonsen[2] points out that the [mediaeval] concept of service was replaced by a concept of 'rights' in the seventeenth century. John Locke believed that free individuals had a right to their own space and a right of property in things with which men had mixed their labor. As diseases began to be defined in England by Thomas Sydenham (the 'English Hippocrates') so doctors, by studying them, had developed a right or authority. Prevention and treatment were applied on 'doctors orders'. The patient must therefore put him/herself completely in the hands of the doctor who 'owns his/her disease'. Paternalism became inevitable. 'The era of Lockean rights in medical practice came to an end in 1946 with the enactment of the National Health Service'.

Philosophical and Legal Ideas

It is difficult and probably pointless to trace the origin of the broad sweeps of philosophical and legal ideas which have followed in the wake of the European Enlightenment. It is sufficient to state that there remains a significant groundswell of earlier religious belief among a wide range of health care professionals, which sees 'Enlightenment thinking' as a major threat.[3] Probably developing from the civil rights movement in the United States of America in the 1960s, concepts of individual rights and patient rights have gradually permeated through British society and into the health care system. There is now an increasing recognition by doctors that patients cannot be taken for granted. They are autonomous individuals who hold certain rights, including the right to control the types of medical treatment they are prepared to accept. These rights are symbolized in the process of consent which, to be legally valid, must include a sufficient sharing of information to allow the patient to make an informed choice. The cultural development of the service, however, still puts a greater emphasis on the patient's signature to undertake a particular procedure than upon explaining what the procedure involves, together with its benefits and disadvantages.

The concept of a legal contract between patient and doctor is by no means a new one. The concept is clearly set out in the Hippocratic Corpus. The Hippocratic writer makes it clear that in this contract the doctor undertakes to promote the patient's improvement and hopefully healing. Patients in their turn undertake to follow the treatments which the doctor has recommended. In recent years this concept of a legal contract has however itself come under challenge. Many have appeared to argue that, whilst the doctor has a duty to undertake any treatment which may be beneficial to the patient, there is no complementary responsibility on the patient to assist with the process. The patient's right to treatment seems to outweigh all other considerations. Thus suggestions that smokers should give up the practice before being offered various forms of cardiac surgery, has received widespread criticism. Even though the scientific evidence points unequivocally to short term and long term benefits, it has still been argued that there is no obligation upon the patient to contribute to his own recovery and certainly such a contribution should not become a condition of treatment. Similar questions arise in the removal of skin tattoos and gender reassignment operations, in all of which the absolute authority of patient rights over all other ethical considerations still seems to be widely canvassed. Agich[4] however points out that 'the concept of autonomy ... is really a limited political/legal concept that is woefully incomplete for the purposes of ethical theory'. He rejects the idea that autonomy 'trumps' all other considerations and finds it unhelpful in the care of the elderly, many of whom may be losing their decision making powers and may need some decisions taking for them.

In the United Kingdom a response to this doctrine of individual rights has been expressed through the political initiative of *The Patient's Charter*. Introduced by politicians, the intention is to set out to patients what rights they can expect to enjoy from services provided by public bodies. These may include the right to choose one's own doctor; the right to have a second or even third opinion; the right not to be kept waiting, etc. It is difficult to quarrel with such laudable concepts. It is surely right that patients should know the services which it is hoped to make available to them. It strengthens the relentless fight with the past historical model of paternalism, in which all the rights lie with the doctor and few, if any, have belonged to the patient. Nevertheless, there seems to have been an insufficient recognition that rights also bring responsibilities; that defining the rights of one party to the transaction, without defining the rights of other parties to the transaction, is inherently unfair and likely to lead to friction and frustration. Even worse has been a preoccupation with rights which can be measured, rather than services which are less tangible in nature. The initiative has ground into the sand of interminable arguments about the length of waiting lists and how quickly a patient can be seen. Other factors, such as the quality of medical care provided, have faded into the background. Moreover, have patient's rights been enhanced if they are weighed and measured within a few minutes of arriving at the outpatient clinic, but then wait over an hour for the medical consultation which was the main purpose of their visit? It can be seen, however, that patients' rights have been a key factor in the development of the paradigm shift.

Medical Technology

The advances in medical technology in the last fifty years are evident to all and have themselves created new ethical problems which doctors and society as a whole must address. Moreover, there are worrying parallels with the Nazi era, which leave no room for complacency. That era was characterized by the application of specific technologies to the pursuit of political objectives. There is increasing concern that the growth in technologies over the last fifty years is now beginning to drive a system which, once harnessed to a political philosophy, would become unstoppable and create far worse problems than have ever previously been faced. Simon Davies,[5] in a book appropriately entitled *Big Brother*, outlines a whole series of technological threats, which seem increasingly to be accepted as normal. The incorporation of machine parts to enable the body to function less inefficiently, brings the science fiction nightmare of 'Cybermen' nearer to reality. Personal privacy is being eroded in frightening ways by increasing demands that individual citizens be numbered and categorized. Personal health information is increasingly leaking into other agencies. The Department of Health in the United Kingdom has recently introduced a system which allows identifiable patient information to be freely transmitted throughout the National Health Service (NHS), in order to operate the 'internal market' of the present health care system. The privatization of some services within the National Health Service and the private funding of new developments in the NHS are again creating situations in which highly personal and confidential information is leaking into the hands of insurance companies, pharmaceutical and other companies, interested in keeping detailed databases of individuals. In response to professional criticisms of the NHS computer network a feasibility study was undertaken to look at encrypting such material during transmission. The proposals which emerged created a system which was designed to be freely accessible to the security services!

The ethical approach of health care workers depends fundamentally on the issue of consent. If individuals have freely consented to this exchange of information about themselves, there can be no criticism of it. Indeed there may be occasional benefits. Ready access to a patient's medical history when s/he arrives, unconscious, in an emergency department may be life saving, although the evidence is currently lacking. However, in its recent circular announcing the new network the Department of Health continued to insist that the very act of signing up for medical care in the United Kingdom 'assumes' that the individual has consented to the release of personal health information for whatsoever purpose health service managers consider to be in the patient's best interests, or those of the Service. There is no provision whatsoever for a patient who specifically objects to the release of such information. No doubt such a patient would be reassured at the time that their wishes would be respected, but in reality such an assurance would be valueless.

Simon Davies also examines the increasing use of camera surveillance, often as a more efficient and less expensive way of policing neighborhoods. Yet this technology is gradually eroding personal private space at an alarming rate. Similarly, the telephone system no longer gives personal confidentiality. Cellular phones can be overheard by others and electronic surveillance within cable systems has existed for many years.

It is hardly surprising therefore that there is increasing suspicion of technology in all its forms and of medical technology in particular. Medical technology has brought great benefits to individual patients, but has often led down paths which the majority of citizens do not wish to travel. Artificial fertility is the classic example, but the development of xeno-transplantation and the incorporation of machinery into human tissue, to which reference has already been made, are other examples. *Institutions* have been slow to respond to these concerns.

The Influence of Institutions

The General Medical Council

The General Medical Council (GMC) has a responsibility for supervising undergraduate medical training in the United Kingdom. It is also developing a role in aspects of post graduate and specialist training. The GMC was established in 1858 and provides appropriately qualified medical practitioners with a 'license to practice'. After a brief flurry of interest in medical ethics after the Nuremberg trials, the subject has gradually been crowded out of an increasingly scientifically orientated medical curriculum. Even more worryingly, the practice which was formerly routine in almost all medical schools, of requiring all newly qualified doctors to make some kind of ethical commitment at the time of graduation, seems almost to have disappeared. Perceived as a 'outdated piece of mumbo-jumbo' its purpose and necessity appears to have been forgotten. Thus at the very time when medical advances were creating unprecedented ethical dilemmas, which have attracted the increasing interest of philosophers and lawyers, the profession itself has become singularly ill-equipped to discuss such matters in a coherent, logical way.

The General Medical Council has become increasingly concerned by this apparent gap in undergraduate medical training and has now required all medical schools to review their ethical teaching as part of a more comprehensive review of the curriculum. The GMC has now been given additional powers by Parliament to review the progress of doctors who consistently fall below an acceptable level of performance. Previously its powers were limited to those doctors guilty of gross misconduct on a single or small number of occasions. This power is provoking a wider debate on what makes a good doctor. Galen believed that all medical practitioners should be trained both in medical science and in philosophy.[6] The present preoccupation with Medicine as a science based subject, almost to the exclusion of the humanities, challenges this concept of a broadly educated person. British doctors seem to be bored by the humanities, perhaps by unwitting adherence to Cartesian philosophies, yet Galen's concept of what makes a good doctor has recently received confirmation from an unlikely source. Using the performance ratings required during the five terms in internship (first postgraduate year), some Australian workers at the University of Newcastle, in New South Wales showed that the only factor predictive of high grades in these assessments was the study of the humanities prior to entrance into medical school.[7] The General Medical Council has tried to identify what it believes to make a good doctor. In 1982 it was empowered to set up a professional standards committee to review professional ethics. This committee has now published four attractive booklets (*Good Medical Practice; Advertising; Confidentiality; HIV and AIDS: The Ethical Considerations*), under the general title of *The Duties of a Doctor*. It seems likely that these documents will form the basis of a formal ethical code, to which British doctors have traditionally been opposed.[8]

The Universities

Medical schools within the universities have been slow to respond to the increasing demand for more ethical training for medical students. There is little doubt that the interest is there. Medical students show a keen interest in moral and ethical dilemmas and many voluntarily attend the various medical groups which have been set up to address such issues. Formal recognition within the curriculum has, with some honorable exceptions, been less common. In 1984 a working party was established under the chairmanship of Sir Desmond Pond 'to express and illustrate its understanding of 'medical ethics teaching' and to identify existing teaching arrangements' Its findings were not encouraging.[9] Even where fifteen hours was formally allocated to the subject they were at lunch times. One of an eight hour series was held from 3.30pm on Fridays. This is hardly a time when medical students will be eager to learn! The working party concluded that 'the importance of the subject is clearly reflected in the hour or day set aside for it'.

Some action has undoubtedly resulted from the report but as recently as 1995, a postal survey involving 85% of the Deans of medical schools still found that few formally examined ethics as part of the medical final examinations. Of those that did ethical issues occupied a minor part of the examinations. There was little evidence to suggest that examiners are given any significant instruction to consider ethical issues when assessing students undertaking those examinations. There are signs that this is changing. Three professors of medical ethics are known to have been appointed in recent years and senior lectureships and lectureships are becoming more common. Pressures on the curriculum remain, however, and cynics will point out that unless a subject is formally examined, students are likely to accord it far less importance in undergraduate training.

Among the principal problems is knowing what should be taught and how the teaching should be given. It seems doubtful if formal ethical theory will commend itself to a student body mostly well schooled in the natural sciences rather than the humanities. Moreover, lawyers and philosophers may theorize, but doctors actually have to take the clinical decisions.[10] There are some fundamental differences in these situations. Thus a philosopher may deny that there is any moral difference between active killing and withholding potentially life saving treatment. Almost all doctors, however, accept that the difference is fundamental. Some universities are now incorporating ethical issues into the relevant subject teaching. Many believe, however, that ethics is best taught by experienced clinicians, competent in their field, in the context of bedside clinical teaching. This 'master/apprentice' model seems to offer the most appropriate way forward for the future.

British Medical Association

The contribution of the British Medical Association (BMA) as an *institution* has been in a series of publications, which have increased in number and complexity over the last fifty years. Beginning with a small booklet *Ethics and Members of the Medical Profession*, which was capable of carriage in the doctor's top jacket pocket, a continuous sequence of publications has continued up to the current 374 page book *Medical Ethics Today*. A companion volume, *Rights and Responsibilities of Doctors*, was published in 1988 and is now in its second edition. A whole series of books and booklets have been published on a wide variety of ethical matters in the present decade, not least a major book on doctors' involvement in torture, *Medicine Betrayed*, published in 1992. In addition, members have access to some twenty five guidance notes on specific matters of individual practice. Over the period the unmistakable trend of these documents has been away from paternalism, and towards the concept of autonomy and the patient's right to choose the treatment s/he wishes to receive. The Association has been at the forefront of this changed approach.

Although British doctors have traditionally rejected formal ethical codes, the British Medical Association was instrumental in encouraging the World Medical Association to produce its *Declaration of Geneva* in 1948. In 1995 a resolution was passed at the Annual Representative Meeting of the BMA, stating that all doctors should make a 'formal commitment to an updated Hippocratic Oath'. It is hoped that the work arising from a need to update the original *Declaration*, in order to implement this resolution, will be done in sufficient time to secure the agreement of the World Medical Association to issue a revised declaration on its fiftieth anniversary in 1998. Although most British doctors would not necessarily regard such codes and declarations as binding in all circumstances, there has been concern by statements from doctors involved with oppressive regimes that they have never agreed to abide by any ethical code and cannot therefore be judged to have broken one. Similar sentiments have been expressed by a doctor in the British press.[11] A meeting of all the medical *institutions* in 1994[12] expressed the view that medical graduates should make some kind of formal commitment to ethical values early in their career training.

The British Medical Association has been actively concerned with doctors in oppressive regimes. In 1986 it produced its first report on the involvement of doctors in torture. In 1992 a further working party produced *Medicine Betrayed*, which has now been translated into a number of languages, as a result of its wide ranging review of the responsibilities of doctors in such situations. The BMA has also set up a human rights group to examine the issue again and to produce a further publication. The Association has been closely involved with human rights abuses in Yugoslavia and the present campaign to ban the use of land mines.

The question needs to be asked, although rarely discussed, whether a regime which is restricting health care resources available to all its citizens can reasonably be described as 'oppressive'. As the problem of limited resources becomes daily more evident in health care systems, doctors are constrained in the treatments which they can offer. The apparently endless demand by health care managers for improved efficiency and reduced costs inevitably results in staff reductions. Recently a study[13] of the use of neuroleptics in care homes showed that 25% of residents were receiving such drugs. Yet in 88% of these cases the use of the drug fell outside American guidelines concerning their appropriateness. It is difficult to resist the impression that patients may be controlled by pharmacological means, in order to reduce the number of staff necessary to care for them. Free market philosophies are considered by Stout[14] to represent an important and potential threat to ethical practice and it is at least arguable that doctors have an ethical responsibility to protest and for doctors in other countries to make expressions of support when colleagues in a particular country are 'oppressed' in this way.

Medical Colleges

The medical colleges in the United Kingdom have made a number of contributions to improve the standards of ethical practice over the last 50 years. The following are broadly illustrative:

- research;
- fraud and misconduct in research;
- clinical definitions; and
- action by particular Colleges.

Research

In 1931 guidelines for medical experimentation with humans were promulgated in Germany by the Reich Minister of the Interior, following earlier concerns about scientific methods in Germany.[15] It is curious that no mention of these guidelines was made during the trials at Nuremberg of those Nazi doctors involved in human experiments at Dachau and elsewhere. These experiments have recently been reviewed. Angell[16] concluded that the hypothermia experiments were 'scientifically worthless'. Berger[17] managed to piece together some of the Dachau hypothermia experiments even though the records themselves were destroyed. He concluded that between 200 and 300 victims were involved and that much scientific observation was simply not recorded. At the trials an entirely new code (the *Nuremberg Code*) was formulated whilst the prosecutions were in progress, probably by an American psychiatrist. Yet in the following two decades both American and English doctors working in their own countries flagrantly disregarded the *Nuremberg Code* in their own human research. H.K. Beecher in the USA published his concerns in the New England Journal of Medicine.[18] Pappworth decided to appeal to the general public through his book *Human Guinea Pigs*.[19] The political pressure so generated resulted in the Royal College of Physicians establishing a working party to review the ethical approval of all research undertaken locally on human subjects. Its report recommended the formation of local research ethics committees in every health district and these proposals were immediately implemented by the Department of Health and Social Security. The College has since twice updated these guidelines. Almost twenty years after their establishment, however, these committees are very patchy in their effectiveness. Working practices within the committees often leave much to be desired.[20] The proposals for ethical approval by these committees differed from the *Nuremberg Code* insofar that they allowed research on children and incompetent patients not able to give consent. Since the research committees were largely dominated by medical members, they perpetuate the concept that doctors must primarily decide what scientific research is 'ethical'. It is at least arguable that research on patients unable to give consent requires a higher standard of scientific validity and a reasonable expectation that its findings will in fact subsequently be published.

Fraud and Misconduct in Research

There is increasing evidence that fraud and misconduct in medical research is more common than previously assumed. The Royal Colleges have again been asked to take the lead in establishing a system through which suspicious cases can be investigated.[21] In a situation which would not have been unfamiliar to Pappworth, however, there are powerful groups arguing that such a process is quite unnecessary. Progress is therefore extremely slow.

The drugs industry has, however, been far more vigorous in its approach and has rigorously investigated any incidents drawn to its attention. The General Medical Council has been equally vigorous in imposing heavy penalties on doctors found to be involved in such practices. Erasure from the Medical Register has been the usual penalty.

Clinical Definitions

The Royal Colleges of Physicians were instrumental in producing a definition of 'brain death', when advances in cardio-pulmonary support disguised the fact that an already dead patient was continuing to be ventilated. If only for the purposes of transplantation, it was important to know when the patient could be clearly identified as dead.

More recently, the Royal College of Physicians in London responded to a request from the House of Lords to define the condition known as 'persistent vegetative state'. It has now produced advice concerning the clinical criteria and suggested guidelines for management.

Individual Colleges

Many of these initiatives have either originated in the conference of medical colleges and faculties, or from the Royal College of Physicians in London. The Royal College of Gynaecologists, however, chose medical ethics as its theme for discussion in 1994. The findings of a three day workshop were published in book form[22] for consideration by members and fellows throughout the United Kingdom. The senate of the Royal Colleges of Surgeons has established a working party to produce guidelines on ethical practice in surgery and the Royal College of Radiologists is also considering mechanisms to address the need for ethical guidance. The Royal College of Psychiatrists played an important role in exposing the abuses of Soviet psychiatry. These, by no means comprehensive, examples illustrate that the royal colleges have been an effective *institution* for producing changes in ethical approaches.

In summary, therefore, the recognition of patients' rights has been the principal factor in the United Kingdom, promoting the paradigm shift, with a number of medical institutions playing an important role, both in that process and also through independent initiatives. In contrast, education has played a minor, almost non-existent, role throughout most of the period, although there are welcome signs at the present time that this situation may be about to change.

References

1   Rivett, G (1986), The Development of the London Hospital System 1823-1982. King Edward's Hospital Fund for London, Oxford University Press.

2   Jonsen, Albert R (1990), The New Medicine and the Old Ethics. Cambridge Mass., Harvard University Press, p.95.

3   Peppin, J (1995), Physician Values and Value Neutrality in Bioethics and the Future of Medicine: A Christian Appraisal. Kilner, J F; Cameron, N MdeS; Schiedermayer, D L. Grand Rapids Michegan, W B Eerdmans Publishing Company.

4   Agich, George J (1993), Autonomy and Long Term Care. New York, Oxford University Press, p. 161.

5   Davies, Simon (1996), Big Brother; Britain's Web of Surveillance and the New Technological Order. London, Pan Books.

6   Temkin, Owsei (1991), Hippocrates in a World of Pagans and Christians. Baltimore and London, The John Hopkins University Press.

7   Rolfe, I E; Pearson, S; Powis, D A; and Smith, A J (1995), Time for a review of admission to medical school? *The Lancet* **346** pp1329-1333.

8   Report of the Committee of Inquiry into the Regulation of the Medical Profession (1975), pp91 & 92. London, HMSO Cmnd 6018.

9   Institute of Medical Ethics (1987), Report of a Working Party on the Teaching of Medical Ethics. London, IME Publications.

10   Maclean, A (1993), The Elimination of Morality. London and New York, Routledge.

11   Leigh, J (1993), 'No obligations' letter to *The Independent* newspaper 19th November 1993.

12   British Medical Association (1994), Core Values for the Medical Profession in the 21st Century. Report of a conference held on 3/4 November 1994.

13   McGrath, A M and Jackson, A (1996), Survey of Neuroleptic Prescribing in Residents of Nursing Homes in Glasgow. *British Medical Journal* **312** pp611-612.

14   Stout, J (1988), *Ethics after Babel*. Cambridge, James Clarke & Co.

15   Grodin, A (1992), The Nazi Doctors and the Nuremburg Code. New York, Oxford University Press.

16   Angell, M (1990), The Nazi hypothermia experiments and unethical research today. *New England Journal of Medicine* (editorial) **322** pp1462-4.

17   Berger, R L (1990), Nazi Science - The Dachau hypothermia experiments. *New England Journal of Medicine* **322** pp1435-1440.

18   Beecher, H K (1966), Ethics and Clinical Research. *New England Journal of Medicine* **274** pp1354-1360.

19   Pappworth, M H (1967), Human Guinea Pigs - Experimentation on Man. London, Routledge & Paul.

20 Neuberger, J (1992), Ethics and Health Care - the role of research ethics committees in the United Kingdom *Research Report* 13. London, King's Fund Institute.

21 Lock, S (1995), Lessons from the Pearce affair: Handling scientific fraud. *British Medical Journal* **310** pp1547-8.

22 Bewley, S and Ward, S H - editors (1994), Ethics in Obstetrics and Gynaecology. London, RCOG Press.

19 Paradigm Changes in Health Care Systems and in Relations Between Patients and (Para)medical Professions in Italy

Antonio Spagnolo

Soon after World War II, the recognition of patients' rights was laid down in the constitution of the Republic of Italy in 1947. In particular, Article 32 protects health as a fundamental right of the individual and, in the interest of society, guarantees free treatment to the poor and the right to refuse treatment except when required by a court order; but the law cannot by any means overstep the limits defining respect for human beings.[1] Thus, in the Constitution health has become a fundamental human right to be guaranteed in relations affecting both private life and dealings with public officials. This principle can also be inferred by a number of judgments pronounced by the [*Italian*]*Cour de Cassation* (Supreme Court of Appeals) and the Constitutional Court. One judgment from 1979 especially confirmed the absolute and primary nature of the right to health, in the general sense of the term, as a right to mental and physical integrity, the violation of which ("biological damage") must be indemnified .

Thus, even before the writing of the national code of medical deontology (which was not drawn up until 1954), the personalistic and solidaristic foundation of the Constitution had led to the recognition of several ethical principles which were intended to nurture the nascent health-care system in the form of the broadest social security scheme to inspire all Western countries, though in varying ways, after World War II.

Certainly, the ethical dimension had always been thriving within the medical profession and had been perceptible in Italy even before the war, even though it had been separate from deontology, yet it had limited itself to just a few topics, such as abortion, sexuality, and procreation.

During the first phase of development of the health care system, however, it was not the ethical dimension that emerged, but rather the social one. It aimed more than anything else at pedagogical instruction of health-care personnel in order to encourage attitudes that would increase socialization and the use of this system. The medical profession gradually became propelled by strong impulses along the lines of public welfare and, as the awareness of rights grew, evolved into an essential guarantor of social well-being.[2] The guarantee of the patients' rights was thus entirely left open for interpretation of deontological codes by health-care staff. Still, professional deontology itself had to confront positive norms dictated by the state by formulating a substantial "health law" as health-care assistance began to become more organized.

The public ethical dimension began to emerge noticeably at the end of the 1970s during and after the debates in Parliament about the *Health Reform Act* that led to the founding of the National Health Service.[3] At that time, special emphasis was placed on the idea of a constitutional "right to health" as a fundamental right, which was then written into the Article 1 of the constitutive law of the National Health Service in 1978; patients' rights were also given specific legal content.

All of these events took an unexpected turn with regard to the decentralization of health care by local governments such that the latter enacted local laws in this field pursuant to statute 117 of the civil code. The two principle sources of inspiration for health reform were normative unification in terms of federal law and decentralization guaranteeing the respect and effective protection of localities and autonomous social units. Thus, the significance of legislative norms and regulations increased by degrees to the detriment of the domain reserved for the trust involved in the relationship between health-care personnel and patients, a relationship that is inherent to the pillars of medicine itself. The cause of this shift can be attributed to the "tarnishing" of ethical and deontological values brought about by various social factors, such as the tendency, present in all modern societies, towards greater freedom of expression and a plurality of ethical inspirations.

In addition, in Italy as in other countries, a movement (both in terms of informing the public and making legislative proposals)[4] has evolved in support of "patients' rights", the definition and legitimation of which were a reaction to international human rights documents.[5] This movement is becoming deeply seated within the modern concept of personal health management, a concept that compensates for the "subordinate" role of the patient with regard to the "culturally dominant" role of the physician, transforming the patient into an "active participant," as everyone should be when the improvement of one's own physical, mental, and emotional well-being are involved. On the one hand, this view holds that everyone has a right and the duty to be healthy, i.e. the liberty and dignity of every human being is to be respected and safeguarded within the framework of society;[6] on the other hand, this means attempting to reassess the "subject" of assistance as a function of an improved "quality of life" as of the moment when the patient receives medical assistance.

The movement mentioned above has taken on various forms in Italy, primarily in the "tribunal for patients' rights", which has in recent years drawn up a number of "charters for the ill".[7] These charters are subject to, on the one hand, the influence of local needs arising from specific conditions of assistance, and, on the other, they also comprise general principles. Other movements by voluntary groups have also been active in affirming specific humanitarian principles and the respect of the human being within the scope of medical assistance, even if they do not formulate specific documents extending beyond their mandates.[8]

It should be noted here that the development of the modern health system has led to ever greater levels of well-being and health protection in the broad sense of the word, which in turn implies that the distinction between "needs" and "desires" is at times difficult to make. Hence, the increasing demand in quality and the increasingly complex bureaucracy in conjunction with it have challenged the fundamental role that deontological "rules" have played up until now.

These factors taken as a whole have induced legislators to come up with laws defining more precisely and unambiguously those domains that must be considered as being the "rights" of the citizen within the scope of health care and to transform these domains into "users rights"; i.e. to attempt to replace the "abstract right" of the citizen with a "right that is called for under the conditions provided for by the system used by the citizen".

All of this contrasts sharply with other countries, especially in the English-speaking world, where the focus, at least initially, was on an ethical development of control mechanisms designed to prevent excessive surveillance by the public authorities. In reality, legislative intervention in Italy proved necessary in the face of the serious functional difficulties often occurring in medical centers, such as the neglect of patients or the blatant violation of the principle of respect for human beings. Still, the legislature has been urged to intervene in behalf of the training for health-care workers in order to stress the importance of the education and practice of professional deontology.

Training in medical ethics also has changed over the years: teaching bioethics in an interdisciplinary fashion, which extends the domain of reflection from the professional context to the greater one involving the "biological realm", has joined the teaching of deontology and professional ethics, usually taught by physicians specialized in forensic medicine. Thus, the 1986 bill reforming the organizational structure of university studies in medicine and surgery[9] introduced bioethics as a university subject, initially creating a problem as to the definition of its contents, diversity, and the relations between deontology and medical ethics.

Some distinguished scholars in Italian forensic medicine looked on apprehensively at first when an attempt was made to take bioethics off the *alma mater* of medicolegal thought that had governed it for centuries in Italy. According to them, this act had not taken account of the fact that, in order to deal with the delicate problems of medical ethics, one had to be, above all, a doctor. Thus, they concluded that the teaching of medical deontology alone would have been sufficient not only for the needs of teaching the subject of ethics to doctors, but also as a basis for correct conduct regarding the law.[10] Somewhat later, the dialectic confrontation was allayed in a document (*Il Documento di Erice*) written in 1991 by an interdisciplinary study group composed of teachers of bioethics and forensic medicine.[11] They resolved to provide an instrument of interpretation and explanation stating more clearly the differences and similarities involving bioethics, deontology, and forensic medicine in terms of finality, instruments, nature of competence, and qualification of instructors. Thus, this document provided bioethics with a conclusiveness that could be practiced as a basis for personal conduct, future rights, and future professional codes.

This document, on the other hand, assigned deontology the task of probing into the nature of the medical profession and thus imparting norms and rules of conduct closely linked with the findings of bioethics. Thus, it was decided that it would be more convenient to allocate bioethics instruction to the domain of forensic medicine alongside the instruction of medical deontology.

Certainly, only within the vast field of bioethical considerations could the progressive passage in our country from a medical discipline founded on a paternalistic model to one more open to the "choice" of patient autonomy be perceived.[12]

Along with the debate within bioethics, there has also been some contemplation within the humanities regarding the philosophy of medicine, rather than philosophy in medicine, as being a postulate for the considerations in bioethics. As of the 1980s, enlightened Italian doctors have stressed the need for a new identity for the medical profession in light of the increasing gaps within it engendered by the fragmentation of knowledge and the bureaucratization of medical assistance.

Aware of the fact that adequate training in the fields of biomedicine and clinical medicine is a prerequisite for correct professional practice, in a specific document (*Bioethics and Training in the Health Sector* from September, 1991) the National Committee on Bioethics[13] referred to below recommended that more attention be given to all health-care personnel, whether at the university level or otherwise, by teaching bioethics in their classes on health care. To this end, the Minister of the University of Scientific Research and Technology along with the Minister of Health recently formulated the Decree of July 24, 1996 requiring that 14 of the courses for the University Diploma (UD) be absolved in the Faculty of Medicine and Surgery and that applied bioethics be taught in the final year of study. The decree, however, leaves out for unknown reasons the "basic" instruction in bioethics in the early years, thus only providing for an extremely simplified study of bioethics. It is certainly difficult for the students to learn how to apply ethics and bioethical criteria after one practical course without having been instructed in the fundamentals and ethics theories. The National Committee of Bioethics, incidentally, recommended that students be made aware of the reality of the global health-care system at an early stage; it is thought that such early exposure to the issues would strengthen humanitarian motives and help students to develop an overall view of their patients rather than one that is fragmented into specialties. Some schools of medicine and surgery go beyond the National Committee's recommendations, autonomously teaching bioethics in the first year of studies by stressing the historical and humanistic aspect of the discipline and advancing in subsequent years to specific problems involving deontological or forensic medicine.

The National Committee recommended that such an introduction to bioethics be instituted at the high school level before the actual preparations for the medical profession have begun. Indeed, over the last few years, a considerable number of bioethics courses have been offered to teachers and schoolchildren all the way down to the grade-school level. The training in health-care ethics is rounded off by advanced post-graduate courses in bioethics and by the possibility of earning a doctorate in bioethical and deontological research and medical ethics at some Italian universities.

The contribution of such training in bioethics for doctors was decisive in drawing up a new medical code of deontology (June, 1995).[14] This code differs from others in that it focuses more attention on patients' and citizens' rights and adopts measures based on general bioethics principles founded on the teaching of the inalienable values and primary rights of each individual. In particular, it conspicuously stresses the role of the patient as a co-star in a medical performance, a role that had at times been ruled out by the unacceptable paternalism of traditional ethics. The new code provides for a greater interpersonal relationship between doctors and patients from the moment the doctor begins informing the patient about the diagnosis and the decision for a certain therapy while respecting, as much as possible, the patient's informed and explicit consent.

Some institutions have contributed to formulating a response to the changes that have taken place between health-care personnel and patients, the first and foremost being the centers and scientific institutes of bioethics that have sparked a number of initiatives with regard to university instruction and informing the public.

In Italy, medical morals pronounced by the Catholic Church have also played an important role by exalting the so-called Hippocratic Oath through the concept of the sacredness of human life.

This moral doctrine has been enriched as well by the intervention of the last few pontiffs, such as Pope Pius XII, in his address to doctors, and his successors[15] as a result of three concomitant facts: 1) crimes against humanity, especially those against the innocent, during the last world war; 2) the development of the idea of "human rights", to which the Church also adhered and, as of Pope John XXIII, contributed; and 3) and the development of medical science and technologies in the field of biomedicine.

In its doctrines, the Catholic Church has always respected the benevolent discoveries and the therapeutic resources of medical science and has used them in its hospitals. On the other hand, it has also seen in doctors a sort of sacred representative or "minister of life", as they are called on to help the living, heal the sick, and ease suffering. Quite recently, in 1995, the Pontifical Council for the Pastoral of the Health Services published a *Charter for Health-Care Personnel*.[16] Written in the form of a code of ethics, this document briefly discusses the most important topics in medical ethics and summarizes the teaching of the Catholic Magisterium on this subject. The objective of the charter is to guarantee the ethical fidelity of health-care professionals, i.e. the choices and conduct that shape one's service in behalf of life.

The above-mentioned National Committee on Bioethics, which was set up in 1990 by decree of the president of the Council of Ministers, also played a considerable role. This Committee has produced a number of documents. Beside the ones on ethics training of health-care personnel and the rapport between health-care staff and patients, as mentioned above, there are documents on organ transplants, the final phase of life, experiments on human subjects, medically assisted reproduction, prenatal diagnostic care, as well as other subjects.

In keeping with the tenor of the institutional decree, the National Committee has a number of tasks, not only in the formulation of expert opinions and suggesting ways of solving ethical and legal problems in order to influence the legislature, but also in promoting the formulation of codes of professional conduct. Frankly, up until now, a code has yet to be drafted; instead, there has been a noticeable conflict between the Federation of the Professional Organization of Doctors and the Committee, because the Federation thought that the Committee had touched on questions that strictly concerned the code of professional conduct although this was not in its mandate.

Moreover, the alleged "imbalance" in the structure of the Committee itself has lessened the Committee's authority with regard to public opinion concerning highly ethical issues such as medically assisted reproduction and the status of the human embryo.[17] Because of such problems, to date, instead of there being one set of documents in agreement with each other, the Committee has only produced documents with conflicting arguments.

Recently, a bill for organizing the structure of the National Committee on Bioethics was presented to the Italian Parliament to assure that the Committee have a well-balanced plurality. Said bill was amended several times by subsequent Italian governments. The reason for this was that setting up truly just quotas was viewed as a problem of structure and that it was considered impossible to create organizations that are truly neutral. The mistake that is often made, actually, is that more responsibility is given to an advisory panel than its opinions merit. Instead, such responsibility should be given to the public and the lawmaker who are the targets of the Committee's opinions.[18]

The institution of a number of local ethical committees over the past few years has also redirected our attention to the problem of experiments on human subjects, which has not yet been regulated by any legislation. In particular, Community Directive 91/507 pertaining to the standards of Good Clinical Practice by Italy's Ministry of Health led to the founding of ethics committees for evaluating the protocols of clinical trials.[19] At first, these committees were viewed with some skepticism, especially by physicians; in this case, as well, it must be noted that the committees were chiefly accepted because of the concern for civil and penal responsibility.

Soon the vast discrepancy in the operative procedures adopted by the different local committees could be observed due to the lack of reglementation to define such procedures. In order to overcome this difficulty, a National Federation of Ethics Committees was set up to give the ethics committees themselves accreditation based on their conformity with operative procedures as derived from a number of international guidelines.

Finally, in March of 1996, the military health administration headquarters of the Ministry of National Defense set up an ethics committee which I have the honor to preside. This committee has been commissioned with revising the protocols for biomedical trials to be conducted by the military health administration as well as the protocols for applied diagnostics and therapy in military health activities.[20] Article 1 of this committee's statutes specifies the Nuremberg Code as being one of the documents that should serve as a guide when the committee formulates its expert opinions. This Committee's sphere of activity is particularly interesting in light of the violations committed, even after Nuremberg, regarding the requirement that consent be obtained for experiments conducted on combat troops or soldiers ready for combat. Other problems could arise in addition to those mentioned above: Where do we draw the line between experimentation *per se* and experiments with a specifically therapeutic or prophylactic intent? How can the problem of the role of the military doctor be solved who is faced with military situations that run contrary to professional obligations? There are still other problems.[21]

In conclusion, it seems that Italy's health-care system generally has oriented itself *chiefly* towards research, in which daily (para)medical activities have a clear legal status, rather than towards setting up deontological and ethical guidelines.

Nevertheless, the need for new rules goes beyond governmental and cultural borders and requires that supranational organizations begin to wield their power. Moreover, it is inconceivable that governmental legislation could cover all of the particularities and special situations that often occur in the dealings between health-care personnel and patients. As a result, the ethicodeontological code still is the preferred instrument for new indications in new areas of intervention.

Notes

1. Mariotti P.- Massaraki G.- Rizzi R., *I diritti dei malati*, Giuffré, 1993; Pittau F. (a cura di), *Il diritto alla salute*, Inas-Cisl, 1989.

2. AA.VV., *Guida all'esercizio professionale per i medici-chirurghi e gli odontoiatri*, Torino, Ed. Medico-Scientifiche, 1994 (updated 1996).

3. Legge 23 dicembre 1978, n.833. *Istituzione del Servizio Sanitario Nazionale* (GU n. 360, SO del 28 dic. 1978). Riordino del Servizio Sanitario Nazionale: Decreto Legislativo 1992, n. 502. *Revisione della disciplina in materia sanitaria a norma dell'art. 1 della Legge 23 ottobre 1992, n. 421* (GU n. 305,SO del 30 dicembre 1992) amended by D.L.7 dicembre 1993, n. 517 (GU n. 293, SO del 15 dicembre 1993). Ziglioli R. (a cura di), *Riforma sanitaria e comunità cristiana*, Brezzo di Bedere, Ed. Salcom, 1979.

4. Disegno di Legge n. 1917: *Tutela dei diritti del malato con particolare riguardo alla condizione di degenza.*

5. *Convenzione internazionale relativa ai diritti economici, sociali e culturali* del 1976; *Raccomandazione dell'Assemblea del Consiglio d'Europa sui diritti dei malati e dei morenti* del 1976; *Carta del malato negli ospedali* della Cee. 1979; *Rapporto del Comitato di esperti per i problemi guiridici del settore sanitario* del Consiglio d'Europa, 1984; *Guida Europea di etica e di comportamento professionale medico* della Conferenza internazionale degli ordini dei medici e degli organismi similari, 1980; *Risoluzioni sui diritti dei malati* del Parlamento Europeo, 1984.

6. In accordance with article 32 of the Italian Constitution and article 1 of law n. 833/1978.

7. Tribunale per i Diritti del malato, *Carta dei 33 diritti del cittadino*, Dichiarazioni conclusive della prima sessione pubblica tenutasi a Roma il 29 giugno 1980.

8. Voluntary work is provided for in laws n. 685/1975, n. 833/1978, and n. 266/1991.

9. Tabella XVIII - Corso di Laurea in Medicina e Chirurgia, passed with DPR 28 February 1986, n. 95; Sgreccia E.- Spangnolo A.G., *La bioetica nel corso di laurea in medicina e chirurgia dell'Universita Cattolica del S.Cuore. Esperienze e proposte*, "Medicina e Morale", 1996, n. 4, pp. 639-654.

10. A. Vv., *Atti del XXX Congresso Nazionale della Società Italiana di Medicina Legale e delle Assicurazioni*, XII Convegno di criminologia e psichiatria forense, (a cura di Vimercati, Colonna e Vinci), Bari, 27-30 September 1989, Graphiservice, Bari, 1989, vol. I.

11. Società Italiana di Medicina Legale e delle Assicurazioni, *Il Documento di Erice sui rapporti della Bioetica e della Deontologia Medica con la Medicina Legale*, 53rd Course "New Trends in forensic haematology and genetics. Bioethical problems", (Erice, 18-21 February 1991), in "Medicina e Morale", 1991, 4.

12. Sgreccia E., *Manuale di Bioetica, I. Fondamenti ed etica biomedica*, Milano, Vita e Pensiero, 1994.

13. Comitato Nazionale per la Bioetica, *Bioetica e formazione nel sistema sanitario* (7. September 1991), Presidenza del Consiglio dei Ministri - Dipartimento per l'Informazione e l'Editoria, Roma.

14. Introna F.-Tantalo M.-Colafigli A., *Il Codice di deontologia medica correlato a leggi ed a documenti*, Napoli, Padova, Liviana Medicina, 1992. Iadecola G., *Il nuovo codice di deontologia medica*, Cedma, Padova, 1996.

15. Pio XII, *Discourcsi e radiomessagi*, voll, 1-20, Città del Vaticano, 1959. Giovanni XXIII, *Discorsi, messagi; colloqui del S. Padre Giovanni XXIII*, voll. 1-5, Città del Vaticano, 1967. Paolo VI, *Insegnamenti di Paolo VI*, voll. 1-16, Città del Vaticano, 1979. Giovanni Paolo II, *Isegnamenti di Giovanni Paolo II*, voll. 1-14, Città del Vati-

cano, 1993. Concilio Vatincano II, Constituzione Pastorale *Gaudium et Spes*, in Enchiridion Vaticanum, 1, Dehoniane, Bologna, 1985, 1, nn. 41-43.

16   Pontificio Consiglio della Pastorale per gli operatori sanitari, *Carta degli operatori sanitari*, Città del Vaticano, 1995.

17   Comitato Nazionale per la Bioetica, *La fecondazione assistita. Documenti del Comitato Nazionale per la Bioetica*, Presidenza del Consiglio dei Ministri, Dipartimento per l'Informazione e l'Editoria, 17 febbraio 1995; Comitato Nazionale per la Bioetica, *La statuto dell'embrione umano*, 1996 (in press).

18   Bill n. 782, proposed on 26 June 1996: *Organizzazzione e dicsiplina del Comitato nazionale per la Bioetica*.

19   Decreto Ministeriale del 27 aprile 1992, Gazzetta Ufficiale della Repubblica Italiana n. 139 del 15.6.92.

20   Decreto del Ministro della Difesa del 13 marzo 1996.

21   Spagnolo A.G., *Necessità, opportnità, utilità della istituzione di un Comnitato Etico presso la Direzione Generale della Sanità Minitare*, Giornale di Medicina Militare, 1996 (in press).

20 The Recognition of Patients' Rights, Especially the Mentally Ill, by International Organizations and in the Jurisprudence of the European Convention on Human Rights

Thomaïs Douraki

Introduction

Since very recently, the mentally and physically ill were considered as beings that should be pitied by society. The evolution of this concept and scientific progress have turned them into individuals that, though "different", can be integrated into the community and thus have rights. This is especially true of the mentally ill; the present tendency is to avoid commitment as medical treatment as much as possible by integrating them into society and by giving them the possibility of living their difference within a context where their rights are respected. The idea of commitment as a treatment, does not aim to deprive these patients of their fundamental rights. Deprivation of liberty, event sufficiently important itself, does not justify the limitation of the person's rights.[1,2]

The existing relation between mental illness, compulsoring treatment of the mentally ill, and the law has led to the creation of texts whose purpose is the legal protection of these persons against abuse. ("A fair law about persons of unsound mind, should prevent the illegal confinement of those who are not mad", wrote P.F. Girard in 1883.)

Detention, in the context of the treatment of the mentally ill, has, actually, two main caracteristics:

a) the limitation of the involuntary treatment except as a last resort and in emergency situations; and
b) the periodical review during detention, carried out by competent authorities who, together with the doctors responsible for the treatment, should decide whether the involuntary treatment should be prolonged.

A third characteristic should be added to these two: the present evo-lution towards voluntary treatment that generally replaces forced hospi-talization.

Some texts declare the patient's right to physical and mental integrity as well as the right of the physically or mentally handicapped to receive professional training and reintegrate society (article 15 of the *European Social Charter* of 1961). In addition: the UN's *Declaration of the Rights of the Mentally Ill* states, that these people should not be exploited. The Par-liamentary Assembly of the Council of Europe adopted *Recommendation 779 on the Rights of the Sick and the Dying* on 29 January 1976.

The Hospital Committee of the European Community also adopted the Declaration *Charter of Hospital Patients Rights* in 9 May 1979. How-ever, the relationship between doctor and patient goes beyond the hospital. A *European Guide to Medical Ethics*, drawn up in January 1987 in Paris by representatives of the medical associations of the European Commu-nity, emphasizes the principle that doctors should only use professional knowledge in order to improve or maintain their patient's health.

The World Medical Association adopted a *Declaration on Patient's Rights* in 1981 in Lisbon. It has been amended during the 47th General As-sembly in September 1995 in Bali, Indonesia. This Declaration, which generally confirmed the rights recognized by other texts, has the double merit of reminding us, that doctors must always act according to their con-science and in the best interest of the patient and, that "whenever a law, an act of government, an administration, or an institution deprives patients of their rights, it is the task of doctors to consider if the rights are guaranteed and protected". This perspective has the advantage of putting the accent on the principle of active collaboration and not on the latent antagonism that the affirmation of such rights could entail.

In April 1994, the Parliamentary Assembly of the Council of Europe adopted *Recommendation 1235 on "Psychiatry and Human Rights"*. Re-flecting the spirit of the Committee of Ministers' Recommandations as well as the changes implemented in laws on mental health, this Recom-mendation pays special attention to the legal status of hospitalized mental patients. Finally, the Resolution adopted on 17 December 1991 by the General Assembly of the UN on the "principles for the protection of per-sons with mental illness" gives many details in relation with a number of important rights.

Recommendation 818 (1977) of the Parliamentary Assembly of the Council of Europe recommended that member-states should create welfare commisions, in order to protect the mentally ill by intervening in affairs concerning them - with the power to discharge them if necessary. In its *Mental Health Act* of 1983, United Kingdom also created an institution which did not exist in the law of 1959, the *Mental Health Act* Commission. The Secretary of State for Social Services, should appoint this special authority, including members of the medical and other professions, in or der to protect the rights of the mentally ill, detained against their will. The *Mental Health Act* Commission has no official powers. Its role is to advise the Minister of Health and establish a practical code on obligatory committals and treatment. However, its efficacy, as with all the other British institutions, most certainly depends on the personality of its members.

Right to Treatment and Compulsory Treatment

Right to the Protection of Human Dignity

"Treatment" is usually understood as medical care but also, in a larger sense, as any intervention or examination with the aim of prevention, diagnosis, therapy, or rehabilitation when carried out by or under the supervision of a physician.

The right to treatment stems from the right to health as put forward by various international groups and nationals constitutions. For exemple:

- Article 25 of the *Universal Declaration of Human Rights* of the UN mentions medical care as one of the means of assuring that an individual has "a standard of living, adequate for the health and well-being".
- The preamble of the *World Health Organization's Constitution* and article 12 of the *International Covenant on Civil and Political Rights of the United Nations* speaks of the "best state of health that [one] should be capable of attaining" as a fundamental right that includes the right to treatment in the general sense of the term.
- Article 13 of the *European Social Charter* states the right "to receive social and medical assistance" in the same general meaning.
- The *Charter of Hospital Patients*, which refers to the right of the ill to have access to hospitals equipped for the treatment needed and to proper medical care itself, also states the right to receive treatment.
- This right is also part of the *Declaration of the Rights of the Mentally Handicapped* as well as of the *Declaration of the Rights of the Handicapped*: here, the "mentally ill have a right to medical care and appropriate physical treatment".

In a much larger sense, all handicapped people - physically and mentally - "have the right to medical, psychological, and functional treatment". One can still speak of a "right to treatment" for the ill who wish such treatment; but the "right to treatment" for those who refuse it seems a bit dubious to us. In such a case, the treatment is rather more compulsory, i.e. imposed on patients in a context of deprivation or restriction of their liberty. It is thus more an obligation than a right.[3]

The concept of the mentally ill as a dangerous person is largely used as a criterion for their hospitalization for compulsory treatment: while the "illness" is linked to a "danger for society", involuntary hospitalization is society's answer to such a dangerous behavior.[4]

The idea of "marginalization" caused by the illness, whether physical or mental, has led the authors of many legal texts on health care to consider the ill as beings who must be isolated in their own best interest, but also of course in order to protect society. This being the case, national legislators have used the danger that the ill represent to an overwhelming extent in texts on mental health to justify their forced internment in a psychiatric ward.

Treatment must be ordered with respect of the dignity of the person. This limitation refers to the right of the ill to be treated as a human being according to the regulations of medical deontology. Any intervention that could cause irreversible damage to the health of the mentally ill must be avoided. This includes, according to present conceptions, inhuman treatment in the sense of article 3 of the *European Convention on Human Rights* and similar proclamations by the UN (the *Declaration on the Protection of All People from Torture or other Cruel, Inhuman, and Degrading Treatment*, article 5 of the *Universal Declaration of Human Rights*, article 7 of the *International Convenant on Civil and Political Rights*. The Convention adopted by the General Assembly of the UN the 10 of December 1984 against torture and other cruel, inhuman or degrading treatment), as well as by the Council of Europe (the European Committee instituted by the *European Convention to abolish torture and other forms of inhuman or degrading treatment* (1987), which went into effect the 1st of February 1989). This committee has the right to visit any place of detention without forewarning, including public psychiatric institutions. Private places of detention, i.e. psychiatric clinics, unfortunately are not included in this important preventive control mechanism.

The idea of respect of human dignity includes, among others, the right to a private life, to privacy, to one's own philosophical convictions and religious beliefs. It finds its application in the ways medical acts are executed: they may not contradict the above mentioned values but must include the patient's right to be informed about the type of medical intervention and the possible existence of alternatives to the proposed treatment.

- The "dignity" and "well-being" of the sick are notions which several texts by international organizations make reference to.
- The *Declaration of the Rights of the Handicapped* states their right to have their human dignity respected (article 3).
- The *Declaration of Hawaii*, approved by the General Assembly of the World Psychiatric Association in 1977 and amended in 1983, also evokes "the respect due to the dignity that all human beings" as a condition of treatment of mentally ill.

The right to respect of the human dignity of the sick, has also been mentioned by the Council of Europe in *Recommendation 779* (1976) of the

Parliamentary Assembly relating to the rights of the sick and dying (article 5); *Recommendation (83)2* of the Committee of Ministers on the "Legal protection of persons suffering of mental illness and placed as involuntary patients" (article 10).

From the Nuremberg Code to the European Convention on Human Rights

The *Nuremberg Code* (1947) was followed by a number of very important texts not only on the universal level (*Universal Declaration of Human Rights* (1948), two International Convenants of the UN (1966), the *International Convention on the Elimination of All Forms of Racial Discrimination* (1965), etc.), but also on the regional European level, the most important of which has been undeniably the *European Convention on Human Rights*, which was adopted by the Council of Europe in 1950.

Individuals who consider that their rights protected by the Convention have been violated can bring their case to the European Commission and then to the European Court of Human Rights, both of which are true European juridical courts, whenever they wish to file a complaint about whatever arbitrary attacks on their liberty - including those caused by their own government - have taken place.

This year, we are commemorating the 50th anniversary of the *Nuremberg Code*, a text adopted at the end of the trials against Nazi doctors for the crimes committed against the mentally ill and the handicapped, among others.

The mentally ill - and what group is more vulnerable than they are, especially when they are committed in psychiatric institutions? - are not exceptions to the rule of protection against the arbitrary deprivation of liberty: a real *code of rights for the mentally ill* has come into being, little by little, and influenced the juridical reality of member-states in the field of mental health at the level of European law, where certain domains are quite advanced (for exemple, the three requirements for the lawful detention of the mentally ill) and others are conservative (say, the refusal to admit that the right of the mentally ill to treatment stems as such from the disposition of the Convention that forbade the deprivation of liberty when the three minimum conditions mentioned above are not satisfied).

Requirements of the Compulsory Commitment of the Mentally Ill in Psychiatric Intitutions through the Jurisprudence of the European Court of Human

Paragraph e of article 5 of the *European Convention on Human Rights* mentions five categories of persons whose liberty can be legally restricted. It covers the field of civil law, as well as criminal law, in the sense that deprivation of liberty can take place because of the person's health, or even because the person committed an infraction which can be linked to the illness. This is certainly true for the mentally ill whose illness causes them to become dangerous to themselves and society; restrictions on their liberty have been the subject of special regulations of national legislators. According to article 5, paragraph 1 of the Convention:

> Everyone has the right to liberty and security. No one shall be deprived of his liberty save in the following cases and in accordance with a procedure prescribed by law:
> e) the lawful detention of persons for the prevention of the spreading of infectious diseases, of unsound mind, alcoholics or drug addicts or va⁻ grants...[5]

Until the famous "Vacrancy" case , this paragraph was considered outdated. But recently, it took a particular importance due to the cases of mental health brought to the European Commision and Court of Human Rights. The deprivation of liberty in this paragraph has one main goal: to prevent those concerned from endangering others or themselves due to their health.

Even if article 5, paragraph 1 seems to distinguish "lawfulness" from the "porocedure prescribe by law", the European Court considers that both are the two sides of the same coin, which purpose is to make sure that this right is respected in a democratic society and not arbitrarily violated. In its judgement in the case of *Winterwerp* (Netherlands, 24 October 1979), the Court created a new jurisprudence reaffirmed by subsequent judgements in X (United Kingdom, 5 November 1981), *Luberti* (Italy, 23 February 1984), *Ashingdane* (United Kingdom, 28 May 1985), *Van der Leer* (Netherlands, 21 February 1990), *Wassink* (Netherlands, 27 September 1990), *Koendjibharie* (Netherlands 25 October 1990), and *Herczegfalvy* (Austria, 24 September 1992).

After confirming that the detention of the mentally ill is "lawful", in the sense of being in conformity with the relevant domestic law, - which itself should be in conformity with the Convention, - the Court announced the three minimum conditions which should be satisfied, if the decision to deprive someone of his liberty constitutes a "regular detention":

- a true mental disorder, established by an objective medical expert before the competent national authority;
- this true mental disorder should be of a kind or of a degree, justifiing compulsory confinement; and
- prolonging of the confinement only if the mental disorder seems to persist.

These conditions of the lawfulness of the detention must be present in cases of non-delinquent as well as delinquent mentally ill patients. Three points should be emphasized here:

- The detention is seen as an *ultimum remedium*, to which one should not have recourse unless all other methods of treatment, such as out-patient treatment, failed.
- Relevant national authorities should decide if detention is necessary, paying special attention to the danger which the patients could represent for their own health and for society.
- The three minimum conditions of lawful detention should be satisfied during all the detention period, which means that the patient should have access to periodic review of his mental health situation.

The Court authorizes only one exception to this rule: Emergency cases. These measures, adopted as provisory decisions, can be adopted by authorities other than the official ones referred to above when a summary medical examination calls for detention. Justified by the imperatives of protecting the public from the danger posed by the mentally ill, this special dispensation concerns temporary measures that must be reexamined before becoming definitive on the basis of a decision in line with the conditions of lawful detention in order to insure individual liberty.

The Court considers having jurisdiction to control the decisions of national authorities, following the guidelines of the Convention, examining whether the requirements for the lawfullness of the detention have been respected in the particular case, authorizing the national authorities some margin of appreciation on the way of application, because the are much more close to the national practice and reality.

The three conditions announced by the Court of Human Rights - a true "code of ethics in the field" - that make the compulsory commitment of a patient suffering from mental illnesses lawful have been celebrated as a grand legal victory over the sometimes abusive attitudes of psychiatrists. However, in reading the judgements more carefully, it is clear that the judge, the real guardian of the individual liberty of the mentally ill, but also lacking the knowledge that would permit him to determine when the mental disorder is serious enough to justify the commitment,if the disorder is "real" and if it persists, justifying the prolonging of the internment, will leave it up to the conclusions of the expert psychiatrists.

The Right of the Mentally Ill to Treatment in the Jurisprudenc of the European Convention on Human Rights

In the *Winterwerp* case, the European Commission and Court of Human Rights, had to judge about the right of the mentally ill to a treatment to ameliorate their health. The patient claimed that his detention in a psychiatric hospital was not lawful according to article 5, paragraph 1(e) of the Convention, for the authorities in charge had failed to administer an effective treatment to improve his health and limit the length of his deprivation of liberty: he had only received tranquilizers, but no real psychiatric treatment.

The Commission expressed the opinion later shared by the Court in its judgement that "the right of a patient to appropriate medical treatment " was not as such derived from article 5, paragraph 1(e) of the Convention (judgement of 24 October 1979). In accepting that forced internment in a psychiatric institution must fulfill the therapeutic and social function, the Commission proceeded in its report to formulate a restrictive interpretation of the meaning of article 5, paragraph 1(e) of the Convention, i.e. that in authorizing the restriction of the liberty of a mentally ill patient, the law only dealt with the social function of the protection. In a hardly convincing argument, the Commission admitted that the absence or refusal of treatment could be considered as "inhuman treatment" in the sense of article 3 or contrary to article 18, which forbids the use of restrictions authorized by the Convention to serve ends other than those intended. In fact, depriving mentally ill patients of their liberty for other purposes than treatment could appear as a kind of punishment inflicted to the patients because of their illness.

Along with the modalities of the detention of the mentally ill, the question of the right to treatment was first posed by the Commission and then by the European Court of Human Rights during the case of *Ashingdane vs. United Kingdom*. "Mr. Ashingdane complained that the British authorities concerned had been unduly slow in transferring him from the 'special' psychiatric hospital at Broadmoor to the 'ordinary' hospital at Oakwood, in spite of favourable medical opinions, the reason being the objections of nursing staff, who claimed that the necessary facilities were lacking. The Court found that, in spite of major differences between the régimes in the two hospitals, the applicant had continued to suffer deprivation of liberty in the second and not, as he argued mere restrictions on his liberty of movement".[6]

The question that the European Commission dealt with during Ashingdane's appeal to the European courts was whether the nature and conditions of treatment in a psychiatric clinic, i.e. the place, the environement, and the type of treatment were set down in article 5, pargraph 1(e) of the Convention.

The Commission reaffirmed in its report the point of view shared by the Court in the case of Winterwerp. In its judgement of 26 May 1985, the Court also stated with reference to the prior judgement on the case *Guzzardi vs. Italy*, where it was found that "the difference between deprivation of and restriction upon liberty is nonetheless merely one of degree of intensity and not one of nature or substance" (judgement of 6 November 1980), that the kind of treatment for the mentally ill - such as differences in the living conditions between ordinary hospitals and those with special restrictions - was not to be considered as a change in the nature of the detention, even if the manner of detention in the normal hospital were better suited to treating the patient's illness, and was thus not set down in article

5, paragraph 1(e). One could justifiably ask along with judge Louis Pettiti, who formulated a dissenting opinion, to what end patients could be deprived of their liberty in psychiatric clinics if not to be treated with a view to improving their state of health, the role of the administration being to look for better ways to insure that medical treatment serves this purpose.

During the case of *Jan Nielsen vs. Denmark*, which concerned the compulsory committement of a twelve-year-old child in a psychiatric clinic on his mother's request, the European Commission concluded in a nearly unanimous decision that this was a violation of article 5, paragraph 1 and 4 of the Convention. The Court, however, judged that such measures were inapplicable (*Judgement Nielsen*, 1987).

The commitment of a child who is not mentally ill in an institution for disabled children", far from being derived from the normal use of parental authority or psychiatry, was, in our opinion and in the opinion of several judges who formulated dissenting opinions, not unlike those which served other ends than therapy, and therefore constituted a flagrant abuse. The treatment which the child received in the hospital as well as the conditions under which it was administered, were not typical of treatment for mental illnesses of the psychotic type: no medication was given to the child. Rather, it consisted of environmental therapy and periodic discussions. This being the case, the goal of treatment should only be the attainment of equal opportunities, the development of the patient's participation and autonomy and the reduction of the amount of time spent in the institution for mentally ill children: committing children who, like Nielsen, are not mentally ill to such an clinic most certainly constitutes inadequate treatment for their normal development.

Admittedly, the right to treatment, to readaptation and reintegration to society of the mentally or physically handicapped is not provided for by the *European Convention on Human Rights* and its protocols. One could, however, wonder whether the possible attitudes of rejection, exclusion, and marginalisation of these people by national authorities, all of which is manifested in their indifference and refusal to admit that these patients' difference merits a special place, does not constitute "inhuman and degrading treatment" as defined by article 3 of the Convention or, in light of the inequality of opportunity in professional training, employment, economic, legal and social protection, discriminatory treatment as set down in article 14.

From Article 5 to Article 3 of the European Convention on Human Rights: Prohibition of "Inhuman Treatment"

Unlike the case of *Ashingdane vs. the United Kingdom*, which dealt with the deprivation of liberty in a psychiatric institution, the case of *Herczeg-falvy vs. Austria* (judgement of 24 September 1992, series A, No 244) concerned involuntary psychiatric treatment as such - that is, the forced administration of neuroleptics, the forced confinement of a delinquent mentally ill to a security bed as well as his confinement and isolation.

This was the first time that the European Commission and Court of Human Rights judged on psychiatric treatment from the point of view of article 3 of the *European Convention on Human Rights*, which itself considers torture illegal as well as "all inhuman or degrading treatment". Unlike other freedoms and liberties that are protected by the Convention, the prohibition of torture and inhuman or degrading treatment permits no derogation, i.e. there is no exceptional case or emergency situation that would justify such measures.[7]

In its judgement, the Court considers "that the position of inferiority and powerlessness which is typical of patients confined in psychiatric hospitals" (paragraph 82) mentions the "situation of inferiority and powerlessness" (paragraph 82), their difficulty in contacting the authorities as well as the European Court of Human Rights, a difficulty that is even more important than for someone hospitalized for other health reasons.

The judgement of the Court which considers the forced treatment of the mentally ill as an "inhuman treatment" according to article 3 of the Convention constitutes an important evolution in European law concerning the treatment of patients in psychiatric hospitals.

In addition, the *European Convention for the Prevention of Torture and Inhuman or Degrading Treatment* could influence the interpretation of article 3 of the *European Convention on Human Rights* through its system of visits by its Committee to psychiatric hospitals. With article 3 of the *Convention on Human Rights* as the starting point for the *Convention on Torture*, the Committee on Torture can prevent inhuman treatment or even put an end to it,through recommendations to the government of the member-state concerned.

It would be necessary, however, to define the standards of article 3: the positive obligation of the state to provide means of treatment ("the obligation to act"), an idea which is not foreign to the spirit of the *European Convention on Human Rights*, should be explored as well at a time when there is a great tendency to psychiatrize socially problematic people (the unemployed, etc.).

As for the methods of treatment, those which concern the mentally ill in psychiatric hospitals have been the subject of special attention in international texts. Thus, article 5 paragraph 3 of the Recommendation R (83) 2 of the Committee of the Ministers of the Council of Europe invites the member states to outlaw clinical tests and treatment on the mentally ill that does not have therapeutic value.

The legal measures taken by national legislators have to regulate those of clinical tests that are therapeutic (cf., for example, French law n° 88 - 1138 from 20 December 1988, which deals with the protection of people in biomedical research). The Recommendation makes reference to even less known practices which are generally not admittable in medical science.

The question of experimentation wich undoubtedly advances scientific knowledge, is considered in the context of "appropiate treatment" and the responsibility which doctors have towards their patients. This also goes for such practices as lobotomies and the sterilization of the mentally ill.[8]

As about the control of the ability of the mentally ill and the mentally handicapped committed in institutions for the handicapped to procreate, sterilization appears to be a grave offense against the norms of the *European Convention* (article 3) and other texts adopted by international organizations.[9]

The Parliamentary Assembly of the Council of Europe adopted *Recommendation 1235* (1994), which deals with psychiatry and human rights, in April 1994. The Assembly also proposed to the Committee of Ministers that new rules on various issues (procedures and conditions of placement, problems and abuses in psychiatry, the situation of the interned) be adopted. Concerning treatment, it more explicitly suggested that:

- a distinction should be made between mentally handicapped patients and the insane;[10]
- lobotomies and electroconvulsive therapy should not be carried out unless the expressed written consent has been given by the patient or by someone chosen by the patient to make that decision, a counsellor or a legal guardian, and that the decision should be confirmed by a rules committee that is composed not only of psychiatric experts;[11]
- the treatment administrated to the patient should be followed by a detailed protocol;
- the healthcare personnel should be large enough and well-trained enough to treat the type of illness at hand;
- a "counsellor" from outside the institution should be accessible to the patients without any obstacles. Additionally, a "legal guardian" must be there to protect the interests of minors; and
- an inspection similar to the one by the European Committee for the Prevention of Torture and Inhuman or Degrading Treatment should be instituted.

Research

Research, a field profoundly marked by the atrocities of the Nazi regime since then has become the basis for the Nuremberg Code, the first one to be adopted after W.W.II. It has been the field where the international organizations have undertaken particularly intensive work.[12]

The Convention for the Protection of Human Rights and Dignity of the Human Being concerning applied biology and medicine (*Convention on Bioethics*), which was adpoted by the Council of Europe, formulated the following principle: "Scientific research in the field of biology and medicine is free to be carried out in accordance with the present Convention and other legal measures for the protection of human beings". While affirming the freedom of scientific research, the draft of the Convention also states that this freedom is not absolute: research is limited by human rights and other legal measures for the protection of human beings, such as those that submit research projects to committees of ethics. The Convention also adds a few other limitations:

- The purpose is the protection of "the dignity and identity of human beings."
- The interests and the well-being of human beings must prevail over the interests of society and science.
- Research on in vitro embryos (where allowed by law) cannot be authorized unless the embryos have not developed beyond a fortnight. Human embryos may not be used solely for research purposes.
- No intervention on the human genome may be undertaken except for preventive, therapeutic, or diagnostic reasons, and even then only when it is not intended to affect the genial line.

Concerning medical research on human beings, *Recommendation N°R (90)3 of the Committee of the Ministers of the Council of Europe on medical research on human beings* adds:

- In medical research, the interests and well-being of those who are volunteer to participate in research must always prevail over the interests of society and science.
- The risks taken by those participating in medical research must be reduced to a minimum. The risks may not be disproportionate to the benefits for them and the importance of the purpose of this research.
- During pregnancy or breast-feeding, women cannot participate in medical research from which their health or the health of their children will not benefit directly, unless this research has to serve other women or children who are in this period of life and the findings cannot be attained on women who are not pregnant or breast-feeding.
- Those deprived of their freedom cannot be subjects of medical research unless their health will directly and significantly benefit from it.
- Those who would be suitable for medical research cannot be coerced into participating without their free consent.
- Those participating in medical research may not receive any financial gain from it. Nevertheless, the costs accumulated and the losses made can be refunded and, if needed, a modest compensation may cover the inconveniences caused by the medical research. If the subjects of such a research are not legally accountable, their legal guardians may not receive any remuneration of any kind except to cover their costs.

The consent of the subjects of medical research is a fundamental requirement. Article 7 of the *International Covenant of the UN on Civil and*

Political Rights states that: "No one shall be subjected to torture or to cruel, inhuman or degrading treatment or punishment...In particular, no one shall be subjected to medical or scientific experimentation, without his free consent". The lack of consent would also be a violation of article 3 of the *European Convention on Human Rights*, which protects from torture and inhuman or degrading treatment. *Recommendation N°R (90)3* further develops these principles in the following principles:

- No medical research may be carried out without the expressed, free, and clear, and specific consent of the person to be experimented on. This consent can be retracted at any point during the experiment. Those who participate in the research must be told of their right to retract their consent before the experiment begins.
- Those participating in medical research must be informed of the purpose of this research and of the methodology of the experiment. They must also be informed of the risks that are foreseeable and the inconveniences that are entailed in the research proposed. This information must be sufficiently clear and capable of allowing subjects to give or refuse their consent in full knowledge of the facts.
- Those not legally accountable may not be subjects of medical research unless their legal guardian or authority or authorized representative or someone designated as such according to national law gives this consent. If those incapable of giving their own consent are capable of understanding the situation, their consent is equally required, and no research can be undertaken without this consent. Furthermore, those not legally accountable may not be subjects of medical research unless there is a direct and significant benefit to their health. However, in exceptional cases, national law can authorize research on the legally unaccountable whose health would not directly benefit provided that these individuals do not resist participation and that the research carried out benefit others in the same category as the subjects and that similar scientific results not be obtainable from subjects who do not belong to this category. This is the case for, among others, people suffering from grave mental disturbances for which new medicine for such disorders must be tested for the benefit of the larger category of people who are suffering from the same disorders.
- In emergency situations, when patients are incapable of giving their prior consent, no medical research can be carried out unless the following conditions are fulfilled:
  - the research to be carried out in emergency cases must have been planned;
  - the plan for systematic research must have been approved by an ethics committee;
  - the research must be undertaken for the direct benefit of the health of patient.

The rules concerning the modes of carrying out for research on human subjects that are set out in *Recommendation R (90)3* are the following:

- All medical research must be carried out within a scientific framework.
- All drafts of protocols of medical research must be subjected to ethical evaluation by an independent and interdisciplinary committee.
- Medical research may not be carried out unless satisfactory proof of the safety of the subject of the experiment has been established.
- Medical research must be performed under the direction of a doctor or of someone responsible for the hospital and holding the knowledge and appropriate qualifications to face all eventualities in the hospital. The doctor who is responsible or any other person responsible must have total professional independence and must have the power to stop the research at any moment.
- All information gained about the character of the person participating in medical research must be kept confidential.
- All medical research planned that does not fulfill scientific criteria in its conception and which does not answer the questions posed is unacceptable even if the manner in which it is being carried out represents no risk for the subjects of the research.

This set of rules is supplemented by rules on the indemnification of the subject of the medical experiment: *Recommendation N° R (90)3* states that the subjects of medical experiments and/or those eligible must be indemnified for the damage done during the medical experiment. As about a system that would insure that those injured are indemnified, the states must control if these indemnities are sufficiently guaranteed. Any clause tending to exclude or limit indemnities for the victim from the outset should be null and void.

The protection of the patient consists for the doctor in obtaining "free and informed consent", i.e. consent given without duress of any sort and after having received the most complete and clear possible information. For mental illnesses, handicaps and other mental disturbances, one could ask to what extent the will of the patient is free (the patient rarely has any alternative) and to what extent the patient's capacity to understand the information given is sufficient. Moreover, the fact that in many countries the treatment of mental illnesses can also be carried out when patients are obliged to participate, in other words against their will, complicates the issue considerably.

At the international and domestic level, the rules concerning free and informed consent are well established. In addition to article 7 of the international Convenant and article 3 of the *European Convention on Human Rights*, articles 4 and 5 of the *Convention on Bioethics* state that:

a) no intervention in health care can be carried out on anyone whose free and informed consent has not been given. This consent can be retracted at any time; and

b) no intervention can be carried out on those who are not legally accountable, nor on those who, though legally accountable, possess a
reduced capacity of comprehension unless they would directly benefit and the consent of their legal representative has been given.[13]

The Impact of the Jurisprudence of the European Court of Human Rights on National or International Legal Texts

National legislations have the tendancy to make domestic law in conformity with article 5 of the *European Convention* - especially in granting the
judge, the guardian of individual freedom, the right to discharge mentally
ill patients. The influence of the Court' s jurisprudence in this issue is incontestable. For instance, the Court's judgement on the case of *X vs. the
United Kingdom* led to the amendment of British legislation on mental
health: the present text of the *Mental Health Act* (adopted in September
1983, and hence after the decision of the Court) gives decision-making
power to the Mental Health Review Tribunals. They have order that mentally ill patients should be discharged, with our without restrictions, which
thus makes them "tribunals" in the sense of article 5 paragraph 4 of the
Convention.

In addition, European law, linked to the wishes of the member-states
of the Council of Europe to harmonize their legislation on mental health,
led on the international level to the adoption by the Committee of Ministers of the Council of Europe of *Recommendation (83) 2* on 22 February
1983, concerning the "Legal Protection of Persons suffering from mental
disorder, places as involuntary patients." The Parliamentary Assembly of
the Council of Europe adopted *Recommendation 1235* (1984), concerning
"Psychiatry and Human rights".

On the other hand, during the same period, a Project of Principles that
accompanied the DAES Report constitutes the contribution of the United
Nations to the protection of the rights of those suffering from considerable
mental disturbances just as the rights of minors are protected. This led to
the Resolution of the General Assembly of the United Nations (17 December 1991) on the principles for the protection of these patients and the improving of care for the mentally ill.

The jurisprudential work of the Court in such a sensitive area as
mental health assumes a particular importance at a time when the right to
be ill and live with one's illness is recognized as a human right and any
measure which deprive people of their freedom for health reasons must be
adopted with the greatest precaution.

Finally, the *Convention on Bioethics*, which was adopted by the
Council of Europe and has learned much from the negative events in Nazi
Germany as well as such occurrences in other countries, assigns special
importance to the question of the treatment and protection of the vulnerable, such as the mentally ill, in scientific experiments carried out by re-

searchers. The accent is put on the consent of the patient or legal guardian as well as on the presence of an ethics committee, whose role is to approve research projects on the mentally ill and the vulnerable par excellence after a serious evaluation of the risks and benefits. With this in mind, the guiding light in the conscience of the specialist is, more than anything else, a love for patients, respect of their personalities and their sufferings, without which the application of any texts, as perfect as they may be, would be impossible as long as attitudes and awareness have not been sufficiently developed in order to respect the ethical rules which are all the more important as the mental illness can render them weak and dependent not only on the power of doctors, but also on wide-spread prejudice.

Notes

1   Douraki, T. (1986), 'La Convention Européenne des Droits de l'Homme et le droit à la liberté de certains malades et marginaux': 97 th Volume of the *Bibliothèque de Droit International*, Paris, L.G.D.J., pp. 436.

2   Koch H.G., Reiter-Theil, S., Helmchen, H. (eds.) (1996), *Informed Consent in Psychiatry. European Perspectives of Ethics, Law and Clinical Practice*. Nomos, Baden-Baden.

3   Douraki T.: *Rights of the Mentally Ill.* Research study prepared in collaboration with Prof. Dinah Shelton (Santa Clara University of California) at the International Institute of Human Rights, Strasbourg, AS JUR (43) 41.

4   See Art. Harding T. (1980), *Déviance et Société*, Genève, No. 3, p. 331-348. Du danger, de la dangerosité et de l'usage médical de termes affectivement chargés. See also Baker, E. (1993), 'Dangerousness, Rights and Criminal Justice' in: *Modern Law Review*, 56, p. 546-547.

5   Douraki, T. (1984), 'La Convention Européenne des Droits de l'Homme et la privation de liberté des malades mentaux'. *Revue Hellénique de Droit International*. Athènes, p. 159-83. See also Wachenfeld M. (1992), 'The Human Rights of Mentally Ill in Europe', *Danish Center for Human Rights*, p. 292.

6   28. 5. 1985, Series A no. 93, pp. 19- 20, paras. 40 and 42.

7   Glueman S. (1996), *Social and psychological effects of compulsory treatments* (dealing with mentally healthy people in special mental hospitals in the U.S.S.R.) Torture, Supplementum No. 1.

8   Stone, A. (1975), *Mental Health Act and the Law. A system in transition.* National Institute of mental Health. Center for studies of Crime and Deliquency, Rockville, Maryland, USA.

9   Szasz, T. (1994), 'Psychiatric Diagnosis, psychiatric power and psychiatric abuse'. *Journal of Medical Ethics*, p. 134-38.

10 Szasz, T. (1974), *The Myth of Mental Illness*, Harper and Row, New York.

11 Torrelli, Maurice (1983), *Le médecin et les droits de l'homme*, Berger - Lèvrault, Paris, p. 209. Cambel T., Heginbotham C. ((1991)), *Mental Illness: Prejudice, Discrimination, and the Law*, Dartmouth, USA, p. 253.

12 Annas, G. (1992), *The Rights of Patients*, Humana Press, Totowa, New Jersey, p. 141-158.

13 *Declaration on the protection of patient's rights in Europe*. Amsterdam, March 28-30, 1994, W.H.O. Douraki, T (1992), 'Droits sociaux des handicapés'. Rapport présenté dans le cadre du Congrès International du Mouvement International des Juristes Catholiques, 'Justiciabilité des Droits Sociaux en Europe', Strasbourg, 22-24 nov. 1991. Affari Sociali e Internazionali, No. 1, pp. 277-286.

21 Answers to Change: The Problem of Paradigm Shift in Medical Ethics from the German Perspective

Stella Reiter-Theil

Introduction

The central question this paper addresses is whether the efforts and changes in some areas of the present-day health sector are *adequate* responses to the developments of the last 50 years in the relationship between patients and health care professionals. If this objective is taken seriously, account must be also taken of some of the assumptions implied in the title of the present paper. Speaking of a *paradigm shift* in this context means applying Kuhn's theory of scientific revolutions to medicine and the health sector in general. Doing so also means working under the assumption that such a scientific revolution - or paradigm shift - from an old paradigm to a new one has taken place, or to put it more exactly: to a new paradigm of ethics in medicine and the health sector. This hypothesis is based on many premises and thus requires closer scrutiny. It will also be necessary to outline the normative aspects of this hypothesis in order to be able to judge the adequacy of the answers at all.

The discussion will thus begin with some critical thoughts on the applicability of Kuhn's theory to medicine and medical ethics; a more refined model of the term "paradigm" and its development will be presented. (Medical ethics and ethics of medicine are both meant here in the broadest sense of ethics in medicine and the health sector in general.) Several examples will be used to illustrate where and to what extent signs of a shifting paradigm are to be found; some conclusions will be discussed concerning which steps should be taken to further the changes that seem to be appropriate for the challenges medical ethics poses.

The Theory of Scientific Revolutions and its Applicability to Medicine

Criticism and Modifications

The theory of scientific revolutions as formulated by Thomas S. Kuhn (1995; first published in German in 1967), not only reached the inner circles of scientific philosophy, but also was the starting point for a wide discussion in the various branches of the natural and social sciences. According to Kuhn, scientific research is a form of "puzzle-solving". Thus, science is not organized by theories, but by paradigms, far more complex structures. The sign of a highly developed science is the predominance of one single paradigm; highly developed science is monoparadigmatic. Science as a process is characterized by two phases: 1) so-called "normal" science, in which a predominant paradigm is established and defended within the scientific community; and 2) the paradigm shift, or the scientific revolution, in which a new paradigm takes the place of the old because it offers more effective solutions to the puzzles. This dynamic is triggered off by the appearance of anomalies that cannot be solved by the old paradigm, thus leading to the search for new solutions. Kuhn himself developed this theory further (1978) and stated near the end of his working life that the term could be done away with altogether. This turn was, however, not taken note of by the scientific community, or at any rate his change of heart was not followed. Many scientists clearly still feel that Kuhn's use of the term "paradigm" is fruitful. Therefore, a closer look at the benefits and drawbacks of this way of speaking and thinking must be more closely discussed.

How is the wide-spread resonance of Kuhn's ideas in scientific philosophy and the various natural and social sciences since the 1970s to be understood? To all appearances, this is due to Kuhn's skeptical view of scientific progress, the quest for truth, and rationality in general. Many scientific philosophers and, above all, researchers in the empirical sciences were apparently ready to drop criteria of rationality, truth, and scientific progress, which had been introduced by Logical Empiricism (through the criterion of verification) or Critical Rationalism (through the criterion of falsification). The criteria of Logical Empiricism and Critical Rationalism had proved to be much too narrow, strict, or unrealistic in light of the experience of quotidian research. But Kuhn's emphasis on the "irrational" aspects of science - social, psychological, pragmatic, political, and economic aspects - seem to allow for a more realistic and convincing view of everyday research (Stegmüller, 1973). However, the application of Kuhn's theory to fields other than the traditional natural sciences - such as physics, astronomy, or chemistry - proved to be difficult despite the enthusiasm of the proponents of the theory (Reiter-Theil, 1984). This view is generally shared by von Engelhardt (1987). The difficulties of application can be subsumed in three categories of points of criticism for the transferral of the theory onto the field of medical ethics: 1) in making the so-called normal sciences the essential criterion for developed science, too much importance has been attached to the "conservative" element in Kuhn's work - change is ascribed to irrational processes to a large degree; 2) the theory is hardly applicable to fields with more than one paradigm; and 3) the term "paradigm" is too vague - Kuhn uses the term in 22 different connotations (Masterman, 1974). For these reasons, Kuhn's theory and its central concepts cannot be directly applied to medical ethics in all its complexity: from scientific investigations to clinical practice, teaching, legal and political implementation measures, and public debates. Medical ethics in its largest context is too plural, too heterogeneous to be characterized by a single paradigm. The changes are, in turn, too specific to be generalized. The call for the respect for human rights - including patient rights - is, for instance, too old to be considered the beginning of a completely new paradigm today. An alternative to this would be a three-level model that allows for a differentiation of Kuhn's term "paradigm" as well as of the concept of the paradigm change. In my opinion, this model, first developed by Masterman (1974), enables us to formulate specific hypotheses about the change in paradigm in medical ethics while avoiding far-reaching generalizations on thin ice.

Modifications on the Term "Paradigm": The Three-level Model

Masterman's modifications on Kuhn's "paradigm" open up new possibilities not only for a more concise definition of Kuhn's term, but also for its modified application to fields of science that exhibit several co-existing and co-developing paradigms rather than the one paradigm of a mono-paradigmatic normal science.

Modifications on the term "paradigm"

Table 1   A Three-Component Model

a) *Metaparadigm (metaphysical paradigm)*: abstract, general, *"Weltanschauung"*

b) *Sociological paradigm*: concrete, observable; stimulates application and development of as yet unperfected innovations

c) *Constructed paradigm*: methodological instruments for investigating the metaparadigm; specific rules for research practice

Source: Masterman, 1974

Masterman extracts three components from Kuhn's paradigm: 1) the metaphysical paradigm (metaparadigm) for the abstract, general part of the paradigm contains the *Weltanschauung* and represents in fact more than just a theory; 2) the sociological paradigm, in contrast, is concrete and observable, being the part of the paradigm that stimulates the application and further development of still unperfected innovations; 3) the constructed paradigm concerns the methodological instruments for the scientific examination of assumptions formulated in the metaparadigm (metaphysical paradigm), including specific rules for research practice. This tripartite model itself assumes that these elements occur in a specific order. Masterman claims that the *sociological paradigm* is first visible in the form of pioneers and scientific teams, while the *metaparadigm* only takes shape after such groups have been established; finally, the *constructed paradigm* is formed as the basis of specific research.

Table 2   Sequence of the development of a paradigm

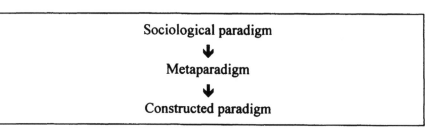

Source: Masterman, 1974

Fatal Polarization between Theory and Practice

In most of the examples from various fields of science, especially astronomy, quoted by Kuhn or Masterman, scientific change begins with the formation of research groups who experiment with a new paradigm before a general theory of this practice has been formulated; this is especially true of research proper and its methods, which are necessary for the realization of a developed normal science within an overriding paradigm. Such a sequence does not, however, hold for medical ethics. Take, for instance, the development from paternalism to the respect for the autonomy of the patient, one of the most often cited examples of the fundamental changes in this area. The picture we get is anything but uniform: medical ethics works in many cases with terms developed from philosophical ethics, especially with terms like the autonomous subject, and it profits from theoretical foundations created to a large extent by (continental) European thinkers, particularly those since the Enlightenment (Pieper, 1992). It is thus clear that in this case theory (the metaparadigm) comes before practice (the sociological paradigm). But the time lapse between theory and practice cannot simply be attributed to the earlier awareness of these concepts in the theoretical sphere. The delay has just as much to do with the lack of communication between "thinkers" and "doers", with missed opportunities and failures by both groups to learn from one another. Experts of theory have tended to disregard practical considerations and develop terminologies that discourage the experts of practice from entering into the dialogue altogether. On the other hand, the medical establishment in Germany has shown little more than a smugness, even concerning the ethical and philosophical reflections in the field, that does not improve the quality of the dialogue either.

If one focuses on the aspect of the developing paradigm in discussions on what the effects of the change in medical ethics should be, three attitudes are suggested: 1) "the old paradigm" (paternalism) is invalid today and must be replaced by something more productive; 2) "the new paradigm" (patient autonomy) has proved to be more effective and must be put into practice in general; and 3) the proponents of the new paradigm must convince, overpower, or at least survive the proponents of the old to further progress. There is no room here for the co-existence of more than one model or for mixed forms and various applications, for a dialogue between theory and practice. Discourse and dissent are polarized in the fight between (two) alternatives, which begin to assume the character of *Weltanschauungen* and disallow any critical and constructive debate. Finally, this view takes no account of the aspect of the temporal sequence that seems to be so important for the establishment of innovations. This raises the interesting question of whether the relatively late acceptance of **recent** - international - medical ethics in German medicine may have to do with this reversal of the sequence of changes. Some examples should illustrate where the sociological phenomenon actually occurred first and where it was followed in the next stage by the metatheoretical underpinnings, as appears to be the rule in scientific research, and where the development appears to be inverted. For the discourse on medical ethics and its establishment in practice, it follows that we should not criticize the practitioners solely for being overly late, hesitant or reluctant to the tried and true old ethical theory. Rather, the attempt should be made to further new practices, to investigate them and thereby reconstruct on this basis the ethical theory in order to use the dynamics of practical innovation for change and combine them with the intellectual and cultural heritage of our liberal arts.

Examples of Change in Fields of Medical Ethics

The Relationship between Health Care Professionals and Patients

In light of the great changes in doctor/patient relations, there has been much talk of a move from paternalism towards conduct oriented around the autonomy of the patient. If one takes a closer look at the situation of medicine and health care professions, one takes on a different, more refined attitude (Gahl, 1995). If we take the tripartite model of the paradigm again, we have the following arrangement: for the component of the sociological paradigm (which occurs as a rule first), at least three models for relations between doctor (health care worker) and patient coexist or compete: 1) the traditional, paternalistic model; 2) the contractual model; and 3) the partnership model, though mixtures of these ideal forms are also to be found (Wolff, 1989). Each of these three models has complex theoretical underpinnings; we accordingly have on the level of the metaparadigm (which usually follows the sociological paradigm) a broad differentiation with long historical roots, especially in philosophy. In the third component, the constructed paradigm (the last phenomenon in the sequence), the stage of development is clearly only slight in so far as developed research on ethical and practical aspects of the realization of one of the concepts for doctor/patient relations is concerned. Here, it is hardly convincing to insist that a complete shift of paradigm has taken place in the field; insisting on a scientific revolution in Kuhn's sense of the term would be reductionist and a normative fallacy as the evaluative judgment has no solid basis. Practice here is regarded as an isolated phenomenon and judged as being insufficient. This normativistic evaluation of practice can hardly be considered other than an arrogant attitude on the side of the ethicists by the practicians themselves. In this way, theory - due to its long history - is played off against practice, which - due to its complexity and relatively new development as a profession - can only pale in comparison with western liberal arts. This position is, however, not acceptable but counter-productive in light of the priority that the practical treating patients has in medicine and the health sector.

Patient Information / Informed Consent

The rise of the rule of the Informed Consent of the patient and its realization is also used as an example of a paradigm shift in the ethics of treating patients; the introduction of informed consent is seen, at the very least, as a stepping stone on the way towards patient autonomy (Sass, 1992). A closer look at the three components of a paradigm shows that such expectations are exaggerated. In the sociological component, we find that the rule has been widely realized in daily dealings with patients, but nevertheless there are many variations between the ideal type and forms of "defensive information" that have little to do with the spirit of the rule (Reiter-Theil, 1997). The theoretical background of informed consent is fully developed as a juridical metaparadigm in legal theory and legislation (Francke, 1994; Kern, Laufs, 1983); but this does not mean that a theory of its practical realization in medicine, beyond certain routines, has been developed. Rather, the legal norm leaves the finding of a solution for the remaining daily problems up to the practitioner and, of course, the patient, which often enough is asking too much of both of them. Here, the domain of a practice-oriented, co-operative ethics of medicine begins. As is to be expected, the constructed paradigm lags behind: witness the state of empirical research on practical questions about how to inform patients and receive their consent, or on operational guidelines for conduct. This may stem from the lack of research devoted explicitly to ethical questions, which would be necessary to link ethical and empirical matters. General methodological guidelines that permit the interweaving of ethical and empirical aspects have, in the meantime, been worked out by various research groups as part of a research program sponsored by the Deutsche Forschungsgemeinschaft (Eckensberger, Gähde, 1993).

Unlike the sequence of paradigm parts set forth in the tripartite model, we are confronted here with the deviation discussed in the first example above: the metaparadigm of informed consent - the philosophy of the autonomous subject and his rights as a patient - has preceded the socio-logical phenomenon, the initiatives of pioneers to educate patients in prac-tice. It can be assumed that such a progression will entail a much more dif-ficult "career" for the implementation of an ethical concept in medicine than would be the case if the concept had arisen from practice and been re-fined by theoretical reconstruction, as Masterman's model proposes. The price of this practice/theory/research line lies in the at least temporary re-nunciation of elaborate theoretical systems and in the reduced complexity of the systems due to reasons of acceptability and adaptation to the de-mands of practice.

Ethical Discourse with Patients: The Patients' Forum on Medical Ethics

There is another form of development and renewal of the relationship be-tween doctor (health care worker) and patient which works differently than informing patients and receiving their consent, though both are based on the respect for the patient's autonomy: the participation of patients in ethi-cal discussions in medicine. One form has been developed within a model project in which patients and their family can discuss selected ethical questions with representatives of the health care system and ethics experts: the Patients' Forum on Medical Ethics (Reiter-Theil, 1995; Reiter-Theil, Hiddemann, 1996). Although the project is still a fledgling, it can still be viewed as an experimental model for a new form of communication with patients. Here, we have the classic process in the sequence of components of a paradigm: the appearance of a sociological paradigm in the form of a research group that develops a model; though it still lacks a metaparadigm in the sense of an elaborate theory, there are various starting points for an ethical reconstruction of the goals and methods for the participation of those concerned in the ethics discourse in medicine (Council of Europe, 1992; Reiter-Theil, 1995; Reiter-Theil, 1997); a special constructed paradigm for research on this model has yet to be developed or adapted (Reiter-Theil, Hiddemann, 1997).

This example, which comprises some five years of experience, allows us to trace a process from its beginnings, in which grass-roots initiatives are organized, to later stages of the development of theories and research based on our findings.

Teaching Ethics in the Health Care Sector

The example of ethics teaching in medical school and other fields related to health care illustrates the heterogeneous and even contradictory situation surrounding the question of a general paradigm shift in medical ethics in Germany. The present situation is best illustrated by the following provocative question: "Teaching ethics in medicine - to be or not to be?" (Reiter-Theil, Hick, in press). But how and to what extent do the development and establishment of ethics classes in various branches of the health sector represent such a paradigm shift in themselves?

There has been a great variety of activities in educational centers, at universities and elsewhere, in Germany and Europe (Bockenheimer-Lucius, Reiter-Theil, 1994; Reiter-Theil, 1997). These initiatives do not, however, represent a paradigm themselves as they are not generally connected to one another or integrated in any of the three components of a paradigm. The most one could say is that there is a polyparadigmatic situation in the sociological component in that differently conceived teaching models with somewhat similar methods have the same objectives without being based on the same requirements. Some of the regional teaching models do have a coherent base that can serve as the foundation for a metaparadigm, but only in this polyparadigmatic situation. A constructed paradigm that takes account of specific research through teaching models is, at best, still being developed; there are, however, still no concrete studies on research on the teaching of ethics, especially on whether aspects of clinical practice are really being dealt with sufficiently in ethics classes (Eigler, 1994), as has been demanded for discussions of pedagogical goals (Kahlke, Reiter-Theil, 1995).

Protecting the Patient in Research through Self-regulation: The Ethics Committee

Lastly, a completely different example of the so-called split paradigm shift should be noted: the establishing of committees for the approval of research projects known as "ethics committees" at medical schools, medical associations (such as the German *Ärztekammer*) and other institutions of self-regulation within the medical profession (Illhardt, 1989, 1995). For some 15 years, this form of protection for the patient and research subject - a sociological paradigm - has been in effect in Germany, with the result that every university clinic and many other institutions have such committees in the meantime - known in the Anglo-American world as "Institutional Review Boards" (Helmchen, 1995; Wiesing, 1993) - which also perform the general function of professional self-regulation and giving political advice (Bundesärztekammer, 1994). Despite the name "ethics committee," one cannot say that an elaborate ethical theory in the sense of a metaparadigm exists as a framework for the institution in which the practical activities were reconstructed; there is little more than procedural rules and references to international decrees, such as the Declaration of Helsinki for the making of decisions on the ethical acceptability of bio-medical research projects on human subjects (Arbeitskreis medizinischer Ethikkommission in der Bundesrepublik Deutschland, 1993). A constructed paradigm has yet to be created; however, the documentation of the work of these committees does hint at some possibilities for research on the functions and effects of ethics committees.

Balance Sheet

The examination of five examples of change in medical ethics in Germany supports the initial hypothesis that the assumption of a general shift in paradigm as such is too general, perhaps even misleading, if not outright wrong. It has been shown that we should usually assume there is a *partial paradigm shift*, of the type that can be meaningfully illustrated using the tripartite model, for important fields of medicine and the health sector in which ethically relevant changes are taking place. Moreover, the analysis of various examples shows that this differentiated way of viewing the shift suggests in which fields work should and can be carried out along these lines. The distinction between the level of practical innovations (1), theoretical reconstruction (2), and the accompaniment and elaboration of research proper (3) provides us with the possibility of moving beyond the common, though unproductive polarization between apparently optimally developed theories, on the one hand, and the seemingly suboptimal, retarded practical realization of these theories, on the other hand, towards a more dynamic, interactive concept in which the sequence from practical innovation, theoretical reconstruction, and the ensuing practical "fine-tuning" in the sense of feedback opens up new perspectives for interdisciplinary co-operation.

Consequences and Challenges for Medical Ethics

On the background of the above analysis and modifications of the term "paradigm" and the examination of examples of change, the initial question must now be readdressed and an answer presented for discussion. The basic question is whether and to what extent in three relevant fields adequate answers have been reached to the - paradigmatic ? - changes in doctor/patient relations resulted 1) in the recognition of patient rights; 2) in the teaching of medical ethics, and 3) on the level of institutions.

The Recognition of Patient Rights

The recognition of patient rights in Germany is guaranteed by the *Arzt-und Arzneimittelgesetz* (law on doctors and medicine), especially concerning the legal basis of informing patients and receiving their consent before treatment. The ethics committees that deal with research projects serve this purpose but do not offer at present any real control over the enforcement of such recommendations in carrying out research, nor can they force researchers to apply their suggestions. Training in medical school can - where such a focus exists - claim to be an adequate response to the changes in doctor/patient relations, though this has not been properly evaluated yet. In all three fields - law, ethics committees, training - it must be assumed that there are contradictory opinions on the "adequacy" of the various responses depending on which discipline or which professional or personal experience the opinion is based on. Between legal experts, on the one hand, and medical practitioners and clinicians, on the other, there are systematic differences in perception and analysis of the legal status and realization of patient rights. This stems, for example, from the clarity of the *limits* of the patient's self-determination to anyone who has worked in an emergency room, though these limits are not legally acceptable at face value (cf. Kettler, Mohr, 1997). In the opinion of many doctors, patient rights have already been taken too far in German law and are perceived as an obstacle to the carrying out of normal medical procedures. This opinion runs counter to the growing calls for absolute autonomy in modern medical ethics, which represents the attitude criticized above that a complete break from the old paradigm is necessary; no account is taken of the reasons why doctors - and patients - might be resisting or refusing to co-operate. Here, we are faced with the *challenge of dialogue* between those concerned and the *furthering of life-long learning* in the profession as well as among patients. This is one of the greatest tasks of the teaching of ethics in medicine in socialization in the health sector as well as in the general education of the population on health issues.

Medical School

In Germany, ethics classes are not required courses in medical school although this has often been seen as a deficiency (Kahlke, Reiter-Theil, 1992); Reiter-Theil, Hick, in press; Sponholz et al., 1995). In light of the diversity of methods and subjects in voluntary classes at medical schools, there can be no talk of a scientifically founded co-ordination of ethics curricula, though the first steps towards a new interdisciplinary discourse on content, methods, and forms of the teaching of ethics in medicine have already been made (Reiter-Theil, 1997; Reiter-Theil, 1993). In line with the heterogeneity of ethics in medicine, there is no visible, uniform theoretical basis for such classes, though there are at least coherent concepts of local groups on a rather pragmatic level (for instance, the *Arbeitskreis Ethik in der Medizin* in Ulm, Germany) and attempts to integrate theory and practice in classes (for instance, the curriculum of ethics in medicine at ZERM in Freiburg, Germany). The adequacy of the various local initiatives and classes can at present only be subjectively judged by those taking part; for a determination of the "usefulness", say, for the later conduct of the participants towards patients in ethically difficult situations, there are not yet any reliable data. The logical *inclusion of the teaching of ethical competence* in medical schools is one of the tasks to be met in Germany at present.

Institutions

The institutionalization of ethics in medicine in Germany has come into being somewhat late compared to other western countries in both politics and universities and still has far to go. There is growing awareness and concern about ethical questions in health care, brought in, for instance by churches, the media, and increasingly by public debate, but the world of medicine itself has only reluctantly shown the need for an open and critical discussion. The foundation of the Academy for Ethics in Medicine e.V. (AEM) was designed as a stop-gap for this hole that was felt in the Anglo-American world to be a "deficit". This interdisciplinary group was able to use a five-year sponsorship by Lower Saxony's VW-*Vorab* starting in 1990 to develop at the University of Göttingen (see the brochure "Akademie für Ethik in der Medizin. Ziele und Arbeitsweise", 1992). After evaluating the achievements, especially of the projects with outside funding, the state of Lower Saxony agreed to continue funding - within certain limits - the project; thus, one can speak of institutionalization (cf. Bockenheimer-Lucius, 1996). As a result of the increasing activities of local groups and the founding of several specialties (for instance, in the form of the renaming of professorships of medical history as professorships of the history and ethics of medicine, Freiburg), the AEM has experienced a shift in function: it is moving from the ground-breaking work of the early years in innovative projects towards a more co-ordinating institution that sees its task primarily in the carrying out of conferences in co-operation with local centers. Along with the founding of the AEM went the establishing of the quarterly "Ethik in der Medizin", which has been appearing since 1989 and, like the "Zeitschrift für Medizinische Ethik", represents an institution of medical ethics in Germany. These forms of institutionalized discourse - the founding and establishing of an academic association beyond the regional level, the formation of local centers, the publication journals - are important steps in the development of a wider, professional debate on ethics in medicine and the health sector and they are, thus, adequate answers to change. They are, however, unspecific about our initial question of whether they address specific changes, say, in doctor/patient relations, quite on the contrary. Indeed, all of these forms of institutionalization taken together are more indebted to the representation of the plural and controversial spectrum than one single method or "paradigm". In the interest of this plurality of doctrines - and the diversity of ethical problems in health care - further competent centers should be set up at universities from which emanate impulses for research and which also offer services like (further) education classes, counseling, and public relations work.

References

Arbeitskreis medizinischer Ethikkommissionen in der Bundesrepublik Deutschland (1993), 'Verfahrensgrundsätze des Arbeitskreises medizinischer Ethikkommissionen in der Bundesrepublik Deutschland'. In: Wagner W. (eds.) *Arzneimittel und Verantwortung. Grundlagen und Methoden der Pharmaethik.* Springer, Berlin, p. 530-533.

Bockenheimer-Lucius G., Reiter-Theil S. (eds.) (1994), 'Themenheft: Unterrichtsmodelle zur Ethik in der Medizin und in den Heilberufen'. *Ethik Med* 6: 659-113.

Bockenheimer-Lucius G. (1996), 'Wechsel in der Geschäftsführung der Akademie für Ethik in der Medizin'. *Ethik Med* 8: 107-109.

Bundesärztekammer (1994), 'Gründung einer Ethik-Kommission'. *Deutsches Ärzteblatt* 91 (43): B-2157.

Eckensberger L.H., Gähde U. (eds.) (1993), *Ethische Norm und empirische Hypothese.* Suhrkamp, Frankfurt a.M.

Eigler J. (1994), 'Ethik als Ausbildungsgegenstand im Studienfach Humanmedizin. Erfahrungen und Wünsche aus klinischer Sicht'. *Z med Ethik* 40, 2: 101-107.

Engelhardt D. von (1987), 'Dauer und Wandel in der Geschichte der medizinischen Ethik'. In: Schlaudraff, U. (ed.), *Ethik in der Medizin.* Tagung der Ev. Akademie Loccum vom 13. bis 15. Dezember 1985, Springer, Berlin, p. 35-44.

Europarat (1992), 'Die Rechte des Kranken'. *Ethik Med* 4, 2: 105-108.

Francke R. (1994), *Ärztliche Berufsfreiheit und Patientenrechte.* Enke, Stuttgart.

Gahl K. (1995), 'Beziehung zwischen Arzt und Patient'. In: Kahlke W., Reiter-Theil S. (Hrsg) *Ethik in der Medizin.* Enke, Stuttgart, p. 23-33.

Helmchen H. (1995), 'Ziele, Beratungsgegenstände und Verfahrensweisen medizinischer Ethikkommissionen'. *Ethik Med* 7: 58-70.

Illhardt F.J. (1995), 'Entscheidungsfindung'. In: Kahlke W., Reiter-Theil S. (eds.) *Ethik in der Medizin.* Enke, Stuttgart, p. 111-119.

Illhardt F.J. (1989), 'Vom Monolog zum Dialog in der Medizin'. In: Wagner W. (eds.) *Medizin - Momente der Veränderung.* Berlin, Springer, p. 103-114.

Kahlke W., Reiter-Theil S. (1995), 'Lernziele für die Auseinandersetzung mit ethischen Problemen'. In: Kahlke W., Reiter-Theil S. (eds.) *Ethik in der Medizin.* Enke, Stuttgart, p. 17-22.

Kern B.R., Laufs A. (1983), *Die ärztliche Aufklärungspflicht.* Springer, Berlin.

Kettler D., Mohr M. (1997), 'Ethische Konflikte in der Notfallmedizin'. *Anaesthesist* 46: 275-281.

Kuhn T.S. (1995), *Die Struktur wissenschaftlicher Revolutionen.* Suhrkamp, Frankfurt a. M. (first German publication 1967; English original *The Structure of Scientific Revolutions*; Chicago, 1962).

Kuhn T.S. (1978), *Die Entstehung des Neuen. Studien zur Struktur der Wissenschaftsgeschichte.* Suhrkamp, Frankfurt a. M.

Masterman M. (1974), 'Die Natur eines Paradigmas'. In: Lakatos I., Musgrave A. (eds.) *Kritik und Erkenntnisfortschritt*. Viehweg, Braunschweig (English original 'The Nature of a Paradigm'. In: Lakatos I., Musgrave A. (eds), *Criticism and the Growth of Knowledge*. Cambridge, p. 39-89.

Pieper A. (1992), *Geschichte der neueren Ethik* 1 und 2. Francke, Tübingen und Basel.

Reiter-Theil S. (1984), 'Wissenschaftstheoretische Grundlagen zur systemorientierten Familientherapie'. In: Brunner E.J. (eds.) *Interaktion in der Familie*. Springer, Berlin, Heidelberg, p. 17-39.

Reiter-Theil S. (1995), 'Von der Ethik in der Psychotherapie zur patientenorientierten Medizinethik. Das Modell Patientenforum Medizinische Ethik'. *Psychosozial* 18: 25-33.

Reiter-Theil S. (1997), 'Ethik in der Onkologie. Grenzen der Verständigung zwischen Arzt und Patient'. *Krankenhaus Arzt* 6/7: 228-235.

Reiter-Theil S. (ed.) (1997), *Vermittlung Medizinischer Ethik. Theorie und Praxis in Europa*. Nomos, Baden-Baden.

Reiter-Theil S. (1998), 'Patientenethik'. In: Korff W., Beck L., Mikat P. (eds.) *Lexikon der Bioethik*, Bertelsmann, Gütersloh, p. 838-840.

Reiter-Theil S., Kahlke W., Dressel R. (1993), 'Vermittlung von Ethik in den Heilberufen - Teachers' Training Course'. *Wiener Medizinische Wochenschrift* 143, *Diskussionsforum Medizinische Ethik* 9/10.

Reiter-Theil S., Hick C. (1998), '(K)ein Platz für Ethik im medizinischen Curriculum? Notwendigkeit und Formen der Vermittlung'. *Z med Ethik* 44: 21-31.

Reiter-Theil S., Hiddemann W. (1996), 'Der Beitrag von Patienten zur Ethik in der Medizin: Problemwahrnehmung, Perspektivenwechsel, Mitverantwortung'. *niedersächsisches ärzteblatt* 6: 2-4.

Reiter-Theil S., Hiddemann W. (1997), 'Das Patientenforum Medizinische Ethik: Ergebnisse eines Modellprojektes'. *Med Klinik* 92, 9: 552-557.

Sass H.-M. (1992), 'Informierte Zustimmung als Vorstufe zur Autonomie des Patienten'. *Medizinethische Materialien* 78.

Sponholz G., Kohler E., Strössler M., Gommel M., Baitsch H. (1995), 'Ethik in der Medizin in der neuen ÄAppO - was Studierende sich wünschen'. *Z med Ethik* 41: 236-241.

Stegmüller W. (1973), *Normale Wissenschaft und wissenschaftliche Revolutionen. Methodologie der Forschungsprogramme oder epistemologische Anarchie?* Springer, Berlin.

Wiesing U. (1993), 'Ethik-Kommissionen in der BRD'. In: Ach JS, Gaidt A (eds.) *Herausforderung der Bioethik*. Frommann-Holzboog, Stuttgart-Bad Cannstatt, p. 235-241.

Wolff H.P. (1989), 'Arzt und Patient'. In: Sass H.-M. (ed.) *Medizin und Ethik*. Reclam, Stuttgart, p. 184-211.

Ethics and Medicine for the 21st Century: The Quest for New Codes

22 Looking for New Codes in the Field of Predictive Medicine

Luís Archer

The 21st century will succeed in writing the complete sequence of the human genome. The resulting knowledge will dramatically enlarge the current possibilities for the prediction of hereditary diseases and other genetic traits. A series of ethical, social and legal problems will then arise, which will demand the establishment of new codes of practice.

Technical Aspects

General Methods for Detection of Genetic Traits

The analysis of a person's genotype may be carried out at different levels: on the individual as a whole (clinical phenotype); on organs, tissues or cells; on gene products (proteins); on chromosomes; or on DNA itself. The latter three levels of analysis are of special interest for our purposes and will be, therefore, further developed. The analysis of a gene expression product can be performed either indirectly or directly. Indirect is the approach of the analysis of specific metabolic modifications of the disease, like in the case of the phenylketonuria. Direct analysis of the phenotypic expression of the mutated gene is used in the case of inborn errors of metabolism and in the hemoglobinopathies. In certain cases, the direct study of the protein, now possible through novel techniques, is more easily informative than gene analysis. This is the case in distrophine (the altered protein in myopathy) or FMRP protein in mental retardation caused by a fragile-X chromosome, among others. Cytogenetic analysis of chromosomes, potentiated by the techniques of *in situ* hybridization, allows the fine detection of anomalies in the chromosome structure. DNA analysis allows, in the first place, the precise localization of genes on chromosome segments and the construction of genetic maps. Physical maps can also be constructed using the recognition sites of restriction enzymes or other markers. Genes can then be isolated, sequenced, cloned and the corresponding proteins characterized. This is happening for a growing number of diseases. When molecular DNA probes become available, they allow the direct diagnosis of the gene mutation (examples are drepanocytosis, X-fragile syndrome, Huntington's disease, etc.). However, for most of the monogenic diseases and due to the great number of possible mutations, direct diagnosis is not possible in practice. An indirect diagnosis is viable with the aid of closely linked polymorphisms which allow the study of the transmission of a gene within a given family.

Predictive medicine

All the above mentioned techniques can be used for different situations of predictive testing. Predictive genetic testing can be performed on single persons, on members of a family at risk, on a population as a whole or only on subsets of it without regard to family history. The systematic search for persons having a given genetic trait is called "genetic screening".

Three main types of predictive testing can be considered: presymptomatic diagnosis of monogenic diseases, diagnosis of predispositions and risk prediction for future generations.

Presymptomatic diagnosis of monogenic diseases detects a genetic disorder long before the onset of debilitating symptoms , with a probability close to 100% for the manifestation of the corresponding disease. There are cases where no prevention or early treatment is possible (Huntington's disease, for instance). There are other cases allowing for early treatment or prevention of complications (like familial polyposis coli).

Presymptomatic diagnosis may be performed at any time during life, including neonatal and prenatal stages, or even earlier in the form of pre-implantation diagnosis. Presymptomatic diagnosis performed in the course of life may refer to diseases which develop only in the carriers of the mutated gene (Huntington's disease or polycystic kidney disease) or to diseases which develop both in carriers and non carriers of the gene. Examples of the latter are several types of hereditary cancers, which represent only 5-10% of the occurrence of that cancer.

Diagnosis of predispositions/susceptibilities to serious diseases only indicates that a given person has a probability of contracting a certain disease which is higher than that of the general population. In a great number of common diseases (cancer, diabetes, cardiovascular diseases) the final morbid phenotype is not simply the product of a gene mutation, but is rather the result of a long chain of genetic and environmental factors. What differs from disease to disease is the relative proportion of these two factors. Prevention can often take place on the environmental factor. Testing of genetic predisposition allows the selection, within the general population, of the persons who carry a predisposition gene. As long as these persons are subjected to special preventive measures, they may live a healthy life. The diagnosis of predispositions can also be done during life, at pre-natal stage or in the embryo before implantation.

Risk prediction for future generations. Balanced chromosome anomalies (translocations, for instance), may be detected and entail the risk of transmitting the anomaly in the unbalanced form. In the case of diseases linked to the X-chromosome (Duchenne myopathy, haemophilia, etc.), diseases resulting from the amplification of trinucleotide repeats, Huntington's disease and others, the probability of healthy carriers to transmit the disease can be determined.

Ethical Problems

Predictive medicine aims at preventing the expression of diseases in persons carrying a morbid genetic trait. Its impact on public health is, therefore, very positive. However, there are areas of misuse which can lead to ethical concerns.

The Genetic Myth

The human genome analysis program tends to create, in the public, the myth of the unlimited capacity of genetics in the prediction of future life and health.

In Greek and Roman mythology the Moirai or Parcae were the inexorable three sisters who were spinning the thread of human life: Clotho (meaning the spinner), Lachesis (meaning the disposer of lots) and Atropos (meaning unalterable fate). In Homer and Hesiod they appear as goddesses of human fate and individual destiny, assigning to everyone his or her inevitable share of good and evil. They seemed to have a general power over events and were always present, spinning the thread of life.

The three Parcae are reincarnated, nowadays, in the genetic machinery of enzymes which spin the double-helical thread of DNA. The present myth announces that this magic thread encodes all our tendencies and wishes, all our future reactions and decisions, all our human destiny and individuality. It strives to make us believe that, if we succeed in deciphering our genome, we can read our future in it, like in a magic glass.

This mythic approach is a dangerous error. Even when the human genome becomes completely deciphered, human life and health remain not fully reducible to genes. Environmental factors, education, human experiences and habits have a decisive impact on gene expression. In addition, psychological motivations, cultural values and historical background also play a role in human health. Even the Greco-Roman myth of the Parcae was leaving some room to human freedom and personal responsibility.

Public education should demythologize the powers of genetics and establish its real limits in the prediction of future diseases and life. The sometimes unproven link between genetic predisposition and disease should be explained.

Informed Consent

In several cases, the prediction of a disease may have deleterious consequences on the tested subject and may conflict with his/her autonomy. Specially in the cases where no prevention or therapy are available, a positive result of a predictive test may cause severe psychological consequences or even suicide, in addition to the possibility of social stigmatization. It is questionable in which cases such predictive tests should be allowed. When allowed, special care should be taken that an extensive information is given to the person involved on the nature, possible results and consequences of the test. Only then, can a free consent be given. In addition, such person should be assisted by competent counseling , before, during and after the test. In any case, the wish not to know should be respected.

In the case of children or other persons incompetent to give informed consent, a common practice allowed their parents or guardians to substitute the needed consent. This practice is, however, being questioned and the limits of parental rights are emphasized. Parents are only entitled to take decisions which are expected to be in favor of their children. They are not entitled to order predictive tests just because they wish to know the genetic makeup of their children. Only if the disease may be declared before adulthood or demands early preventive measures, parents are allowed to request predictive tests.

Confidentiality in Relation to Family Members

When a positive result of a predictive test is obtained, this information may be important for other members of the family in order for them to undergo similar tests and preventive or therapeutic measures. In these cases, the tested person should be strongly urged to allow the communication of the result to those who clinically need this information. If he/she refuses to do that, the doctor is in a difficult dilemma. The doctor either breaks the right to confidentiality or the principle of beneficence towards people in danger who need his/her assistance. The classic answer of medical ethics gives the priority to absolute confidentiality. However, this solution may be questioned and the problem deserves an urgent discussion in the perspective of new Codes for the next century.

In the opinion of the ESLA Working Group:[1] "The principle...of non-disclosure of genetic information should prevail but only up to the point where it would threaten the interests of the individual himself, or would impinge adversely on the interests of others - family members, relatives, fellow employees, the public at large". In the 1994 London Conference on "Parliaments and Screening", Caroline Miles, from the Nuffield Council of Bioethics, mentioned rare cases in which the doctors felt that it was their duty to override the wishes of the screened person and to disclose the genetic information to family members. On this, Caroline Miles said: "We have suggested that this is a matter that needs to be discussed by the professional standard setting bodies of the medical profession - and the nursing profession - with a view to providing guidelines to doctors and nurses".[2] This urgent discussion may lead to a new code for the next century.

Confidentiality in Relation to Employers

Far more stringent criteria have to be followed when the disclosure of genetic information is intended for non-medical reasons. Such is the case when employers request that information.

The problem of the access to employers of predictive genetic data of their potential or actual employees has to be discussed considering the appropriate balance between the rights and interests of the employers, of the employees and of society.

Employers are certainly interested in the genetic data which may ascertain the foreseeable future state of health of the applicants for a job. The reasons for this are several. They are interested in reducing production costs and increasing cost effectiveness of investments. For this purpose, they have to avoid inefficiency or absenteeism of the worker, loss of the training investment by a premature incapacitation of the worker and increased payment of health, invalidity or death insurance contributions.

These interests of the employers are legitimate. In the framework of a market economy which accepts the free enterprise system, the employers are entitled to safeguard the productivity and to look for the best return of their investments. Nevertheless, these legitimate rights must be weighed up against the equally legitimate rights of the employees and of society.

The employees have the right not to know and to oppose, therefore, predictive tests. Even regarding tests already performed, they have the right to privacy and to not being unjustly discriminated. Most importantly, every individual has the right to work, which is a fundamental element of many modern constitutions and international agreements.[3] Work is a need for personal fulfillment and integration in the society, in addition of being, for the vast majority of the population, the main source of income and sustenance. To deny employment for reasons not of incapacity but of a mere prediction of a future disease or predisposition would represent a severe stigmatization. This would be even more unjust than the denial to handicapped persons of the special protection for the enjoyment of their right to work, which is prescribed by most laws.

The right to work should not be denied because of the prediction of a disease. Otherwise, a class of persons would be created who, although currently fit for work, were barred from employment. This discrimination is unjust for the individual and burdensome for society. These persons would have to be maintained from public funds and estimations have shown that they would cost more to the society than what they would to the employer.

For all these reasons, current regulations and doctrine in Europe agree that the rights of the employee, in such cases, should take precedence to the rights of the employer and that the latter is only entitled to inquire about the present, not the future, health conditions of a job applicant. The same position was taken by the draft Bioethics Convention proposed by the Council of Europe, which in its arts. 17 and 18 states that predictive tests can only be performed and the results communicated for health purposes.

A special case deals with certain working environments which can cause mutations originating a genetic disease. This effect can be acting on all kinds of persons, or be specific just to those individuals who have a genetic predisposition.

In the first case, work and safety rules should eliminate or minimize the risks, and genetic monitoring of the workers is advisable to confirm the safety at work. In the second case, it is important to identify the workers possessing a genetic predisposition, so as to limit their access to specific posts involving greater risk. This limitation in their right to work is justified by their right to health. But even in such cases, the testing should be performed on a voluntary basis, under conditions of a fully informed consent. If a worker refuses to undergo the test, his or her contract remains in force.

It is important in the latter cases that the disease keeps being considered as occupational, since in fact its agent is environmental. Genetic monitoring and screening should not be allowed to slip into detection of hereditary diseases in general and lead to discrimination. Even more important is to avoid a selection of resistant workers with the purpose of saving the expenses connected with feasible improvements of the working conditions. It would be greatly unjust to indulge in conditions of low levels of safety at the expenses of the exclusion of a class of the working population.

The rights of society to health should also be considered. There are certain jobs in which the unexpected deterioration of the worker's health could affect the safety of the public or of the fellow employees. A typical example is that of an airline pilot. In these cases, predictive tests (as, for instance, detecting a gene predisposing an individual to heart disease) may help to prevent serious accidents and are ethically justified. However, there is the danger of over-generalizing this principle and using these predictive tests with unjustified frequency. For instance, there are no ethical reasons to justify the exclusion of a person endowed with the gene for Huntington's chorea from being a pilot, as long as he is healthy.[*] In a future Code, regulations and provisions should be made in order to create independent bodies in charge of restricting the requirement of predictive tests for safety reasons to the due proportions and defend the rights of potential or real employees not less than the rights of society to safety.

In agreement with the above mentioned aspects, the Nuffield Council on Bioethics thinks that the exclusion of people from employment opportunities is only acceptable when proven to be absolutely necessary for health or safety reasons. The Council describes, in detail, the strict conditions required for genetic screening of the employees[5] But the Council's Chairman, Patrick Nairne, added in 1994: "This...is the right approach at present; we recommend that the Department of Employment keep the matter under review".[6] This is not an easy issue. New developments may require a new Code for the 21st century.

Confidentiality in Relation to Insurers

The problem of the access to genetic data from the part of insurance companies is not less difficult than that of the employers. In the case of life, health or other personal insurance, there is a conflict of interests between the insurer and the applicant. On the one hand, the insurer is interested in getting as much information as possible on the genetic predisposition and predictive diseases of the applicant, with the purpose of estimating the true extent of his contractual liability and commensurating premiums with health risks of the applicant. This interest of the insurer is justified by the principle of free enterprise, which allows him to conduct his own business as he sees fit. On the other hand, the applicant is interested in obtaining insurance without having to know or to reveal too many of his/her most intimate weaknesses. This interest is justified by the principle of privacy and by the rights not to know, of non-disclosure and of non-discrimination.

In favor of the insurer's position of free enterprise are also social interests of the community, as shown in the fact that, if many predictive tests become easily available and are routinely performed, the cost of the insurance premiums for the individuals showing negative results could become considerably lower and this would increase the general access of the public to insurance. Also in favor of the insurer's position is the fact that insurance contracts come under the category of contracts guided by the utmost of good faith. The applicant should inform the insurer of all circumstances known to him which might have a bearing on the assessment of the risk. This is why, in current insurance practice, insurers gather relevant information from the applicants through health questionnaires (family history, etc.) and medical examinations, without a general opposition of the applicants. The question only became acute with the prospect of including, in the medical examinations, genetic and predictive tests, which are considered as man's most intimate bastion.

The reluctance of the applicant in being tested or revealing information of genetic nature is justified by the right not to know, by the freedom of decision concerning what personal information should be disclosed, to whom and when, and by the right of not being discriminated.

The respect for the wish not to know, especially in the so delicate area of predictive genetics, having profound psychological-emotional impact on the affected persons, is generally accepted and, therefore, the right not to undergo predictive tests should prevail against the interests of the insurer.

In respect to the predictive tests already performed by the applicant, it has been sometimes assumed that their results should necessarily be disclosed to the insurer. This, however, may cause that two persons with the same genetic deficiency may be treated differently, just because one underwent a predictive test and the other not. As a matter of fact, it is known that many people who wished to undergo a predictive test did not ask for it just to avoid insurance complications.

However, the obligation to disclose the results of previous genetic tests is, in itself, questionable. Such obligation comes from the duty of contract loyalty and the requirements of good faith: both parties in the contract should share the same information. But this obligation may conflict with the individual's self-determination as regards the confidential information he/she chooses to pass on: "Recent European legal thinking advocates that the way out of this apparently unsolvable problem is to recognize that the interest of the insured should take precedence...The solution advocated by this current of opinion is based on an appeal to certain constitutional values of the social and democratic rule of law, where human dignity and the free development of personality are viewed as being clearly superior to other subordinate legal interests and values".[7] The same author proposes that legislation is passed to protect the applicant's right of non-disclosing genetic information, without having the insurance contract rejected or affected by premium surcharges.

The recent solution adopted in several European countries has been the establishment of a temporary moratorium, during which the governments and insurance companies should discuss the future use of genetic information. In the U.S., several insurance companies lost recently interest in requesting predictive tests, probably because they were not cost-effective. But the situation may change with future biotechnological progress. A continuing dialogue is necessary.

The individual right to refuse the use of the results of predictive tests for non-medical purposes may come into conflict, in the next century, with the economic mechanisms of our liberal societies. Society has then to seriously decide on the role of solidarity in its collective organization.[8] Legislation should not be postponed until predictive testing becomes a widespread practice for insurance. Much before that, the threat that genetic information may be misused should lead to an early declaration on the inadmissibility of any obligation from the part of the insurance applicant to disclose genetic information.

Privacy and confidentiality rights may be threatened by the overwhelming progress in genetic data informatization. *Data Protection Acts* regulate this matter. But their efficacy should be continuously evaluated. People should be informed that they have the right to demand that their blood samples are destroyed immediately after the results are obtained. Otherwise the samples might be used later for different purposes. In view of the fast development of data processing, a new *Code* might be needed, in the future, for data protection.

Eugenics

In its new forms, eugenics may also be a danger in predictive medicine, and deserves to be discussed. In terms of the new technologies, eugenics may be redefined as any action which aims at lowering the risk of a genetic disease by reducing the frequency of carriers of the corresponding gene in the population.[9] In this sense, it would fall under eugenic actions the abortion of a heterozygous but healthy fetus, able to give rise to a person who, although completely healthy, would be carrier of a genetic disease. There are, in fact, requests for abortion in such cases of predictive diseases for future generations. It would also be considered close to eugenics to recommend abortion of fetuses affected by genes of late-onset diseases, able therefore to give rise to persons who would live a normal life for 40 or more years. The same can be said about embryos or fetuses carrying genes of predisposition or susceptibility to develop certain diseases. In the North of England, selection of *in vitro* embryos has been performed, destroying upon preimplantation diagnosis the embryos showing the presence of predisposition genes for a late-onset disease carried by the mother. These are clearly eugenic practices.

These practices are inscribed in a general tendency and pressure towards the utopian right to a completely healthy genome. "Many women or couples feel that genetic health almost becomes a condition that a child must fulfill; should it not meet the normative expectations of parents and society - norms that no one can rationally justify - it is his or her 'bad luck'".[10] This tendency towards the right of a fully healthy genome is scientifically utopic because there is evidence that every human person carries several defective genes in a heterozygotic state.[11] In addition, the so called "bad" genes confer, in several cases, protection against other diseases. Man shows a nice balance between the risk factors and the protective factors.

The most serious eugenic danger of predictive testing resides in the possibility that it might start being used, in the future, to eliminate healthy embryos or fetuses whose characteristics do not fit the personal wishes of the parents. This would violate fundamental rights, in addition of opposing the biodiversity of our species. This is why the Council of Europe passed a Recommendation in 1990 proposing that prenatal diagnosis and screening are only approved for medical reasons.[12] Also the Pompidou *Report* presented to the European Parliament on February 2, 1994 insists "on the risk of eugenics by selection of fetuses". This Report proposes that: "le diagnostique pré-natal ne puisse avoir pour objet que de diagnostiquer, de prévenir ou de traiter une affection d'une particulière gravité et soit indissociable d'un conseil génétique documenté et correctement conduit".[13] More recently, the new French Law of 1994[14] limits the prenatal diagnosis to the cases of risk of a "particularly serious disease". Article L 162.16 of the *Health Code* introduced by the new Law defines that "le diagnostic prénatal s'entend à des pratiques médicales ayant pour but de détecter *in utero* chez l'embryon ou le foetus une affection d'une particulière gravité". This disposition means that, in principle, the access to the prenatal diagnosis is limited to the cases of risk of those diseases susceptible to legally justify abortion.[15] In this way, the misuse of predictive testing for choosing children "à la carte" is thought to be prevented.

Towards a New Code

Predictive medicine is a relatively new field, especially developed by the recent progresses of molecular biology and human genetics. Its ethical evaluation has been codified in a variety of norms, some of which are the following: *Report* by the U.S. President's Commission for the Study of Ethical Problems in Medicine and Biomedical and Behavioral Research (1983); *Chancen und Risiken* (Bericht der gemeinsamen Arbeitsgruppe des Bundesministers für Forschung und Technologie und des Bundesministers der Justiz, München, 1984-1986); *Resolution from the European Parliament A2-327/88* on the ethical and legal problems of genetic engineering (1988); *Report on Genetic Screening: Ethical Issues*, Nuffield Council of Bioethics (1993); *Outline of a Declaration on the Human Genome and its Protection in Relation to Human Dignity and Human Rights*, UNESCO International Bioethics Committee, 1995; *Draft European Convention on Bioethics*, Council of Europe, 1995.

All these and other documents are the final result of a great number of reports prepared by specialists, as well as of intensive discussion. Some points of these documents are overlapping, others are complementary. It would be desirable to boil them down to a limited number of sharp statements, which could constitute a new *Code* of the future.

The legal status of such a new *Code* could be discussed. It might, like a E.U. Directive, be binding to the undersigned countries, so as to force them to transpose its decisions to the national legislations. Or it might, like a Convention from the Council of Europe, be legally binding by itself in all member states. Or it might have the moral power and independence of a unanimous Declaration, without any legally binding character.

Another question is which Institution would candidate to elaborate such a new Code. We could think of UNESCO, WHO or CIOMS. Certainly, the appropriate range of countries involved would be an important element for this decision. The main objective is that, for new fields such as predictive medicine, we become able to overcome the unavoidable multiplicity of analytical documents and come to the synthesis and simplicity of just a "*new code*".

References

1   Working Group on the Ethical, Social and Legal Aspects of Human Genome Analysis, European Commission, Report of 31 December 1991, point 3.2.1.

2   Miles C. (1995), 'Genetic screening-2' in *Parliaments and Screening - Ethical and social problems arising from testing and screening for HIV and genetic disease,* Ed. by Wayland Kennet, John Libbey Eurotext, Paris, p.68.

3   de Sola C. (1995), 'Privacy and Genetic Data. Cases of Conflict (II)', *Law and the Human Genome Review* 2: 147-156.

4   Berg K. (1993), 'People who are healthy should be treated as healthy persons whatever their future disease risks are'. *Revue Internationale de Droit Économique,* 1: p.131.

5   *Genetic Screening: Ethical Issues,* Nuffield Council on Bioethics, 28, Bedford Square, London, WC1 3EG, 1993.

6   Nairne P. (1995), 'Genetic screening-1', in *Parliaments and Screening - Ethical and social problems arising from testing and screening for HIV and genetic disease,* Ed. by Wayland Kennet, John Libbey Eurotext, Paris, p.62.

7   Yanes, P. (1995), 'Personal Insurance and Genetic Information', *Law and the Human Genome Review* 2: 166.

8   Comité Consultatif National pour les Sciences de la Vie et de la Santé (1995), *Génétique et Médicine: de la prédiction à la prévention. Avis. Rapports. (N° 46),* Paris.

9   Papiernik É. (1992), 'Vers un Nouvel Eugénisme?' et *Vers un Anti-destin?: Patrimoine Génétique et Droits de l'Humanité,* sous la direction de François Gros et Gérard Huber, Ed. Odile Jacob, Paris, pp. 116.

10   Haker H. (1993), 'Human Genome Analysis and Eugenics', in *Ethics of Human Genome Analysis : European Perspectives,* Hille Haker, Richard Hearn and Klaus Steigleder eds., Attempto Verlag Tübingen, p. 305.

11   Müller H.J. (1950), 'Our Load of Mutation', *Am. J. Hum. Genet.* 2: 111-176. Vogel F. (1979), 'Our Load of Mutation: reappraisal of an old problem', *Proc. R. Soc. London* B 205:77-90.

12   *Recommendation n° R(90) 13,* adopted by the Council of Ministers of the Council of Europe in 21 June 1990.

13   Pompidou A., Rapport présenté au nom de la Commission "Energie, Recherche et Technologie" du Parlement Européen, sur les aspects éthiques des nouvelles technologies biomédicales, en particulier le DPN. Le 2 février 1994 (A3-0057/94).

14   *Act 94.654* of 29 July 1994.

15   Lenoir N. (1994), 'Aspects juridiques et éthiques du diagnostic prénatal: le droit et les pratiques en vigueur en France et dans divers autres pays'. In *Analyse Génétique humaine et Protection de la Personnalité,* Publications de l'Institut suisse de droit comparé 25, pags. 29-55, Zürich.

23 Allocation of Limited Resources and Equity

Göran Hermerén

Organization and System

In the main bulk of this paper, I will call attention to some key conceptual, empirical and normative problems concerning setting limits, making priorities and allocating resources for health care. Before we go into these problems, however, we have to pay attention to the organization of health care in the relevant countries as well as to a number of aspects of the welfare system in those countries.

Some factors are particularly important in this context. They include the extent to which private production of health care exists, how health care is financed, if patients have been granted any rights or guarantees to receive certain hospital care freely or within a certain time limit, how the health insurance system is construed, the existence of political decisions as to the patients' right to choose hospital and doctor, and so forth.

Recent changes in the organization and financing of the health care system can have great consequences for the resource allocation problems. Moreover, if these aspects of the organization and financing of the system are not made explicit, data from different countries may be misunderstood, and talking at cross-purposes will almost inevitably arise.

Three Emerging New Areas since 1964

Since 1964, when the declaration of Helsinki was first adopted by the World Medical Assembly, medicine has changed considerably. New areas have emerged, which present partly new ethical challenges to us.

The Declaration of Helsinki, as the earlier Nuremberg code, focused on how to prevent harm to human individuals in research, in the first place atrocities committed by individuals against individuals, as in the research performed in the Nazi concentration camps, on, for example, how cold water a human being can survive in. Hence the focus was on individual rights. This was, of course, necessary and important at the time, and the fact that also other issues emerge today does not detract from the value and historical importance of these codes.

The contemporary discussion of ethical problems in certain areas of health care and medicine, like epidemiology, genetic (pre-symptomatic) testing, and resource allocation raise partly new issues. There is a shift of perspective from the individualistic starting point underlying these earlier codes to a more societal one, where solidarity, justice and altruism emerge as some of the key concepts.

The basic similarity between the three emerging new areas is that the choice between various possible courses of action open to the agents will have consequences for more than one individual. Therefore, particular problems arise with the interpretation and application of the requirement of free and informed consent. Who is to give the free and informed consent? When? And on what grounds?

In predictive, pre-symptomatic genetic testing, the family or the society at large is directly involved, as are future generations of families at risk. If some members of a family with increased risk of getting a certain genetic disease want to be tested, and others refuse, whose autonomy should be respected? Should some members of a family have the right to veto a test of other members of the family, even if these members would benefit from the test? There is an extensive literature on these problems.

In epidemiology, those who are infected by certain diseases can spread their infections to others. Those with certain genetic predispositions can die prematurely, if exposed to hazardous working conditions or pollution in air and water. Consideration for the integrity and welfare of some groups may then clash with the obligation to do good and minimize harm, i.e., with consideration for the welfare and integrity of others. The interest of workers may clash with those of the owners or managers. What is good for those who are infected may clash with what is good for their relatives and friends. A recent discussion of some of the ethical problems in this area, with references to others, may be found in.[1]

In discussions of resource allocation and setting limits, many problems concern justice between different groups, between generations, and sometimes within a single life. Here concepts like equity, need and solidarity will play an important role. But how are these concepts to be interpreted? And if the needs of one individual (or group) conflict with the needs of another individual (or group), whose needs should be satisfied? On what grounds?

In all these three areas, there is a clear tension between a health policy perspective based on considerations of justice and the obligation to do good and to avoid harm rather than an individual consumer rights perspective based on the duty to respect autonomy and integrity.

There are guidelines in epidemiological research,[2,3] and guidelines for genetic testing in specific areas are emerging. Should there also be guidelines for resource allocation? In other words, do the new developments in medicine mean that in these areas, and particularly for problems concerning resource allocation, international codes and guidelines are possible and desirable - to supplement the earlier codes mentioned above? This will be discussed at the end of this paper. But first we have to comment on the nature of the resource allocation problem and some of the ethical issues it raises.

The Problems

It is important to clarify both the nature of the problems we are discussing, and the starting points or premises for the discussion of this problem. When this is done, we have to examine the steps from these premises to the conclusions drawn. At least, this is so, if we want to understand what is going on today and want to have a fair chance to predict what the problems will be during the first decades of the next century.

Needless to say, this is particularly urgent if - against the background of our discussion of the Nuremberg code and the declaration of Helsinki - we want to encourage thinking on possible guidelines for allocation of limited resources during the next decades. In that case it will be necessary to clarify the goals and identify the obstacles more or less blocking the road to these goals.

Allocation of resources takes place on different levels. Various stakeholders and agents are involved, formally and informally, and their responsibilities are not the same. Hence the agents and stakeholders need to be made explicit, and this also holds for their roles, how their roles are perceived by themselves and by others. Who should decide about priorities and resource allocation? This question does not have one answer, because it tries to answer several different problems at the same time. The answer varies with the allocation problem.

It is particularly important to separate problems arising in the clinical setting from others. In the clinic, a doctor meets a patient and has to decide what diagnostic and therapeutic measures that patient should be offered. Also the time of the doctor is a limited resource. How long should he see the patient, and which patients should be asked to see him or her again? A doctor may face dozens of such problems each day, and has to make a quick decision every time on the basis of incomplete and sometimes uncertain evidence.

The problem facing those working with the budget of a hospital or county council is very different. On the basis of extensive and carefully reviewed evidence concerning needs, costs and effects - at least in theory - they once a year have to decide how much money should be allocated to different clinics and different activities. If the evidence is perceived to be incomplete and uncertain, there is ample time to check it and supplement it with new data.

On a still more general level, of course, problems of resource allocation arise when the parliament of a country decides on how much of the budget should go into military defense, education, health care, culture, sports, courts and justice, transportation, road construction, fights against unemployment, etc.

In practice, limits are set in several ways, which can, and probably need to, be combined in order to have the desired effect: (i) allocating resources to the clinics, hospitals and county councils by political decisions on several levels as indicated above, and (ii) directing the flow of patients into the hospital system, for example, by organizational reforms of the interaction between primary care and specialist care in hospitals, by health care guarantees, by differentiating fees and changing the extent to which certain health care is to be paid for by patients themselves, etc.

Many agents and stakeholders clearly have different roles in these strategies. Hence, there is not one problem of setting limits but many. Accordingly, a first important task is to clarify these problems, partly empirical, partly conceptual and partly normative, and to indicate their relations to each other.

Principles and Variations

Many earlier attempts to solve the vexing problems of resource allocation and setting limits in health care, or of providing guidelines for how to handle such problems, like the Oregon approach,[4] are based on DRG (diagnose related groups) or some such concepts. But diagnoses and diagnostic methods vary in sensitivity and specificity. Sometimes flaws are discovered in them, sometimes they are improved. Therefore lists based on DRGs have to be revised often.

More importantly, even disregarding these problems, there are important variations within each group of people with the same diagnosis. The suffering varies for people with the same diagnosis, both at different points of time (or different stages in the development of a disease) and at the same time or stage of development. Sometimes the suffering caused by a particular disease in almost unbearable, sometimes it is possible to alleviate the pain or to learn to live with it.

For these reasons, an approach based on principles is better than an approach based on DRG or similar concepts. Moreover, we have to look for solutions which are not only for those on Medicaid and similar programs but cover the entire population, that is, for solutions which cannot be accused of inequity (of not being offered for all in a fair manner).

Particularly at the clinical level, principles have to be put into practice by applying them to the situation at hand. In that way, it is possible to take due consideration to variations within groups, using and interpreting the principles as road signs, pointing in a certain direction, not as a substitute for thinking.

But which (normative) principles should be used when resources are to be allocated and limits are to be set? The principles can be stated in very different ways, which I will now briefly comment on and then discuss in some more detail in what follows.

Three Approaches

Decisions on ethically contested issues are based on premises of various kinds, both factual information and normative principles. In the context of resource allocation, there are a number of obviously relevant factual premises. They include, for example, information concerning the health care options available (needless to say, they are not the same in the third world and in western Europe), the cost and efficiency of these diagnostic and therapeutic options, the waiting time for certain treatments, as well as the needs of the population at large. Unfortunately, the certainty of our knowledge of these important aspects varies considerably.

Even so, the conclusions drawn from a description of these and other facts can vary, depending on the norms and values taken for granted or explicitly used. If talking at cross-purposes is to be avoided, it is important to be explicit also as to the normative starting points. The values and cultural traditions even in countries in Europe are not always the same. Of course, this can account for some of the differences of their health care systems and in the services offered to their citizens.

I will here distinguish between three main types of normative approaches to these problems. They focus on goals, rights and markets respectively, and therefore these approaches could be called goal-oriented, rights-oriented and market-oriented. To avoid misunderstandings, I would like to stress that I do not assume (i) that these approaches are exhaustive; (ii) that they exclude each other; and (iii) that one of them is "correct" and the others are mistaken.

Thus, there are other approaches, and the only thing I want to claim is that the three approaches to be discussed in more detail below represent important and different attempts to solve the problems of resource allocation, all of which have their advocates.

Moreover, certain elements from some of the approaches can be combined with certain elements from some of the others, as I shall try to show below. This is particularly true of the need-oriented and the right-oriented approaches. Thus they do not exclude each other, though as a whole they are quite distinct and may yield different results when applied to the same problem.

Finally, and more importantly, I will not argue that there is only one correct solution. There are three different approaches each with its pros or cons. In one political, economic and social situation, the pros of a particular solution may outweigh the cons, in another situation it may be the other way around, though I shall not hide which one I prefer, at least for the part of the world in which I live.

Focus on Goals

The first questions concerning any goal-oriented approach are clearly: Which goal? And whose goal? Here I propose that the starting point should be the goals of medicine and health care.

Unfortunately, none of these goals are uncontroversial. Each of them can be stated and interpreted in several ways. Concerning both medicine and health care, there are families of goals, more or less closely related. The important thing is to be explicit and make clear which particular formulation and interpretation of these goals that is used as a starting point.

My general idea is that the basic goal of medicine is humanitarian, that is to help those who suffer, and to use the resources (human, economic, etc.) as effectively as possible. If resources are wasted, then it may be impossible to help others. But per se, the basic goal of medicine has no economic dimension.

To be somewhat more specific, we may distinguish between medical and political goals of the health care system. Albert Jonsen, Mark Siegler and William Winslade[5] have suggested the following goals for health care:

- restoration of health;
- relief of symptoms (including physical distress and psychological suffering);
- restoration of function and maintenance of compromised functions;
- saving or prolonging of life;
- education and counseling of patients regarding their condition and its prognosis; and
- avoiding harm to the patient in the course of care.

There are potential conflicts between some of these goals, for example, between prolonging life and avoiding harm to the patient. But these conflicts will not be discussed here. Nor shall I discuss the many different problems and possibilities of establishing a ranking order between these goals. Thus, the authors, quite correctly in my view, make clear that there are tensions between several of these goals, and that several different ranking orders between them are possible. But this is at least a start, which illustrates one possible set of medical goals, as good as any that I have seen in the literature, though it is by no means above criticism. For instance, it might be argued that 2 and 3 could be regarded as subsets of, or included in, 1, and that 6 falls a bit outside a list of independent goals.

But it is important to see that they can be supplemented by political goals for the health care system as a whole, such as:

- to see to it that what the health care system can offer is distributed to the citizens in a fair way, that is, according to need rather than according to social position or economic power;

- maintaining and strengthening the confidence of the general public in the health care system;
- making the system function in a cost-efficient way, so that every invested dollar (mark or crown) results in as much good care as possible; and
- to maintain and improve the quality of health care concerning diagnostics, treatment, follow up and prevention, including the way in which the staff in general relates to patients.

Ethical Points of Departure

Clearly, one must not confuse (a) the normative points of departure explicitly stated in government reports or guidelines from national or other ethics committees with (b) the implicit starting points actually used by different decisionmakers. People may or may not be aware of the latter. The explicit and implicit starting points concerning values and norms of a particular individual or group may coincide, more or less, but they do not always do so.

To illustrate the normative premises of a goal-oriented approach, I will mention briefly the ethical point of departure in the recent Swedish government commission report on priorities and resource allocation[6,7] - and later contrast them with a few others, which may be more appealing to people coming from other countries, where the welfare politics has a different foundation, and where individualistic rather than collective solutions prevail. The three main principles in the Swedish model include:

- *Principle 1: human dignity.* All people are equal in dignity, regardless of personal characteristics and functions in society. Therefore, they have the same human rights and the same right to get these rights respected.
- *Principle 2: need and solidarity.* The resources available should be spent on the individual or activity most in need of them.
- *Principle 3: cost-efficiency.* When choosing between different fields of activity or measures, a reasonable relation between costs and effect, measured in improved health and improved quality of life, should be aimed for.

These principles have been placed in ranking order, in such a way that the principle of human dignity takes precedence over the principle of need and solidarity, and the principle of cost-efficiency is subordinate to both the others.

These general principles have to be supplemented by more specific guidelines developed within the different specialties (oncology, heart surgery, kidney transplantation, psychiatry, etc.). These guidelines should specify the effects of various interventions along the three dimensions discussed in the next section below. They should also take into account the quality of life of the patients, and pay attention to variations within the groups (all patients suffering from the same disease do not suffer equally, and an early diagnosis sometimes makes a considerable difference). Complications and risks with various forms of treatment should be indicated, as well as the probability of the effects on patients belonging to different subcategories.

If such more specific guidelines are developed, two problems need careful attention:

- the *consistency* problem: "are there any inconsistencies between these specific guidelines and the general principles?"; and
- the *commensurability* problem: "are the medical interventions and their effects comparable in different areas, such as psychiatry, long-term care, obstetrics, surgery and oncology?"

General Comments on Some Concepts of the Principles

These principles all contain vague expressions. In this section, I propose to comment briefly on some ways of clarifying the principles.

The second principle will in practice be very important. What is need? Can it be measured? Here we must distinguish between definitions and criteria of need on the one hand, methods of measuring needs on the other, and finally valuing needs, i.e. whether (the satisfaction of) certain needs are good, bad or indifferent.

As to the crucial concept of need, I will only say here that it is not limited to medical needs in a strict sense; also social and psychological needs are included. This means that my discussion will not be based on a narrow medical conception of disease but rather on a concept of need related to welfare and quality of life.

But here it is important to distinguish between the need (of an individual or a group) of better *health,* for example, defined in terms of increased life expectancy, and the need of better *health care.* Obviously, the latter may be a means to the former, but it is not the only means. Since our topic is allocation of limited resources in health care, it is the latter concept that is relevant in this context.

Need in this sense is to be distinguished from demand. The needs of a person are elaborated in a dialogue with the doctor, where the patient relates his problems, the doctor examines the symptoms, and proposes different alternative therapeutic measures, which the patient can accept, refuse or ask for more information about, etc.

Need obviously has to do with, and is partly determined by, the seriousness of the condition. If A's condition is more serious than B's, and A would suffer more than B if he did not get care, A is clearly in greater need of help than B. But different people can experience and respond to the same condition in different ways, which should be taken into account. If the need is the same, the treatment should be the same, regardless of where in the country the patient lives and of his or her personal characteristics, economic situation and social functions.

Nevertheless, it should be possible to clarify the needs of the patient and the seriousness of the condition along several dimensions, as has been suggested e.g. in:[8]

- the degree of physical and psychological pain, suffering, and anguish;
- the degree of physical, psychological and social reduction of function (functional disability or disturbance), measured in ability to cope with problems in daily life; and
- the risk for death, invalidity, serious pain or suffering in case treatment is delayed or no treatment is offered.

Research and development concerning ways of measuring and interpreting needs along these and similar dimensions are obviously important, given this view. So are clinical studies and critical examinations of the cost-efficiency of diagnostic and therapeutic measures, as well as regular and systematic studies of the needs of the population at large.

The third principle presupposes that costs and effects of the interventions can be measured and the relations between them estimated, at least on an ordinal scale.

As to measurement of expected effects of medical interventions, they could be measured along the three dimensions mentioned above, and in principle be specified in quantitative terms (How extensive are the effects?), in probability terms (What is the likelihood that the intervention has any effect?), in risk terms (Which, if any, is the risk to the patient's health, if the intervention is postponed?), and in epistemic terms (How well do we know the uncertainty of the evaluations and judgments?).

Decisions concerning the order of priority between effective measures are always difficult to make and to accept. If such decisions are based on commonly accepted ethical principles, this will facilitate understanding by the general public, including hopefully also those affected, and will help to sustain confidence and trust in publicly funded health care.

In our part of the world, this obviously presupposes that the political process in which resources are distributed to different activities on several levels is a democratic one and has been accepted by the majority of citizens in the country. This is necessary in order to facilitate acceptance and legitimacy for the inevitable but difficult decisions which have to be made, when limits are set and resources are scarce.

Under what conditions does a person have the right to be a patient? Criteria of inclusion and exclusion (of treatment) need to be developed democratically and fairly, and if possible justified in the light of generally accepted theories of fair distribution of scarce resources. This is particularly true for the relations between the seriousness of the condition, the effects of the intervention (as well as the effects of a non-intervention), and the costs.

These ethical starting points could be contrasted with a number of other alternative ones, for example, defined in terms of autonomy and demand (let the market decide what health care it wants and is prepared to pay for), maximizing expected utility, or others. Such contrasts and comparisons should sharpen our awareness of the significance of the ethical starting points.

Cost-efficiency, Research and Resources

To know if a certain treatment is cost-effective, clinical studies have to be made. At present, only a small part of the medical treatments currently offered have been evaluated in scientific clinical trials. The figure of 20 % is sometimes mentioned in this context, others regard it as too optimistic.

This would seem to mean that more resources have to be spent - and paradoxically, that you have to spend money in order to save money. Besides, new treatments are invented all the time, so we would never, even if we did spend much more money than we do today on clinical research and evaluation, be able to evaluate all treatments in a scientific way.

However, systematic studies of the cost-effectiveness of certain treatments carried out in Sweden by SBU (Statens beredning för utvärdering av medicinsk metodik) suggest that (a) some treatments actually used are ineffective, others are even counterproductive, i.e. cause harm, and (b) if inefficient and counterproductive methods were abandoned, more money would be saved than the evaluation of these methods has cost. And this money could be used to help others to get better treatment.

Thus, it is true that the third principle would, at least at the outset, increase the costs. But this cost should be regarded as an investment. The evidence available suggests that this investment would pay off before long. It is important to underline this, because when resources are scarce, it is always tempting to cut down on research. To do so, however, would not be to use the resources in a rational way.

Conflicts Between General Principles and Praxis

The three principles above may appear very general, with little analytical bite, as it were. Yet it is not too difficult to show that they clash with what is current practice also in a welfare country like Sweden. I have tried to do this elsewhere.[9] Besides, the situation might vary from country to country. It should be interesting to check what clashes there are between current practice and these and other principles in several different countries.

It will have to suffice to say that some of the critical issues, at least in Sweden, concern negative discrimination of the elderly, positive discrimination of harms caused by football and other sports activities. They also include terminal care, prevention and treatment of chronic diseases, patient's rights to receive certain kinds of treatment within fixed time limits, the combination of DRG and the buy and sell system introduced in parts of Swedish hospital care.

Still other critical issues include the extent to which patients have a right to choose between hospitals, doctors, and alternative treatments, as well as the right for doctors and physiotherapists to establish a clinic or a practice anywhere in the country.

I will now proceed to make a number of more specific comments on issues raised by these principles by contrasting them with other approaches and discussing if and to what extent they exclude each other. I will then comment on the relations between, for example, needs and rights, demand and the role of the general public, as well as demand and market forces.

Focus on Rights

Another approach to the problem of resource allocation is based on rights. The precise relation between the two approaches depend on exactly how the goals and rights involved are construed and what they are based on. Anyway here, as in the first approach, the obvious questions that need to be faced at the outset include: which rights? And whose rights?

As to the last question, several constructions are possible. Are we talking about the rights of human beings, for example, as specified in the UN Declaration of Human Rights, or about the rights of citizens of a certain country, as specified partly in the laws and rules of that country, or of the rights of patients, as indicated by guidelines of hospitals, county councils and professional organizations?

And how are these rights to be understood: as claim rights, liberty rights or as rights to say no - that is, to prohibit others to do certain things to you and your body without first obtaining your informed consent?

In Norway and in several other countries there is a growing interest in specifying patients' rights, and the patients' rights movement is clearly gaining momentum, even if there are considerable differences between the ideas behind the patient charters, proposed bills, and so forth, in different countries.

Obviously, there is a tension between an approach based on principles of the sort advocated earlier and certain rights in the form of guarantees to patients. This tension will be discussed briefly in the first subsections below. But this does not exclude that certain elements in the goal- and need-oriented approaches can be combined with some elements in the rights-oriented approach, as I will then try to show. A certain appeal to rights is clearly built-in into the first principle above.

Guarantees and Principles

Do guarantees imply need? Does need imply guarantees? None of these questions could in my view be answered in the affirmative.

As mentioned in the introduction, in some countries citizens are granted certain rights. They may be guaranteed to receive certain treatment free of charge, or to receive it within a certain time after the diagnosis has been carried out. This policy exists, for example, in both Norway and Sweden.

Such guarantees, of course, mean that certain priorities have been introduced in the system of health care. Patients covered by such guarantees are in a favorable position in comparison to persons without such guarantees. Particularly, if guarantees of this sort are introduced in areas where it is easy to measure the effects, and for tactical political reasons, there may be clashes between such guarantees and priorities based on principles of the sort advocated here. This has been the case in Sweden.

Obviously, it will create confusion if politicians and health care authorities speak with double tongue, as it were, and deliver contradictory messages. Therefore, two alternatives suggest themselves. The first is, obviously, to abolish all such guarantees, and to work with a consistent set of principles. The second one is to expand the guarantees to include all patients and all treatments eventually.

The latter approach would in effect mean that all problems of setting limits and allocating resources would have to be solved *within* such a system of guarantees. This is hardly a viable strategy. It would most certainly be very inflexible and face obvious difficulties of handling changes when new and more efficient methods of treatment are developed as well as the problems raised by variations within groups with the same diagnosis.

But the Swedish parliament, very unwisely in my view, choose neither of these strategies. It expanded the existing guarantees to include also a few others. This means that they did not solve the problems they had already created of inconsistencies between current guarantees and generally accepted principles. Instead they added to their number by creating new problems.

It is inevitable that if not all diagnoses and treatments are covered by guarantees, but only some, those which are not covered will be at disadvantage. More often than not, people with diagnoses and needs not covered by a guarantee will be treated after those covered by a guarantee when resources are scarce - particularly if hospitals have to pay or can be sued if patients have to wait for treatment longer than the time specified in the guarantee. However, to avoid oversimplification, a more careful discussion of the relations between needs and rights is necessary.

Needs and Rights

The emphasis on needs here does not mean that a need-based system of guidelines for resource allocation, like the system mentioned above, is incompatible with, or excludes a system based on patients' rights, at least not entirely. As already mentioned, the principle of human dignity, as interpreted here, contains explicit references to rights.

But to describe the relation between needs and rights in the three principles stated above, we must distinguish between different kinds of rights.

First of all, individuals also in the system advocated here have the right to a quick and correct diagnosis. Without such a diagnosis, it is not possible to decide what they suffer from, how severe their disease is, and what they need in terms of treatment and care - and hence to decide what priority, if any, should be given to the treatment of their condition.

Second, patients also in this system have the right to say no to any treatment suggested by their doctor. Obvious exceptions include patients who are legally incapable or incompetent.

But none of these rights are strictly legal rights in the sense that violations of them make it possible for dissatisfied patients or relatives to sue doctors or health care administrators, at least not in Sweden. If such a system were introduced, we would - as experiences from the US suggest - introduce a system which lawyers would benefit (and even profit) from. It would lead to higher costs with little benefits to large groups of patients, the hospital, and the state.

Focus on the Market

Market oriented approaches can be more or less radical, depending on what restrictions, if any, are put on the market forces. In the extreme versions, no restrictions at all are put on the market. Let people get what they are willing to pay for, and the invisible hand referred to by Adam Smith will in the end solve all resource allocation problems and set the limits where they should be set.

Other versions include giving people a check on a certain sum when they are born. This check can used to pay for whatever health care they want during their life time. But the length of people's lives vary, and so does their ability to plan and foresee what is going to happen to them. Besides, sickness and misfortunes do not affect people equally, or in relation to their capacity to plan and save.

The objections to extreme market-oriented versions are only too obvious: they will lead to a health care system, where only those services are offered which people with money are willing *and able* to pay for. If some people have virtually no money, they will not be able to get any health care at all. If others have lots of money, they may ask for health care services for themselves for which there may not even be any medical reason. This may clearly lead to an extremely inequitable system.

Such extreme versions are hardly interesting and have few advocates today. But there are more interesting versions, when health care is offered on a market which is regulated in some detail, or when patients may have to share the costs for certain exclusive treatments. The more patients have to pay for less exclusive treatments, the more we are approaching the extreme forms of market oriented solutions.

Extreme market-oriented approaches are based on the assumption that health care is like soap or any other merchandise which is sold on a market. Therefore the customer (or consumer rights) perspective is appropriate. The crucial question is the extent to which the analogy holds between seeking the help of a doctor and e.g. buying a new car (choosing between different models on the basis of what you can afford and on the information available about these cars).

This analogy, of course, is criticized by those who advocate the first two approaches, that is, by those who claim that in a welfare state access to health care is a right, as well as by those who claim that the basic goal of health care is humanitarian.

A neo-liberal might think that it is the right of the rich to use their money in whatever way they please and buy all the service they want, including in vitro fertilization and plastic surgery, as long as they: (a) pay the full cost for this and (b) do not deprive anyone else of the possibility to get access to health care. However, one should not underestimate the difficulty of demonstrating that these two clauses (a) and (b) are satisfied; the costs of health care services can be estimated in several ways, particularly if the training of doctors and other health care staff has been subsidized by the state.

But for the reasons to be outlined below, also the goal-oriented approaches have to accommodate certain features of the market approach - certainly, in all of western Europe, there has recently been a strong political pressure in that direction. A desire to increase the freedom of the patient has been stressed by spokesmen of many political movements.

A clear distinction between those who order (commission) health care services and those who provide them in the system may certainly help to improve efficiency, if the internal accounting system and bureaucracy can be kept under control. Some same goes for competition between those who provide the services, provided the quality of the services can be maintained.

But the danger of confusing a means to reach a certain goal with one of these goals should be observed. To save money is not one of the goals of health care. But in order to be able to help as many as possible, resources should be used in a cost-effective way.

Demand and the Role of the Public

The general public has to have a voice in the discussion of resource allocation problems. This is essential for the confidence in the system, particularly if the health of the country is financed by taxes - as well as for the willingness to pay, if the health care system is based in market forces in one form or another.

However, the role of the public can vary, and is indeed very different, in countries with different political systems. In countries with representative democracy, the general public has a voice via their elected politicians in county councils and parliaments. The politicians elected can influence resource allocation problems particularly on the political-administrative level and the general political level, i.e. when resources are allocated to different activities, hospitals, etc.

Also mass media have an important role to play here, as a channel for the voice of the general public. This, of course, is important in a democratic society. Saying this is not to say or suggest that this role is never misused. Massmedia tend to focus on individual cases. There are examples from several countries, including both Norway and Sweden, where doctors and politicians have taken a certain decision and, for example, said no to a heart transplant abroad. Then the family of the patient has contacted the media. With reports about the suffering of the individual patient the media sometimes managed to stir the opinion of the general public in such a way that the politicians have not always been able to resist it. They have therefore changed their earlier decision even when they realized that the new decision was against their better judgment or inconsistent with principles they had agreed on before.

In these ways, some public input to allocation issues is secured, a political process is established for handling conflicts over allocation issues. Doctors should not have a monopoly on expressing views and deciding resource allocation issues on the political levels. Monitoring could be devised, as well as a board of complaint, if this is considered necessary or desirable.

In the clinical setting, however, the need of a patient has to be established in the dialogue earlier described between doctor and patient. Here, politicians and mass-media should not interfere.

Individuals, at least in Sweden, do not have the right to demand a certain treatment. But they are according to the *Health Care Act* (HSL) entitled to refuse some or all of the treatments proposed by the doctor. Suppose the public had a voice in the sense that patients would be given a right to demand a certain treatment. This would certainly not solve the problem of resource allocation in a situation with scarce resources, since there are reasons to believe that many people would want the best and most exclusive treatment for themselves and their relatives, regardless of the costs.

Moreover, one must not underestimate the psychological difficulty for a doctor in a clinical situation to look his or her patient straight into the face and say that there is a treatment the doctor believes would help, but the doctor cannot give it to his or her patient for economic reasons; the clinic cannot afford it; or other patients need the treatment better.

The clash between doing so and one of the clauses in the Declaration of Geneva, adopted by the World Medical Association in 1948 and amended in 1983, should be noted: "The health of my patient will be my first consideration". Besides, who is the doctor's patient? This is a problem I will return to later.

Demand and Market Forces

There is a place for people to express what they want to have in any free society, and in principle for others to try to satisfy such demands, provided they are not indecent, offensive or against generally accepted moral views. But the right to express a request or a demand does not necessarily entail an obligation for others, in particular for doctors, to satisfy this request or demand.

Requests and demands have to be examined critically, and weighed against each other, especially when resources are limited. They should be tested against evidence concerning the needs of the person making the request or the demand, as well as against known facts concerning the needs of other people (and there should perhaps also be an obligation to find out what these needs are).

Besides, it should be remembered that in many western countries today doctors are encouraged to compete for patients because of the financing and accounting system used in health care in some countries. The same goes for hospitals. Then there is the temptation to give the patient what the patients demands, in order to keep the customer happy, as it were, even if this means to violate the principles stated earlier, for example, by giving the patient something the patient does not need, or spending resources on persons with lesser need than those waiting for treatment.

Since resources are limited, this means that a practice of giving treatment to people who do not always need it is encouraged, while others - as a consequence of this - cannot be given the treatment they need, due to scarce resources. There is a right to die, to put it brutally, but not a right to receive adequate treatment.

For this reason it is essential to emphasize the importance of the need-based approach and to use it as a bulwark against the commercial tendencies plaguing much of contemporary health care in the western world. And the main reason for this, as stressed earlier, is the essentially humanitarian goal of health care, to help those who are in distress and suffer, i.e., cure when possible, and when this is not possible, to alleviate symptoms, and when this is not possible, to comfort.

Studies in the history of medicine will be necessary in order to decide if and to what extent doctors' obligations to groups is new, and whether the individualistic approach so conspicuous today is a fairly recent phenomenon. Certainly, this phenomenon is parallel to, and is stimulated by, other changes in our contemporary societies. Besides, there are strong economic forces pressing individual doctors and the entire health care system in many western countries in this market-oriented direction, which favors individualism.

Today, it is generally taken for granted that the doctor's first duty is to his patient. This is also suggested in the Declaration of Geneva. But who is this patient? The person who seeks the help of the doctor and can get to his clinic? Then we take for granted that those with most urgent needs are also those who are able to get to the clinic or the hospital, sit in the doctor's waiting room and seek his help. If this assumption, on the other hand, is rejected, this is bound to have important consequences for the practice of medicine and for the allocation of health care resources, in Europe as well as in the developing countries.

Present Trends

Priorities have always been made, and resources have always been allocated to health care in one way or other. But the underlying principles, and the justification, have rarely been made explicit. What is new is the public awareness of this, and their interest in the issues.

This has to do not only with the emergence of high tech medicine but also with a number of other factors, such as demographic changes in the structure of the population (in the first place, more elderly people), better education, democratization of values, and so forth.

Such developments have helped to increase the gap between ideal and reality, between need and possibility, or between the health that care can be offered, given the resources available today, and the health care that could be offered, if our resources in time, buildings, people and money were unlimited.

If priorities and setting limits are unavoidable, the extent to which tragic choices may be necessary can be diminished by a combination of a number of strategies, including:

- specification;
- effectivization;
- rationalization;
- increasement of fees;
- raise of taxes;
- lowering of standards; and
- redefinition of the task of the health care system.

By *specification* I mean development of specific guidelines within different fields of health care, as discussed above. Apart from everything else, this process may have important educational effects in increasing the awareness of the people involved of various relevant aspects of these problems. But important though this is, it alone will not solve the problems. Hence, other strategies are also needed.

In this context, *effectivization* presupposes evaluation of methods of treatment, and not using inefficient ones. By *rationalization* I mean better planning and use of hospital facilities (rooms), medical staff and equipment, so that no rooms in hospitals are empty, staff always have meaningful work to do, and expensive equipment are used as many hours a day as possible.

To increase the fees patients have to pay can obviously be combined with the strategy that in certain cases, for example, for exclusive therapy or for contested cases like IVF (in vitro fertilization) and biosynthetic growth hormone, patients have to pay a larger share of the actual costs, not just a standard fee. It has also been discussed whether this should be applied to certain treatments for elderly people; age as a basis of discrimination has been a hotly debated issue in many countries.[10,11,12]

If standards are lowered, this means that not all needs can be met, only the most basic ones. At least, this is so in theory. Whether this is so also in practice, is hard to know.

Redefinition of the task of the health care system is another obvious strategy. There is clearly something to be said for the principles (a) that people should as soon as possible be directed to those who can help them best; and (b) that people in the welfare sector, including nurses, doctors, curators, psychologists, and so forth, should be ask to do what they are best qualified for. In that way resources are used as cost-effectively as possible.

But the danger is, of course, that those who need help are sent to some other sector of the welfare area, which may be just as short of funds as the health care system.

The Future

In the future, the various stakeholders and agents on the health care arena will have to define their goals, and discuss the strategies and means to achieve these goals. It is important to observe that questions of value do not only arise in connection with the goals but also in the choice between different strategies to achieve these goals.

The lengthy discussions spent in the working party preparing the bioethics convention of the Council of Europe on the wording of the clause about "equitable access to health care", or alternatively "equity of health care", "equality of access", "equality of opportunity", "access according to need", etc. and other principles relevant to the issues discussed here, supports this contention.

Needless to say, the outcome of the political debate on the future of health care will to a large extent depend on what courses of action will be taken by individuals, patient organizations, the health care staff and their organizations, the media, the county councils and their equivalents, hospital boards, national boards of health care, as well as by the government.

The interaction between these agents will vary from country to country, depending on the political system.

Some of the issues discussed here have been further penetrated at an international conference in Stockholm sponsored by WHO and governments in the Nordic countries in 13th through 16th October, 1996. This conference, among other things, had to address conflicts in and between the various norms systems in and behind the organization and financing of the health care services, to clarify the role of health care in the general welfare politics in different countries, to define the specific competence of health care staff (as opposed to the competence of the staff of others parts of the welfare sector), and to discuss how general principles of the sort mentioned here are to be implemented to have an effect on hospital care at all levels.

The Need for International Declarations

Is there a need for international guidelines for allocation of health care resources? This must, at the present time, at least in my view, remain an open question. Societies are very different, also in the economic resources they spend on health care and the standard of living; the "natural span of life", a concept introduced into the debate concerning setting limits by Daniel Callahan,[13] certainly means different things in different parts of the world.

But there is more to it than that. The reason for leaving this question open is not only the many differences between the ways in which the health care systems in different countries are organized and financed (as mentioned in the opening paragraph of the paper), but also the cultural differences. Obviously, there are also important political differences between the systems and decision procedures in the European countries, and even more so if we take a global perspective.

Thus, European guidelines might be desirable, in view of the increasing medical tourism between countries in Europe. But whether such guidelines also are politically possible and feasible remains a more difficult question, which can be discussed in a constructive way only after a great deal of political debate and comparative research.

Analogously, discussion of possible guidelines and research on how they are in fact interpreted and applied, could be desirable, but this does not necessarily mean that a world wide binding code in principles for resource allocation is possible.

Of course, it might be possible to agree on the importance of meeting the needs of the population and on considering the severity of the diseases as important principles for distribution of health care resources, provided it is left to the various countries to interpret what this means and to decide on when, how, and by whom the needs of individuals and groups are to be estimated.

Research Areas

There are many areas in which research on problems of the sort discussed here is possible and desirable. Needless to say, and unfortunately, there are also research areas which may be desirable but not possible, or possible but not desirable.

These research areas include the following two main approaches: case studies and comparative investigations of how such problems of resource allocation are handled in practice in a number of specific areas, for example concerning transplantation and organ donation, now or in the past.

In particular, the following issues need to be studied systematically, and in a comparative and historical perspective: which, and whose, interests are at stake? Who decides what issues on which level? What is decided at each particular level in the countries or health care system studies? How are the decisions justified, that is, which facts and values are explicitly or implicitly used to justify the decisions taken? To what extent are the decisions taken formally, and to what extent informally? Which are the key concepts in the decisions and the justifications of them? Which, if any, guidelines are used and how are they interpreted and applied by decision-makers on different levels in the health care system?

Another set of questions, of course, concerns not the issues per se but the debate about the issues - and the relations between the debate and the stand taken on various issues: how is the debate, if any, carried on? Who is taking the initiative to the debate? Which individuals, groups or organizations are taking part in the debate? Which particular issues are being debated? Which are not? Which are the key concepts in these debates? How are the key concepts used and interpreted in the debate?

Systematic, comparative and historic research may thus be illuminating not only for those who want to understand contemporary medicine and health care policy but also for decision-makers today.

Notes

1   Hermerén G. (1996), 'Ethics, epidemiology, and the role of ethics experts'. *Nord. J Psychiatry*; 50 (June).

2   Etiska riktlinjer för epidemiologisk forskning. Befolkningens hälsa ett övergripande krav (1994), *Läkartidningen*, 91:4783-6.

3   Last J.M. (1991), 'Epidemiology and ethics'. In: *Ethics and epidemiology: international guidelines*. Proceedings of the XXVth CIOMS Conference, Geneva, Switzerland, 7-9 November 1990, edited by Bankowski, Z. Bryant, JH. & Last, JM. Geneva: CIOMS, repr 1993:14-28.

4   Health Services Commission (1992) *Prioritized List of Health Services*, Portland, Oregon.

5   Kilner J.F. (1990), *Who Lives? Who Dies? Ethical Criteria in Patient Selection*, New Haven & London: Yale University Press.

6   *Prioritering i sundhedsvæsendet*, (1996)Copenhagen: *Det etiske råd*.

7   Westrin C-G. Nilstun T. (1994), 'The ethics of data utilization: a comparison between epidemiology and journalism'. *Brit Medical J,* 308: 522-3.
8   Pedersen KM. et al. (1995), *Et bedre sundhedsvæsen - men hvordan?* Copenhagen: Lægeforeningens forlag.
9   Hermerén G. (1994), *Prioriteringar och etiska konflikter,* SPRIDA, Stockholm: SPRI.
10   Binstock RH. & Post SG. (eds) (1991), *Too Old for Health Care?* Baltimore & London: Johns Hopkins University Press.
11   Daniels N. (1988), *Am I My Parents' Keeper? An Essay on Justice Between the Young and the Old,* New York & Oxford: Oxford University Press.
12   Nilstun T. & Ohlsson, R. (1995), 'Should Health Care Be Rationed By Age?' *Scandinavian Journal of Social Medicine,* 23 (2): 81-84.
13   Callahan D. (1987), *Setting Limits. Medical Goals in an Aging Society,* New York: Simon & Schuster.

References

Allebeck P. (1990), 'Ethical aspects on epidemiological research', in: *Ethics in Medicine,* edited by Allebeck, P. Jansson, B. New York: Raven Press, 151-157.

Beauchamp T. & Childress JF. (1994), *Principles of Biomedical Ethics,* Fourth edition, New York: Oxford University Press.

Choices in Health Care (1992), A Report by the Government Committee on Choices in Health Care, The Netherlands,.

Daniels N. (1985), *Just Health Care,* Cambridge: Cambridge University Press.

Det svårfångade människovärdet. (1991), Stockholm: Statens Medicinsk-etiska råd.

Eddy D. (1990), 'Clinical decision making from theory to practice. Practice policies - Guidelines for methods', *JAMA* 263: 1839-41.

Hedenius I. (1982), *Om människovärde,* Stockholm: Bonniers.

International guidelines for ethical review of epidemiological studies, Geneva: CIOMS, 1991.

Jonsen A.R., Siegler M. & Winslade W.J. (1982), *Clinical Ethics,* New York: Macmillan.

Kjellstrand C.M. (1988), 'Giving Life-Giving Death. Ethical Problems of High-technology Medicine', Stockholm *Acta Medica Scandinavica,* (suppl.) 725.

Liss P.E. (1993), *Health Care Need. Meaning and Measurement.* Aldershot, Avebury.

National Advisory committee on Core Health and Disability Support Service: Your Health and the public Health. (1992), New Zealand.

Nordenfelt L. (1991), 'Livskvalitet och hälsa'. *Teori och kritik.* Stockholm: Almqvist & Wiksell.

Priorities in Health Care. Ethics, economy, implementation. Final Report by the Swedish Parliamentary Priorities Commission. (1995) Stockholm: SOU:5.

Retningslinjer for prioriteringer innen norsk helsetjeneste. Oslo: NOU 1987:23.

Veatch R. (1986), *The Foundations of Justice. Why the Retarded and the Rest of Us Have Claims to Equality,* New York: Oxford University Press.

Vårdens svåra val. Rapport från utredningen om prioriteringar inom hälso- och sjukvården, Stockholm: SOU 1993:93.

Vårdens svåra val. Slutrapport från utredningen om prioriteringar inom hälso- och sjukvården, Stockholm: SOU 1995:95.

24 The Equitable Allocation of Limited Resources

Carmen Rauch, Jean-Paul Moatti
and Jean-François Mattéï

> L'originalité propre aux problèmes éthiques en politique réside donc dans le moyen spécifique de la **violence légitime** comme telle, dont disposent les groupements humains.
>
> — Max Weber[*]

Medicine, Justice, and Politics

The importance of politics in the fair distribution of resources allocated to the health sector no longer needs to be proved. The recent increase in the control of social security accounts taken by the French Parliament is evidence enough. Thus, the notion of justice has taken on a particular acuteness.

At the same time, political philosophy and philosophy in general are raising their heads again. A work like John Rawls *Theory of Justice*[1] deals with the issues on a global level! Hans Jonas' *Responsibility Principle*[2] argues that people need to reflect on the "responsibility" they have to take their fate into their own hands, and he insists that politics must play the determining role! J.J. Rousseau's *Discours sur l'origine de l'inégalité parmi des hommes*[3] has also retained its import, and his *Contrat Social*[4] is still an important reference work. And of course economists are consulted and their different theories studied closely.

The former director of the health insurance firm for salaried workers in France, G. Johanet, made a ruling that leaves no room for an appeal on leaving the organization in 1993: "Refusing any economical approach in a sector that spends 1.4 million francs [± US$ 280,000] a minute is not ethical".[5] Up to now, doctors have been little preoccupied with economic problems, as there is nothing in the Hippocratic Oath about finances except that the poor should be lavished with care for free.

Moreover, the medical profession to a great extent is involved in the battle against the **injustice** of fate or the biological history of every human being. Medical research aims to sharpen man's knowledge of man even further in order to remedy the inequalities better. The profound meaning of this knowledge is thus an attempt to create a better life for all people in a solidarity movement with the most destitute. In this same spirit, there has been a development in Europe since the end of the 19th century in politics in which the costs of health care have been carried by the state in order to prevent a situation as morally scandalous as a law primarily reserved for the rich (L. Séve).[6] After 1838, the French state took charge of the mentally insane and in 1898 of worker's compensation after injuries. Along the same lines, Bismarc's impetus gives Germany its first state health insurance, and in 1942 England follows suit with the creation of the Welfare State. In 1920, France's Ministry of Health was called into existence, as was the Social Security system in 1945.

Presently, despite or because of the fact that medicine is at the center of biotechnological innovations and a forerunner in the race for knowledge about human beings, the field of medicine has reached a point where a majority of the questions it poses to mankind converge.

Ethics, Codes, and Laws

The fundamental ethical question within the domain of bioethics could be formulated as philosopher and MP Lady Mary Warnock once put it: "Must we do everything that is technically possible?" This question can be approached from a **moral** as well as an **economic** vantage point, and there has already been a cursory answer given at the national level in the so-called "bioethical" laws passed in France in July 1994.[7]

These texts, which directly concern medical practice, make deontological codes more precise in certain domains where they had been made ineffective by the spectacular advances in biotechnology. But above all, they provide such founding principles as respect for the dignity of human beings and the non-commercialization of the human body or laws on filiation which our civilization is based on.

These problems are within the jurisdiction of ethics and thus belong to the realm of philosophy, not to mention the development of the sciences and technology; they also concern, to an extent that cannot be overlooked, the field of economy and, last but not least, politics itself. In addition, we should not forget that medicine itself has been very quick to take account of the phenomenon of the global village through such organizations as the World Health Organization or the World Medical Association. Thus, it is important that there is a concerted international effort to formulate ethical codes and laws concerning the practice of medicine.

Within the present context of confrontation between cultures that are now more in contact with one another than ever before, different models of society are implicitly clashing with one another. Our occidental society, to which we are attached in various ways (which are not the subject of this paper), will have to measure out with the greatest possible pertinence the necessary respect for a certain kind of individualism, without which no one would be able to pursue and realize their dreams and ambitions; on the other hand, we must also be able to renounce this personal freedom when the "public good" would benefit greatly from our doing so - what many today are calling solidarity. "In light of the grim outlook that the despotism of egoism offers, solidarity holds the future".[8] It is invigorating to subscribe to this optimistic affirmation of Lucien Sève's!

Only a national debate in which the issues are clearly discussed within the spirit of taking responsibility for everyone, oneself and all the others - only such a debate in which every citizen has to face questions democratically will be able to establish a new contract uniting the French with their social net. The role that Politics and the Law play is critical here.

The Apories of Relation: Ethics and Money

"Ethics has no worse enemy than money", Professor Jean Bernard never ceased to repeat! Why this phrase?

To begin with, there is an inherent rejection of ethics in the notion of *profit*, particularly in a field such as the health sector. The first contradiction quickly becomes apparent: *profit is justified* by economic considerations as it has less to do with a fixed allowance than a just remuneration for risks taken with an investment. Second, therapy is coordinated by the evolution of research. This gives us the second contradiction: research is expensive and necessitates the collaboration of pharmaceutical laboratories, who then have to make a profit to survive. Third and more shockingly, according to the logic of insurance companies, modifications in an individual's chances of survival have a price tag. Last but not least, there is a fatal conflict between the interests of the individual and those of society. Sir Anthony Eden summed it up well in 1942 when he said, "Everyone is in favor of general economies and individual expenses".[9]

All in all, an ethically acceptable solution within a system primarily founded on the market economy can be found as long as the human body is not commercialized in any way, shape, or form. The principle is strongly defended, as we have seen, by the French law of July 1994, which was amended to the Civil Code. It is intended to be above all a defender of a certain concept of man; it opposes the pressure from financial lobbies with the "force" of the Law.

These "questions of money" must be viewed from two angles: on the one hand, the logics of the market economy tends to favor the reification of man, while on the other hand there are problems linked with the equitable distribution of resources that are becoming more and more scarce in the health sector.

In fact, the importance of ethics and deontology within the medical profession has, among other things, profoundly ethical roots having to do with the structural impossibility of the production of medical care for the mar-

ket. The consumer is incapable of judging the quality of the care offered by
the market. The doctor is supposed to act as the "moral representative" for
his client when giving prescriptions; doctors are expected to make the
same choices that patients themselves would make if they knew the facts
equally well as the doctor.[10]

The concerns about protecting oneself from potential failures in one's
role as counselor, about protecting patients against being abusively exploited by the doctor's monopoly on information and, inversely, doctors
against unfair practices by other doctors or "non-rational" complaints by
unsatisfied customers - all of this justifies the regulatory intervention of the
State and the development of socialized systems of health insurance.[11] And
it certainly explains the universal importance of the self-regulation of the
medical profession, which makes reference in its deontological codes to
ethics in looking for a guarantee for the relationship of "mutual confidence" between doctor and patient.

Here, nothing beats a good education. As Nicole Questiaux put it to the
Comité Consultatif National d'Éthique (CCNE): "...there is a problem of
access to the basic knowledge in the field of health education. This is an
important aspect of a medical eduction. The schools play a major role here,
as they will have to more and more". Shortly after which, she adds: "The
CCNE sees itself obliged to affirm *that a population oriented at solidarity
must understand what this solidarity is based on. And yet, there is, for
various reasons, a lack of explanations*" (Progrès Technique, Santé et
Modèle de Societé. Mai 1996). At this point, she repeats: "reflecting on
ethics can help us greatly in determining what everyone's responsibility is
in making these decisions."[12]

The Difficulty of Equitably Allocating Limited Resources

From Hammurabi's code of laws, through the Hippocratic Oath and the
Prayer of Maimonides, up to recent Nuremberg Code, the medical profession has always been "surrounded" by ethical demands.

Decreed in 1947, the Nuremberg Code established the limits of human
experiments within the domain of science and medicine where the discov-
ery of anti-biotics (sulphonamides, amino-glucosides, penicillin) and
therapeutic studies were concerned.

Fifty years later, after so many international accords - all of them heirs
of the Nuremberg Code - the debate is more and more centered on biomedical ethics that deals with new fields such as the removal and transferral of organs, artificial insemination, the therapeutic uses of molecular biology, neurosciences, and the equitable allocation of limited resources.

Like other industrialized nations, France's health sector has been taking
an ever-increasing part of the federal pie. Between 1960 and 1991, the
percentage of the total budget taken up by the health services rose from
4.2% to over 9%.[13] This constant increase in the portion of the entire

budget ear-marked for the health sector among those industrialized nations with a state-run health service has reached the point where the entire project is jeopardized. Our limited resources force us to make difficult decisions. The refusal of treatment for economic reasons appears at first glance to be contrary to the Hippocratic Oath. The doctor primarily "representing" a patient has a hard time reconciling his profession with what is expected of him as a "representative" of society.[14]

Nonetheless, it is important to remember than the traditional, absolute distinction between medical ethics and economics rules out the possibility of a real debate on the efficiency, the equity, and the legitimacy of the criteria - be they implicit or explicit - used to allot resources in the different health systems. The regulation of these resources by the market being completely inadequate, one must, for the sake of the debate's clarity, examine the various criteria used by the medical profession in allocating scarce items in order to throw light on the diverse forms of collective ethics that underlie them.

In the present economic situation we are facing the danger that ethics might become a means for the medical profession to get control of the debate on the Welfare State and may serve as a distraction to the choices that reality forces on our systems of health and our means of spreading out and increasing access to medical innovations.

One could say that the lack of transparency reveals the kind of approach denounced by Max Weber in which politics reserves the right to be the arbitrator of value judgements at the collective level, leaving the doctor to make individual choices concerning the well-being of people. This will never do. The questions that must be openly discussed are as follows:

- the health criteria for value judgements (either implicit or explicit) concerning the reallocation of resources
- are they efficient: do they allow the members of a collective body to get the most out of the resources used by medicine and the health services?
- are they equitable: how are the costs and advantages of health care spread across the population?
- are they legitimate: are the decision-making processes through which resources are reallocated generally accepted and acceptable? (One should take note at this point of a new concept: the 'reponsibilization' of the ill.)

In general, insurance - especially health insurance - is based on the principle of the regrouping of individual risks in order to play the law of the numbers. The two grand principles behind the "philosophy" of systems of health insurance are the notions of efficacy and equity. Public and private insurance companies presently have these modes in common at the present.

The principle of efficacy within insurance is based on a logic in which generally low-risk people who are objectively interested in no longer being insured by a system in which the mean risk is higher are regrouped. A system of purely private insurance companies is thus inevitably doomed to increase the inequalities in coverage according to revenue and state of health.[15] The opposite is an egalitarian, collective ethics "according to the principle of justice" proposed by John Rawls that "makes judgments according to a thing's usefulness to the person who's the worst off in this situation" and gives priority in the distribution of scarce items to "those who are at the lowest level of well-being today". The existence of a single, obligatory health insurance for everyone, along with a system of mutual coverage, has assured France of a more satisfying logical distribution from the point of view of equity for the time being. But the debts run up over the last few years force us to rethink the field of "legitimate medicine," as difficult as it is to distinguish the border between luxury medicine and medical care.

Ideas that are difficult to rationalize, like emergency situations or the subjectivity of "desires" and the needs of each person, only complicate the problem further.

The present alternatives for a rationalization of medical practice (by means of mandatory protocols, the maximizing of epidemiological objective in public health, or the equalization of marginal costs by QALY) are the products of a questionable utilitarian ethics. An interactive utilization of economic calculation coupled with the evaluation of medical strategies and health programs should clarify the consequences of various ethical value systems on medical decisions.

In fact, there are four factors at work here that are able to regulate the system satisfactorily: the mode of financing (by the parliament), the individual responsibility of the user, the collective regulation of risks by those who have the right to help from the health sector, and a more efficient organization of services offered.

Conclusion

Composed as it is of individuals, society contains both a holistic and an individual current. Society can only develop - and individuals only assert themselves - if they rely on both currents, which constitute an integrating axis[16] that can only be derived from universals in a society where church and state are separated.

Renouncing the principle of universals, as the relativists would have us do, would be tantamount to renouncing the possibility of an open dialogue. This very dialogue is part of the foundation of the "social fabric" everyone wishes to keep intact. All the same, abandoning the principle of universality, the lone guarantee of an ethics based on human beings - as difficult as it would be to respect - would open the door to the law of nature which, in lieu of a moral law, certainly works well according to its own logic.[17]

The equitable redistribution of limited resources will remain one of the greatest problems in ethics for years to come. Responsible citizens who demand long-term policies from short-sighted politicians, along with the respect for universally valid human values, will prevent our age from becoming one of tragic choices.

Notes

*   Weber M. (1959), 'Le savant et le politique'. *Plon* (10/18) p. 179.

1   Rawls J. (1987), *Théory de la Justice*. Éd. du Seuil, Paris. Orig.: Rawls, J. *A Theory of Justice*. Oxford Univ. Press, 1988.

2   Jonas H. (1993), *Le principe responsibilité*. Éd. Cerf, Paris.

3   Rousseau J.J. (1963), *Discours sur l'origine de l'inégalité parmi des hommes* (1e éd. 1755). Union Générale d'Édition, Coll. 10/18, Paris.

4   Rousseau J.J. (1963), *Le contrat social* (1e éd. 1762). Union Générale d'Édition, Coll. 10/18, Paris.

5   Mainoni D'Intignano B. (1994), 'Conflits d'éthique en médecine'. Commentaires, *Printemps*, nr. 65: p. 95

6   Séve L. (1994), *Pour une critique de la raison bioéthique*. Éd. Odile Jacob, Paris, p. 299.

7   Mattei J.-F. (1994), 'La vie en questions: pour une éthique biomédicale'. *Rapport au Primier Ministre*. La Documentation Française, Paris.

8   Séve L. (1994), *Pour une critique de la raison bioéthique*. Éd. Odile Jacob, Paris, p. 307.

9   Michel L. (1993), 'Éthique et répartition des ressources'. *Le Supplement*, nr. 185: p. 134.

10   Arrow K.J. (1963), 'Uncertainty and the welfare economics of medical care'. *American Economic Review*, 53: 941-973.

11   Le Net M. 'Le prix de la vie humaine'. *La Documentation Française*, Paris, 1978.

12   Questiaux N. (1996), 'Progrès Technique, Santé et Modèle de Societé'. *Rapport au CCNE*, Mai 1996.

13   Moatti J.P., Huard P. (1995), 'La juste évaluation des dépenses de santé'. *Pour la Science*, nr. 218: p. 34.

14   Moatti J.P. (1991), 'Éthique médicale, économie de la santé; les choix implicites'. *Annales des Mines*, Juillet-Août: p. 75.

15   Moatti J.P., Le Coroller A.G. (1996), *Éthique et Économie de la Santé*, nr. 2.

16   Chaunu P. (1980), *Histoire et foi*. Éd. France Empire, Paris, p. 81.

17   Kremer-Marietti, A. (1987), *L'Éthique*. PUF, Coll. Que Sais-je? Paris, p. 125.

25 Transcultural Medical Ethics and Human Rights·

Robert Baker

The document we now refer to as the Nuremberg Code was an artifact of a specific time and place; it was manufactured in a decidedly *ad hoc* manner to justify the legally dubious but morally necessary *ex post facto* criminal conviction of sixteen specific individuals. How, in retrospect, can we today treat this "Code" as anything other than a convenient legal fiction? How can this, or any other code, legal or otherwise, validly condemn actions committed *prior* to its formulation? Or, to put the same question more abstractly, how can a code, moral or otherwise, have transtemporal validity? And, to ask a parallel question, how can words formulated by three American state supreme court judges at Nuremberg in 1947 to justify twenty-three specific court decisions (sixteen convictions), be applicable outside of American legal-moral culture? By what right, other than the right of the victor, did these judges apply American (or Anglo-American) moral-judicial concepts to German nationals? And even if the judges' ruling somehow applied to German nationals, what validity could their Code have for other European countries? Or outside of European culture? Is not the imposition of this Code on other cultures simply a matter of American cultural imperialism? How could the Nuremberg Code have transcultural validity? How can any code have transcultural validity?

In our postmodern, pluralist, multicultural age, perhaps the easiest way to answer these questions is to deny the validity of all transcultural and transnational norms. If we have learned anything, the postmodernist claims, it is that every age, every culture, every subculture defines its own norms of morality and law. And properly so, multiculturalists suggest: no age, no culture, no subculture, has the prerogative, much less the right, to impose its moral vision upon any other. The ideal of universal human rights, postmodernists tell us, is an artifact of modernity, of the European Enlightenment, and these artifacts readily deconstruct under the critical gaze of the postmodernist critique. Ours, multiculturalists assure us, is an age of pluralism, an age in which multiple perspectives assert their properly equal place. In this postmodern multiculturalist age, no one, and certainly no three American state court judges presiding over ad hoc proceedings at Nuremberg in 1947, can set standards binding upon other times and other cultures.

Yet the Nuremberg Code has defined standards for human subjects research that seem to be, if not universal, then at least transcultural; and no one, no multiculturalist, no postmodernist, seriously suggests that the sixteen convictions at Nuremberg ought to be invalidated because American justice lacked moral or legal authority. This raw fact suggests that whatever modicum of truth there may be in the postmodernist critique of Enlightenment universal moral standards, or the multiculturalist assertion of the equality of all cultures, it is not the whole truth, nor even a truth that, in practical terms, defines everyday moral workings in our global village. It must somehow be possible to recognize differences in cultural and subcultural perspectives and yet still articulate and embrace a conception of transcultural moral norms, including the ideal of human rights. In this essay I attempt to articulate and defend a theoretical account, a frankly philosophical account, of that possibility. Using the Nuremberg Code as a case in point, I shall demonstrate that even though a codes of ethics may be a response to a discrete set of problems that arose at a particular junction in a specific society at one definite time, the norms articulated in such a code may nonetheless become binding upon actions performed at other times, places, and culture, that is, they may become transculturally valid. I believe that it is imperative, as we cross the threshold into the twenty-first century, with its promise of ever newer and more powerful technologies, to appreciate the very real potential, and the equally real limitations, of transculturally valid codes of ethics.

Conflict as the Basis of Transcultural Validity

The analysis that I offer here, while it is quite naturally read as emanating from the American pragmatist tradition, actually grows out of an attempt to understand the history of medical ethics from a theoretical perspective developed by such philosophers as David Gauthier (1986), Robert Nozick (1974), and John Rawls (1971). I read these philosophers as, in various ways, reasserting Enlightenment ideals of moral reason in the face of the irrationalist, subjectivist, pluralist, particularist, multicultural predilections of the postwar era. Most of these philosophers have also reanimated the metaphor of the social contract (originally proposed by such seventeenth- and eighteenth-century philosophers as Hobbes, Kant, Locke, Rousseau, and Spinoza) to illustrate the claim that moral and legal norms are valid (that is, have normative force) precisely because those whom they would bind either have, or would have, rational grounds for assenting to them. The most riveting corollaries of this theory, and certainly the corollaries with the most revolutionary impact, are the presumption of the equality of contractors, the legitimating role of assent, and the correlative delegitimation of any morality or law to which an agent could not rationally give assent - or to put the same point as it might have been put in the more flamboyant language of the eighteenth century, the deduction of inalienable human rights universally binding upon all societies.

Less often remarked, but nonetheless implicit in the metaphor of the social contract, is the presumption that, as in any other contract, the need to articulate formal agreement presupposes an absence of trust and implies a recognition that the interests of the parties may well be in conflict; for were there no conflict, there would be no need to state terms of agreement. What is noteworthy about the presumption of underlying conflict is that it *inverts* the conventional wisdom that a common morality, a common set of laws, or even a transcultural, or a transnational, or a transtemporal code, must rest upon a common set of interests, values, or principles. From a contractarian perspective, conflict, not consensus, underlies morality and law; common conflicts thus provide the basis of common laws, even when cultures are quite different. In this sense, postmodernists misjudge the Enlightenment; such philosophers as Hobbes and Spinoza never denied the subjective, pluralist, nature of interests, or perspectives, or values. On the contrary, they predicated their philosophies upon a frank recognition of a natural state of pluralism and discord; they presumed conflicting interests and irreconcilable values. For the classic contractarian, even minor matters of manners, and certainly major moral codes or systems of law, are essentially attempts to resolve underlying conflicts. Universal morality, insofar as it is achievable, rests on the common nature of conflict, not upon any prior consensus about moral precepts or principles. In this essay I explore this contractarian conception of universality predicated upon common conflict. More specifically, I shall try to demonstrate that the Nuremberg Code can be read as an attempt to address conflict, and that the shared experience of these conflicts provided a basis for the Code's transcultural validity.

Codes and Conflicts

On the contractarian analysis any particular moral code, or codification of law, should be analyzable as an attempt to resolve some underlying conflict. This proposition is, at least in part, empirical, and hence partially testable. Since our subject is the Nuremberg Code, it is not unreasonable to ask the historical question: do known codes of medical ethics really address conflict? Codes, of course, are those formulations of etiquette, ethics and law that stipulate (and often enumerate) proper and improper *actions* (but need not, and generally do not, deal with such things as the character of the actor, or the specifics of individual cases). The oldest and most famous formalization of medical morality in Western medicine, the Hippocratic Oath, is a code (although, unlike the Nuremberg, the duties stipulated in the Oath are not enumerated). On a contractarian analysis, therefore, we should be able to read the Hippocratic Oath as an attempt to resolve some set of conflicts.

Can the Oath be read as a social contract, that is, as an attempt to address and resolve conflicts? Easily. Even a cursory appraisal readily reveals that the Oath addresses conflicts between indentured apprentices and their master-teachers, between physicians and patients, and between society and physicians. Consider, for example, the Oath's prohibition of any action "abusing the bodies of man or woman, bond or free". The prohibition addresses a fundamental conflict between the medical practitioner's need for access to the patient's body (for purposes of diagnosis and treatment) and patient-family-societal values of modesty, sexual exclusivity and privacy. The norm, moreover, attempts to resolve the conflict, and thereby to legitimate the physical examination of patients by physicians, by blocking a sexual conception of the physician- patient encounter, that is by constructing the patient-physician relationship in asexual terms. (A companion norm of confidentiality also protects the patient's modesty and privacy.)

Moreover, to continue the contractarian analysis, these norms are rationally conserved in formal medical ethics just insofar as they continue to resolve the conflicts that they address. The Confucian medical ethics of classic Chinese culture, for example, had no need to stipulate or to conserve a specific norm to resolve this particular conflict because it turned to technology instead: female patients were able to satisfy the diagnostic needs of their (male) physicians by using anatomical dolls as vicarious representatives for their bodies when they explained their symptoms. In the West, however, we rely on a norm of asexuality to legitimate the physical examination of the body, and so we conserved this norm in our medical ethics. Thus the apparent immutability and "universality" of the norms of asexuality (and confidentiality) is really a function of the persistence of the underlying conflict they address, and their continued efficacy in resolving it.

The Nuremberg Code

A parallel analysis of the Nuremberg Code generates the insight that the "universality" of the ten prohibitions stipulated in the code rests on their ability to legitimate medical research on human subjects in the face of underlying conflict between researcher and subject - especially vulnerable, stigmatized, captive or condemned subjects. The conflict arises because, as the judges expressly remark, while it is important to protect human subjects, it is also necessary to legitimate "permissible" medical experiments.

Permissible Medical Experiments

The great weight of evidence before us is to the effect that certain types of medical experiments on human beings, when kept within reasonably well-defined bounds, conform to the ethics of the medical profession generally. The protagonists of the practice of human experimentation justify their views on the basis that such experiments yield results for the good of society that are unprocurable by other methods or means of study. All agree, however, that certain basic principles must be observed in order to satisfy moral, ethical, and legal concepts (Katz, 1972, p. 305).[1]

This need for legitimization noted, the judges proceed to enumerate ten basic actions that a researcher must undertake to conduct permissible medical experiments upon human subjects, starting with the "absolutely essential" action of receiving "the voluntary consent of the human subject". As the judges point out, in the first and longest article in the Code, by "voluntary consent" they mean that the subject must be capable of free choice and informed, that is, given "sufficient knowledge and comprehension of the elements of the subject matter involved as to enable him to make an understanding and enlightened decision". Thus, just as the norm prohibiting "abuse of...bodies" in the Hippocratic Oath legitimates physical examination, the ten norms prohibiting abuse of human subjects in the Nuremberg Code legitimate - and were consciously designed to legitimate or make "permissible" - medical experiments on human subjects.

Questions about the permissibility of medical experiments on humans had been placed before the Nuremberg Court by the defense, which had adduced persuasive evidence that physicians in America and other allied countries did not always restrict their experiments to volunteers. In support of this claim they cited papers published in eminently respectable medical journals that reported research in which it was apparent that people had been subjected to experiments without their knowledge or consent. One could not condemn German physicians, the defense argued compellingly, without simultaneously indicting the entire medical research enterprise in America and throughout the world. To counter these charges, the prosecution (and ultimately the judges) turned to two American medical advisers, Colonel Leo Alexander, MD (a neurologist and psychiatrist who had treated concentration camp survivors and who acted as an advisor to the US Secretary of War) and Professor Andrew C. Ivy (former scientific director of the Naval Medical Research Institute at Bethesda Maryland and the official observer for the American Medical Association). Both testified with relatively clean hands about American military medical practice, for the American military typically adhered to the traditions of volunteerism and auto-experimentation initially established by Walter Reed. Yet, as the defense was to force Professor Ivy to admit, at no time prior to the Nuremberg indictments had the American military, nor any official representative of American medicine (such as the American Medical Association), nor any international medical society formally stated this ideal of "volunteerism", nor was there an explicit policy restricting research to voluntary subjects - although in American law any unconsented medical intervention was considered a battery. (There was, however, no requirement that consent be documented, or even that the consenter be *informed* about the risks of the intervention.[2])

The judges (and the expert medical witnesses) had a problem. They understood all too well the threat of delegitimation posed by the defense arguments; as Ivy later wrote, to admit to "the performance of experiments on human subjects without their consent", even upon subjects already "condemned to die", "would undermine the faith that ordinary patients have in the profession" (Ivy, 1947). But the defense argument was well-documented, and, except for a hastily adopted American Medical Association (AMA) policy statement adopted at Professor Ivy's insistence on December 11, 1946 - that is, *after* the Nuremberg trials had begun - the *only* official statements on the research "ethics of the medical profession" had been German. Ivy tried to introduce the German regulations into the proceedings, but the defense objected, quite properly, that these were administrative directives that had no standing in German *criminal* law and were thus not relevant to the *criminal* proceedings being conducted by the Nuremberg Court.

Hence the Court's quandary. The defendants' conduct had been morally outrageous. It demanded condemnation. (Indeed, the 1943 Declaration on German Atrocities had officially proclaimed that anyone guilty of atrocities would be punished.) Yet the defense case was factually and legally sound. During the period that the defendants performed their experiments, neither the American Medical Association's Code of Ethics, nor any international code of medical ethics, nor, for that matter, the Hippocratic Oath, required, or even recommended, informed consent as a prerequisite for morally permissible experiments on humans. Moreover, despite a long-standing tradition of auto-experimentation and volunteerism, it was evident that some American researchers had, at times, performed experiments on human subjects without informing them or receiving their consent, and that these experiments were published in respected medical journals. Finally, although Anglo-American law clearly condemned unconsented medical investigations as assaults, the Anglo-American law of assault was inapplicable to German nationals acting on German territory operating under the laws of the Third Reich. Despite certain readings of a few lines in the Hippocratic corpus, it appeared that, however atrocious these outrages perpetrated in the name of medical science might have been, no previously stated moral or legal principles would provide a clear justification for condemning them - except, as it turned out, certain Prussian and German administrative issues in 1900 and 1931.

Pre-war German medical science had been the most advanced in the world. Not unnaturally, therefore, it was German society that first formally recognized and responded to the dangers of research on human subjects. The issue surfaced as scandal. In 1896 it was discovered that Albert Neisser, a professor of dermatology and venereology, had "inoculated" children and adolescents with an experimental "immunizing" serum drawn from syphitics, without informing them or their parents.[3] In the 1930s another scandal shocked the German public when they learned that 75 children had died because their pediatricians injected them with an experimental tuberculosis vaccine - again without the children's or their parent's knowledge or consent. In response to these scandals, German governmental bodies issued regulations designed to untangle he conflated roles of care-giver and scientific investigator, in part by differentiating investigation from treatment, in part by requiring physicians to inform to their patients when they are undertaking the investigator role, and, most importantly, by requiring patient consent as a prerequisite for initiating any investigations requiring human subjects (Grodin, 1992). It was the Germans, therefore, who first invented the idea of using the informed voluntary consent of the subject as the mechanism for untangling the roles of researcher from therapist, and for guaranteeing the knowing and voluntary participation of humans subjected to scientific research. This "disambiguating" mechanism, informed consent, fit positivist legal doctrine well, and received moral support, as it were, from the Kantian concept of autonomy. It was a fittingly German solution to the problems created by the advances of German medical science.

The Nuremberg Court was ultimately to "universalize" these German solutions by stripping them of their cultural context. Both Doctors Alexander and Ivy sent memos to the judges and to the prosecution outlining possible regulations governing research on human subjects. Ivy's memo restated the three rules he had persuaded the AMA to adopt in 1946 (informed consent of the subjects, proper medical supervision, and prior experiments on animals); Alexander's memo condenses and simplifies the elaborate fourteen-point 1931 German Reich Health Council rules into six points (informed voluntary consent of the subject; humanitarian intent of the experimenter; exclusion of fatal or disabling interventions; proper supervision; humanitarian benefits that outweigh any risks to the subjects; scientific-grounding and a basis in animal experiments). The prosecution reiterated several of the Alexander-Ivy rules in his summation, thus officially putting before the Judges the Alexander and the Ivy memos. The Court's judgment reformulates the summarized Alexander-Ivy memos as a Code of ten principles -*ten* being an authoritatively resonant number in Judaeo-Christian culture - governing "the moral, ethical and legal" requirements of permissible medical experimentation on which "all agree". These two words, "all agree" seemed to refer neither to Alexander's memo, nor to Ivy's, nor to the prosecution's summary, nor to the 1931 German Reich Health Council's regulations, nor to the AMA's standards, but to some "universal", and hence atemporal, concord on standards for research on human subjects, which, by virtue of its universality, could and did provide the judges with grounds for convicting sixteen individuals for morally and legally impermissible research on human subjects. Paradoxically, the Court's ad hoc decision would actually achieve the "universality" it had fabricated, or, as I should prefer to characterize it, the Nuremberg Code eventually attained transcultural validity.

Universalizing the Nuremberg Code: The First Attempts

Bioethicists and historians often ponder the two decade "lag" between the pronouncement of a universal set of research standards at Nuremberg and the implementation of these standards in America and elsewhere. To talk of a "lag", however, is to read history backwards and thus to beg the question of how an ad hoc, legally problematic amalgamation of American idealism and surreptitiously appropriated German standards, that had never been "accepted" outside of Germany or America, became a truly "universal" standard. The real question is not why the Code was not immediately applied, but how did it achieve its "universality"? Conventional wisdom would have it that a code can achieve transcultural or universal validity only if it rests on transculturally or universally shared precepts, principles or values. The unconventional position that I have been advancing inverts this analysis: it is the commonality, not of principles and values, but of problems and conflicts, and the correlative need for a solution, that prompts one culture to accept a conflict-resolving norm invented by another. The Nuremberg Code offered a resolution to a set of conflicts surrounding medical research on human subjects; on a contractarian analysis the norms it formulated could not - and would not - be accepted as solutions until the conflicts it addressed were recognized as problems. So the first question one must address is how and when did various societies come to recognize that medical research on human subjects posed a problem.

Perhaps not unexpectedly, since the Nuremberg Court was a US military court, the problematic nature of research on human subjects was almost immediately recognized by the upper echelons of the America military and of the United States government, and they tried to implement the Nuremberg Code almost immediately. The *Advisory Committee on Human Radiation Experiments* reports that as early as 1947, key administrators at the Atomic Energy Commission and other branches of the US government, and in the military itself, attempted to reformulate the Nuremberg Code as administrative regulations applicable to all government-supported experimentation on human subjects. Memos, rules, and regulations were drafted, often disseminated, and sometimes implemented (Advisory Committee, Chapter 1, 1996).

Internationally, there was a parallel attempt to implement the Nuremberg Code. In 1948 the World Medical Association (WMA) issued a new version of the Hippocratic Oath that required physicians to respect the laws of humanity (on which the Nuremberg Code had been based). In 1954, it issued formal *Principles for those in Research and Experimentation*, that reiterated the main themes of the Nuremberg Code, particularly their requirement that "each person who submits to experimentation be informed of the nature of, the reasons for, and the risk of the proposed experiment...and... consent...in writing". The WMA's *Principles* were designed to implement the Nuremberg Code in the clinical context, and, even as it preserved the core idea of informed consent, nonetheless accommodated the needs of clinical researchers by empowering surrogates to consent on behalf of incapacitated patients - thereby legitimating research on those who lacked capacity to consent, or to volunteer themselves as subjects. A year later the Public Health Council of the Netherlands issued guidelines that also attempted to implement and enforce the WMA *Principles* in clinical contexts through the institution of local research councils (later to be called institutional review boards, or IRBs).

Inertia tended to stall the impetus for change, both internationally and in America. The new regulations tended to be received as bureaucratic impositions, or as an unduly formalistic idealism, rather than as a needed reform. World-wide, researchers argued the case for Nazi exceptionalism. It was not *German* physicians but *Nazi* physicians who had abused the role of medicine. The Nazis were no longer with us and so there was no need for special codes addressing research on human subjects. Historian David Rothman notes that the prevailing American perception of the Nuremberg Code was that the defendants "were Nazis first and last; by definition nothing they did, and no code drawn up in response to them, was relevant to the United States" (Rothman, pp. 62-63). Jay Katz, author of the influential legal compendium *Experimentation With Human Beings*, also reports that at the time the Nuremberg Code was thought to be "a good code for barbarians but an unnecessary code for ordinary physicians" (Advisory Committee, p. 86); and, indeed, at that time ordinary American physicians agreed, "these codes [were] necessary for barbarians but [not for] fine upstanding people" (Advisory Committee, p. 86).

Resistance in the Research Community

The research community resisted the Nuremberg reforms on all fronts. They argued that if Nuremberg-type restrictions were needed at all, they should apply only to so-called "non-therapeutic experiments," that is, to those experiments that conferred no potential "therapeutic" benefit to subjects. "Therapeutic research" ought to be exempt from informed consent and most other Nuremberg restrictions. Underlying the researcher's rhetoric of "therapeutic research" was a real issue. Practically all medical research on human subjects is performed with the aim of developing new therapies and occurs in clinical environments. Thus were so-called "therapeutic research" exempted from Nuremberg-type restrictions, almost all medical research could proceed unimpeded by external regulation - or by requirements of *informed* consent. For all practical purposes, a therapeutic exemption would free researchers from the strictures of external regulation - it would also deprive most human subjects of the informed consent protections required in the 1947 Nuremberg Code and the 1954 WMA Principles.

In the US the issue was joined in 1961. Fittingly, the place was America's premier research university, Harvard. As we noted earlier, the upper echelons of the American government and military had been receptive to the Nuremberg Code from the very first. In 1954 the Army Office of the Surgeon General reissued the Nuremberg Code as a set of rules regulating all military and all military-funded research on human subjects, including, as it turned out, research at the Harvard Medical School. The Harvard researchers objected. At a June 8, 1962 meeting, the Board of Administrators of Harvard Medical School, responding to the complaints of the medical faculty, rejected the Surgeon General's 1954 regulations as overly-stringent. The Harvard Board adopted in its place a set of principles drafted by Dr. Henry Beecher that emphasized that in therapeutic contexts obtaining informed consent may be "folly...difficult...to the point of impossible". Therapy required, not formalism, but a "special relationship of trust between subject or patient and investigator". On July 12, 1962, representatives from Harvard met with the Army Surgeon General, and, Harvard, being Harvard, gained permission to exempt itself from the Surgeon General's Regulations; it had its own principles inserted into its contract with the US Army. In the aftermath, the US Surgeon General's Office officially revised its regulations on human subjects research to accommodate the Harvard position, that is, it officially recognized an exemption for so-called "therapeutic" research.

Helsinki I and The Triumph of Virtue Ethics

Researchers around the globe were sounding similar themes. In 1963 both the British Medical Association and the British Medical Research Council (MRC) issued research guidelines exempting "therapeutic experiments" from stringent constraints of informed consent:

> Provided...the medical attendant is satisfied...that a particular new procedure will contribute to the benefit of that particular patient...he may *assume* the patient's consent to the same extent as he would were the procedure entirely established practice. (Medical Research Council of Great Britain, p. 263)

The World Medical Association itself introduced a strong therapeutic exemption at its meeting in Helsinki in 1964 (the research guidelines they issued are often referred to as the Declaration of Helsinki, or Helsinki I, to differentiate them from later declarations). Priorities had clearly shifted. Where Nuremberg had offered itself as a universal code of ethics and law, Helsinki I presented itself simply as a "guide to each doctor in clinical research". This guidance, like the Nuremberg Code itself, rested on something "fundamental", but where the Nuremberg Code had declared the "voluntary consent of the human subject" to be "essential", Helsinki I declared a fundamental "distinction between ... therapeutic and ... purely scientific ... research". Helsinki I then affirms that "the doctor must be free to use a new therapeutic measure if in *his* judgment it offers hope of saving life, re-establishing health, or alleviating pain" (*emphasis added*). Although "his" judgment is clearly paramount, Helsinki I urges clinicians, "If at all possible, consistent with the patient's psychology, [to] obtain the patient's freely given consent after the patient had been given a full explanation". Thus, in a little over one and one-half decades, the rights of the patient-subject, that had been so firmly pronounced at Nuremberg, had been eroded down to a conditional prerogative of the clinician-researcher. As one might anticipate, Helsinki I was immediately and enthusiastically endorsed by researchers around the globe, including the American Medical Association, the American Society for Clinical Investigation, and the American Federation for Clinical Research.

Helsinki I, like the Harvard Principles and the British guidelines, presupposed that the therapeutic relationship would automatically predominate over the scientist-subject relationship; it also presupposed that the conscience and sense of personal honor and integrity of the decent (that is non-Nazi) therapist-researcher provided a reasonable safeguard against abuse. Henry Beecher justified the Harvard Principles by expounding upon the expediency of virtue:

> The best approach concerns the character, wisdom, experience, honesty, imaginativeness and sense of responsibility of the investigator who in all cases of doubt or where serious consequences might remotely occur, will call in his peers and get the benefit of his counsel. (Advisory Committee, p. 91)[4]

Beecher here expressly states the implicit presumption of researchers everywhere: that an ethic of individual virtue, that is, the ethic of honor that has historically been associated with elites in Western culture, was appropriate to medical researchers and would moreover *best* resolve the underlying conflation of the roles of researcher and therapist.

The Inadequacy of Virtue

Evidence of the inefficacy of an elitist virtue ethic of honor was accumulating even before the ink dried on the Declaration of Helsinki. Ironically, the victims were again Jews; this time, however, the perpetrator was a gentleman who was self-evidently neither a "barbarian", nor a Nazi, nor any sort of "fringe researcher". He was an eminently respectable medical scientist, a member of the research elite, who was engaged in important, cutting-edge scientific research (for which he was later awarded the presidency of the American Cancer Society). His name, Dr. Chester Southam; his home base, the Sloan-Kettering Institute - the Harvard of cancer research. The experiments in question were part of a series that Southam was conducting to challenge the widely-accepted viral theory of cancer. Southam's hypothesis was that, while viruses might be responsible for some cancers, tumors tended to develop only in organisms with impaired immune systems. To confirm this hypothesis Southam conducted a series of experiments designed to demonstrate that an organism will reject implants of live cancer cells, even if it is fatigued, or has just undergone surgery, or is dying - unless its immune system is impaired.

Southam's data was derived from research on humans as well as animals. Who were his subjects? Prisoners, women who had just undergone hysterectomies, and dying patients. Southam and his colleagues typically obtained consent from patients or their surrogates, but they seldom informed them of the cancerous nature of the cells to be implanted - often characterizing the implants as "tests for immunity". Apparently no one objected to Southam's experiments until 1963, when he and his colleagues began to experiment on dying patients at Brooklyn Jewish Chronic Disease Hospital. Jews had reason to remember Nuremberg and two young Jewish physicians protested to the hospital's trustees, citing the Nuremberg Code. Eventually one of the trustees, again Jewish, and again motivated by the Nuremberg precedent, took the case to the *New York Times,* and ultimately to the New York State Board of Regents - which suspended Southam's license to practice medicine for a year. (This suspension, however, did not impress the researchers at the American Cancer Society, who proceeded to award Southam its presidency (See Katz, pp.11-65)).

What is important about the Southam case was not merely his duplicity, nor the arrogance of the medical research elite who embraced him as their representative, even after his methods of recruiting "volunteers" became public knowledge, but the evident failure of the virtue ethic to protect human subjects. The American Cancer Society may have missed this point, but it was not lost on the administrators at the US Public Health Service who had funded Southam's research. They began to reassess the case for regulation. In 1965, the Director of the National Institutes of Health (NIH) recommended a system of *mandatory* peer review for all research funded by the NIH or by the Public Health Service to assure an *independent* determination that the rights of research subjects were being respect and that the instruments of informed consent were approptiate. It was now evident to those funding medical research that the research elite could not police itself, that, at a minimum, honor must be accountable to peer review.

One of their own, Henry Beecher, came to the same conclusion, based, in part, on the Southam case. In a process of public recantation memorably portrayed by David Rothman (1992), Beecher "blew the whistle" on his fellow researchers, and even on himself, first at a professional meeting in March 1965, and later in an article published in the *New England Journal of Medicine* (Beecher, 1966; note this article that had earlier been rejected by the *Journal of the American Medical Association,* or *JAMA*). The article analyzed the treatment of human subjects reported in twenty-two research papers published in such leading medical journals as *Circulation, JAMA, Journal of Clinical Investigation,* and the *New England Journal of Medicine* between 1948 and 1965. These papers had been written by eminent researchers at the Harvard Medical School, the National Institutes of Health, Sloan-Kettering, and other elite institutions; and they had been funded by the National Institutes of Health, the Surgeon General's Office, the US Armed Forces, the US Public Health Service, as well as by Merck, Parke-Davis, and other leading pharmaceutical companies - and they all involved morally questionable practices, such as injecting live cancer implants into patients without their knowledge. Beecher, as he to his credit publicly admitted, had been wrong: virtue ethics was inadequate, the elite could not police itself.

In 1967, the British whistle-blower Dr. M. H. Papworth demonstrated that the British research elite and National Health Service hospitals were as incapable of self-policing as their American counterparts. And the scandals kept unfolding. In the early 1970s it was revealed that between 1932 and 1972 the US Public Health Service center at Tuskegee conducted a study on the effects of untreated syphilis, without informing the subjects that they had syphilis. The study was continued in the post-war era, even though effective treatments for the disease were by then inexpensive and readily available. What made this experiment especially scandalous was that the researchers were, for the most part, whites, while the subjects were uniformly black. Almost simultaneously came the revelation that researchers at an institution for the mentally handicapped in New York, called Willowbrook, had deliberately infected inmates with hepatitis. It began to appear that the voice of conscience in the affluent, middle-aged, white, male, well-educated elite who made up the American medical research establishment tended to be silent about the rights of research subjects who were poor, or elderly, or black, or Jewish, or post-reproductively female, or uneducated, or in prison, or mentally handicapped. The victims of American medical science, like the victims of German medical science, seemed to mirror the prejudices of the scientific elite.

The Bioethical Rebirth of the Nuremberg Code

The American research scandals of the 1970s prompted the formation of a number of investigative committees, including the National Commission for the Protection of Human Subjects of Biomedical and Behavioral Research (1974-1979). The Belmont Report, issued by the Committee (1979), was ultimately to underwrite the "universality" of the Nuremberg Code, but, just as importantly, a young philosopher serving on the Committee's staff, Tom Beauchamp, was to co-author a textbook in which the virtue ethic of the clinical-research elite was rechristened "paternalism", and subjected to a powerful philosophical challenge. Beauchamp and his co-author, James Childress, argued (1979) that moral disputes in medicine were best understood in terms of the conflict between four fundamental principles: autonomy, beneficence, non-maleficence (not harming), and justice. The virtue ethics of the clinical-research elite tended to prioritize in favor of beneficence and to presume, "paternalistically", that clinicians, by virtue of their expertise and experience, could unilaterally determine the best interests of their patients. Yet, Beauchamp and Childress argued compellingly, clinicians could offer no valid reasons for prioritizing beneficence over autonomy, nor for the perplexing claim that they could determine their patients' interests better than their patients themselves.

Reread in the light of this "bioethical" critique, the Nuremberg Code was readily reconceptualized as a defense of patient-subject autonomy (Beauchamp and Childress, 1979, pp. 62-64). And so, ironically, a Code written in the late 1940s, based on a German administrative law of 1931, which, in turn, refined a Prussian precursor from 1900, came to be appropriated as a foundational document of a bioethics reform movement initially centered in American in the 1970s. Ironically, once it was reconceptualized as "bioethics", the European research elite tried to resist "bioethical" reform by branding it as American cultural imperialism. Ideals of "autonomy", and "informed consent", that had been invented in Prussia, even the ideal "human rights", perhaps the proudest achievement of the European Enlightenment, had somehow been reconceptualized as uniquely American. Despite appeals to intellectual chauvinism, bioethical ideals of informed consent were codified and implemented around the globe. The US Government officially re-endorsed Nuremberg-type regulations in a series of policy statements from 1965 onwards (Department of Health Education and Welfare Guidelines, 1971; Department of Health and Human Subjects, 1991); internationally, there was a parallel re-endorsement of Nuremberg starting with Helsinki II (Tokyo, 1975), Helsinki III (Venice, 1983), Helsinki IV (Hong Kong, 1989), the Council of Europe (Recommendation No. R (90) 3, 1990) and the Council for International Organizations of Medical Science and World Health Organization Guidelines (CIOMS, 1982, 1993 - all of these documents are in the Appendix to the *Encyclopedia of Bioethics*, Reich, 1978, 1995).

A Functional Reanalysis of the Nuremberg Code's Universality

The conventional wisdom has been that global, or universal, or transcultural, codes presuppose shared principles or values; the unconventional position that I have been developing this paper is that transcultural validity presupposes common conflicts, not common principles or values. Moreover, as the failure of Helsinki I and other post-Nuremberg researcher virtue ethics demonstrates, a code that does not resolve the conflicts it addresses will lose its validity. Generalizing further from our experience with the Nuremberg Code and its successors, it would appear that a moral code or statement of moral principles may be accepted as "transculturally valid" between two or more cultures if it: (1) addresses fundamental conflicts common to these cultures; (2) it correctly identifies either (i) the range of cooperative solutions acceptable to the participants affected in these cultures and/or (ii) protects primary goods that non-negotiable for participants (that is, fundamental human rights); and (3) the solutions are effective in resolving the conflicts. Notice that all the successful successors to the Nuremberg Code both address and successfully resolve the conflicts identified by the Nuremberg Court. Thus all the new regulations carefully identify the conflicting interests of researcher and therapist and they force the researcher to differentiate between the two roles - both by explaining to potential subjects the nature, and the risks, and the benefits of the proposed research, and by obtaining consent. The newer regulations, however, refined the Nuremberg code in three fundamental respects. They recognize a need to experiment upon incapacitated subjects, and thus permit surrogates to consent on their behalf. They acknowledge that the therapeutic context requires different standards than non-therapeutic contexts, in part because the subjects themselves might benefit, but also because the conflation of the researcher-therapists roles heightens risks of abuse for patient-subjects. And, perhaps most importantly, the new codes reflect the failed foray into virtue ethics; they require researchers to seek prior approval for their research design, consent procedures, and similar matters from a committee of peers and (often) community representatives. The burden of proof has shifted: researchers seeking to avoid the constraints of informed consent now had to justify themselves to their peers and to community representatives.

Of deeper signficance is that all these Nuremberg-style codes "autonomy" is given higher priority than any other value, or, if you will, the rights of individual patients and/or subjects are given priority over the need for medical knowledge. Why? A historicist might answer that autonomy receives priority because the 'ur-text' for all research codes was written in Prussia, reflecting the Kantian influence on German culture; a historicist might also observe that the Nuremberg Code was rewritten by Americans, whose culture places a premium on ideals of self-determination. These answers misread the question. It draws our attention to possible factors influencing the Prussian code of 1900 or the Nuremberg Code of 1947, but it does not explain the transcultural validity of the codes; it does not explain the reasons why such a code was accepted by the British, despite their proclivities towards utilitarianism, or by the Dutch, despite their notions of solidarity, or by the Japanese, whose traditional medical ethics is based upon Confucianism. The phenomenon that needs explaining is the transcultural prioritization of "patient-subject autonomy" above "medical knowledge". To explain this phenomenon we need to look beyond the historical origins of the Code to its function.

Here again, the metaphor of the social contract is illuminating: for the metaphor symbolizes, not only an understanding of the normative power of morality and law in terms of an agreement between those whom they would bind, but also the insight that certain goods are non-negotiable. Traditionally, contractarians have characterized these non-negotiable goods as "rights", or "inalienable rights", or "natural rights", or "human rights". The American philosopher John Rawls, however, introduced the more flexible notion of "primary goods" to accommodate the contextualization of non-negotiable goods within and between cultures. The basic idea is that within any cultural sphere certain goods are non-negotiable - perhaps because they are considered essential to self-respect or to a meaningful existence. Thus for any given culture, or sub-culture, certain goods will be considered more primary than others, and some will be considered so primary that they are non-negotiable; these nonnegotiable goods will have the status of "rights". The specification of primary goods may vary within and between cultures, but, while different cultures may designate different goods as non-negotiable or "primary", some goods will be designated as primary in each culture, and thus, in a sense, there is a culture-relative concept of primary goods, or rights. Moreover, where different cultures concur on the primacy of certain goods, there will be a transcultural conception of rights, and were all cultures to concur on the primacy of certain goods, there would be universal rights.

What I should like to suggest is that the near-global embrace of Nuremberg-like codes for almost a century (that is, since they were first invented in Prussian in 1900) indicates at least this: that any culture that values the prevention and cure of disease, disability, and suffering strongly enough to have developed a scientific medicine, will treat these as primary and will, therefore, try to preclude the assimilation of the physician-patient relationship into the investigator-subject relationship. For in any culture that accepts scientific medicine, people enter into the role of patient in the belief that by so doing they will increase their chances of recovery, not make them worse. They entrust themselves to healthcare professionals because they believe that the medical science with serve them, not that they will serve medical science - or advance the careers of scientific researchers. From the perspective of patients, therapy is primary, medical science is secondary. When, therefore, clinician-researchers like Neisser and Southam invert these priorities by placing their patients at needless risk through surreptitious inoculations, their actions called into question the underlying rationale for both the therapy and science. Patients value medical science primarily because it promises to enhance the efficacy of future therapy; consequently any science that undermines effective therapy will be seen as valueless. By subverting the therapeutic relationship medical science delegitimates itself.

Beauchamp and the other bioethics reformers of the 1970s not only "disambiguated" the roles of therapist and researcher, they developed a conceptual framework to support this distinction and articulated it in a discourse about "autonomy" and "paternalism" that positively-valued "patients' rights" and "informed consent". Their discourse mirrored, in a scholarly way, the more deeply visceral public reaction to the "scandalous" violation of the primacy of therapy. There was, it should be remarked, nothing cerebral about the reaction of the Prussian public in the 1890s, or the American public in the 1970s, or the global public in 1947 to the trespasses of researchers: the public was outraged. Why? Physicians are, in a sense, priests of the body. We reveal our selves to our physicians much as an earlier age entrusted its soul to priests. We trust them both to shepherd us through this incarnation and into the next. And if we have become skeptical about the next incarnation, we rely all the more heavily on the physician to guide us through this one. The trespasses of the researchers were thus more than scandal, they were sacrilege.

At Nuremberg, the trespasses of the physicians required a separate trial at which "the Case Against the Nazi Physicians" was heard by a separate tribunal, independently of all other war crimes. What made this trial special was not merely the horrible acts that had been done, but that *doctors* had done them. Their actions inverted our expectations: doctors are compassionate, not dispassionate; they heal, they do not harm; they save life, they do not destroy it. Whatever rules or regulations may, or may not, have been in place at the time, these *doctors* had violated a fundamental obligation. They should not have needed a formalism, a rule, a law, to tell them that they had trespassed upon a primary good and thus had violated the fundamental terms, not merely of a given societal conception of the physician-patient contract, but of any possible contract. They had trespassed upon what I have referred to as a "primary good" and what was traditionally called a "human right". Any such trespass is transtemporal and can be condemned even when there is no formal rule of morality or law expressly forbidding it.

The analysis advanced to this point is that any culture that accepts scientific medicine will be forced to differentiate the role of therapist from that of researcher, that such a cultue will also prioritize therapy over research, and that, in this sense, it will accept the idea of patient-subject rights. Postmodernists and multiculturalists might object, however, that while this may be true in the European cultural sphere, when we impose "informed consent" and such notions *outside* of Western culture, we flaunt the anthropologically-correct observation that concepts such as "individual rights", or "autonomy", or "self-determination", have often not been articulated, and may even be incapable of articulation, in other cultures. Should not we show our respect for other cultures, the postmodernist and the multiculturalist ask, by refraining from imposing Western rituals of "informed consent" on other societies?

I presented this argument, in outline, at the preliminary workshop conference held at the Albert-Ludwigs-Universität, Freiburg, preliminary to the larger conference to be held there in 1997. Predictably, those who favored the idea of human rights received it warmly; others were politely skeptical, suggesting that it was "Eurocentric" (a curious term to apply to a Bronx-born New Yorker), and thus inapplicable in Asia and other non-

European cultural spheres. Anecdote can never replace analysis but it can enhance it. As it happened there was only one Asian participating at the workshop conference, Professor Rhito Kimura, who directs the Asian Bioethics Program at the Kennedy Institute of Ethics. As a risk-taking New Yorker, I turned to Professor Kimura and asked him whether my analysis was consistent with the Japanese experience. He replied that initially Japanese physicians regarded bioethics generally, and the idea of informed consent in particular, as unnecessary, intrusive, alien, and utterly irrelevant to the Japanese medicine. Yet in the aftermath of the international reforms of the 1970s and 1980s, the idea permeated Japanese medical cultural to such an extent that the expression: "In-form-ed-(o) Con-sen-t- (o)" is now a standard term in the *Japanese* language. To reiterate, this anecdote does not confirm my analysis; however, it does suggest that it can not be dismissed by labeling it "Eurocentric", or "American cultural imperialism".

Postmodernists and multiculturalists often write about ethics in a way that suggests that it serves little or no rational social function (other than the an expression of group solidarity or an assertion of claims to privilege or power). I have tried to suggest that a more careful, historically contextualized, structural analysis of the discourse of "informed consent", "autonomy", and "rights" reveals that this discourse is a part of our global culture precisely because it serves the transcultural need to differentiate therapy from research and to assert the primacy of the former over the latter. The internationalization of medical science has thus necessitated a globalization of medical ethics. There are, of course, some cultures that have no medical science, and so have had little reason to distinguish between therapy and research. But even if we put aside, for a moment, the fact that any researcher as part of the global community of science would be accountable to the CIMOS or the Helsinki III standards, researchers would have no reason whatsoever to believe that a culture that did *not* embrace the ideals of science would be *more* willing to risk the health and life of its members to further these ideals than cultures that actually embraced them. The post-Nuremberg codes are thus transculturally valid in all cultures, irrespective of whether or not the culture embraces the norms and ideals of medical science.

Notes

* The analysis offered in this paper has been sharpened and enriched at the workshop at Albert-Ludwigs-Universität, by written comments from my workshop colleagues and from my colleagues at the Center for Bioethics of the University of Pennsylvania and at Union College. I should like to acknowledge the perceptive remarks of Ronald Carson, Paul Honigmann, Stuart Horner, Rihito Kimura, David Rothman, and William Winslade. I should also like to thank Karl-Heinz Leven, Donald Light, Jon Merz, Jonathan Moreno, Linda Patrik, and Maurice de Wachter for their reflective written comments on various drafts of this paper. Finally, I should like to thank Ulrich Tröhler

for inviting me to analyze the possibility of transcultural validity in the context of the Nuremberg Code - and for being a gracious host.

1 The 1931 Reichgesundheitsrat, opens with a similar statement: "In order that medical science may continue to advance, the initiation in appropriate cases of therapy involving new and as yet insufficiently tested means cannot be avoided...scientific subjects involving human subjects cannot be completely excluded...as this would hinder or even prevent progress in the diagnosis, treatment, and prevention of disease" (Annas, 1992, p. 130; also *Deutshe Medizinische Wochenschrift* 1931, p. 509).

2 Anglo-American malpractice law arose from the law of battery, hence the operative notion was *voluntary*. The notion that voluntary consent had to be *informed* is specific to the medical context. Thus even Justice Cardozo's classic formulation of the pre-Nuremberg American legal conception of consent in medicine states that "every human being of adult years and sound mind has a right to determine what shall be done with his own body; and a surgeon who performs an operation without his patient's consent commits an assault" (*Scholendorff v Society of New York Hospital*, 211 N.Y. 2d (914) - note the absence of any requirement that consent be *informed*. It was not until 1957, a decade after the Nuremberg Code, that the notion that consent must be *informed* entered into American case law (*Salgo v, Leland Stanford, Jr. University Board of* Trustees, 317 P.2d 170 (1957); see also William Winslade's discussion, in Chapter x, as well as Faden and Beauchamp, 1986). Ironically, therefore, the 1931 German analysis of the relevance of *informed* consent to research on human subjects was considerably more advanced than anything in Anglo-American ethical or legal theory at the time of the Nuremberg trial, and, compounding the irony, the Nuremberg Court may be the first court to introduce the idea of *informed* consent into Anglo-American law, and, as it turned out, into American medical ethics.

3 Karl-Heinz Leven has pointed out to me that the Neisser incident is often presented misleadingly. The point at issue was really rather subtle. In 1892, Dr. Neisser had injected "zellfreies Serum", that is, serum *without* cells of syphilitics, in an attempt to discover a method of immunizing people against syphilis. Four of Neissers eight patients later became syphilitic, but since they were prostitutes Neisser presumed that they had attracted the infection in "natural ways". Nonetheless, Neisser mentioned the theoretical possibility that they could have been infected by his injection when he published his research, and it was that remark that caused the scandal. On December 29, 1900, Dr. Neisser was fined of 300 German marks by the *Koenigliche Diszplinarhoffuer Nicht-richterliche Beamte* because he had experimented upon people without their consent. See Barbara Elkeles: *Der moralische Diskurs über das medizinische Menschenexperiment im 19 Jahrhundert*, Stuttgart, Jena, New York: G. Fischer, 1996, pp. 180-217).

4 As Beecher later comments (Beecher, 1970, p. 218), the idea of "peer review" in morally problematic cases was first proposed by Thomas Percival in *Medical Ethics* (1803); this was the first code of medical ethics written in English, and the first English-language work to use the expression "medical ethics". Percival, however, required *mandatory* peer review; thus Beecher's original position was more lenient than Percival's.

References

Advisory Committee on Human Radiation Experiments (1996), *Final Report of the Advisory Committee on Human Radiation Experiments*, Oxford University Press, New York.

Annas G., Grodin M. (1992), *The Nazi Doctors and the Nuremberg Code*, Oxford University Press, New York.

Beauchamp T., Childress J. (1979, 1983, 1989, 1994), *Principles of Biomedical Ethics*, Oxford University Press, New York.

Beecher H. (1966), 'Ethics and Clinical Research', *New England Journal of Medicine*, Vol. 274, pp. 1354-1360.

Beecher H. (1966) (a), 'Beecher's Code: Some Guiding Principles for Clinical Investigation', in Beecher, 1970, pp. 289-292.

Beecher H. (1970), *Research and the Individual: Human Studies*, Little, Brown and Company, Boston MA.

British Medical Association (1962), 'Experimental Research on Human Beings', in Beecher, (1970), p. 268.

Faden R., Beauchamp T. (1986), *A History and Theory of Informed Consent*, Oxford University Press, New York.

Gauthier D. (1986), *Morals By Agreement*, Oxford University Press, Oxford.

Grodin M. (1992), 'Historical Origins of the Nuremberg Code', in Annas and Grodin, 1992, pp. 121-144.

Harvard Medical School (1965), *Harvard Medical School Code*, in Beecher, 1970, pp. 283-284.

Ivy A. (1947), 'Nazi War Crimes of A Medical Nature', *Federation Bulletin*, vol. 13, pp. 133-146.

Katz J. (1972), Experimentation with Human Beings, Yale University Press, New Haven.

Medical Research Council of Great Britain (1963), 'Responsibility in Investigations on Human Subjects', in Beecher, 1970, pp. 262-267.

National Commission for the Protection of Human Subjects of Biomedical and Behavioral Research (1979), *The Belmont Report*, DHEW Publication No. OS 78-0014.

Nozick R. (1974), *Anarchy, State and Utopia*, Basic Books, New York.

Papworth M. H. (1967), *Human Guinea Pigs, Experimentation on Man*, Routledge and Kegan Paul, London.

Public Health Council of the Netherlands (1955), 'Report on Human Experimentation', in Beecher, 1970, p. 241.

Rawls J. (1971), *A Theory of Justice*, Harvard University Press, Cambridge, MA.

Reich W.T. (1978, 1995), *Encyclopedia of Bioethics*, Macmillan, New York.

Rothman D. (1991), *Strangers at the Bedside*, Basic Books, New York.

World Medical Association (1964), 'Declaration of Helsiniki (Helsinki I)', in Beecher, 1970, p. 277-279.

World Medical Association (1954), 'Principles for those in Research and Experimentation', in Beecher, 1970, p. 240.

26 Medical Ethics and Human Rights in South America

Horacio Riquelme

Introduction

In the so-called developing nations of South America, such as Argentina, Chile, and Uruguay, the state of medical ethics is a complex matter consisting of basically three coexisting currents that are explicitly based on ethical approaches to thinking and acting:

a) a bioethical dimension concerning the important aspect of the analysis of the consequences of technology and of shifting boundaries in medicine (organ transplants, biotechnology, human reproduction);

b) a social-medical dimension, namely the toll that poverty still takes in the form of structural violence (insufficient facilities and treatment) on a large part of the population;[1] and

c) a human rights dimension, as the time of the military dictatorships still effects us latently and the consequences for individuals and society of the organized use of violence are slowly becoming visible.

These three dimensions of ethics in medicine in South America are embedded in independent structures[2] and develop parallel to one another. Deontology in medicine (ethics as a required course) is admittedly witnessing a revival at the present both academically and professionally (in 1992 in Uruguay, for instance, two volumes of medical-ethical norms, codes, and explanations for students and working people were published[3]). No academic authorities in the countries of this study have, however, seen themselves in a position to introduce a synthesis of these three approaches. Probably, the events under the military dictatorships heightened awareness of the ethical fragility of medical practice; it is also likely that the non-confrontationality that arose at that time still affects even the representatives of quite similar views of ethics in medicine.

The societal experience of the last twenty years in South America have shown that medical practice there has been influenced by the totalitarian rule to a great extent and that many ethical axioms have been regularly broken in the process, as if they only contained compliant declarations of intent rather than fundamental principles of professional ethics - principles that are well known to those working in the health sector of the three

332

countries looked at and have been ratified by many international conventions and codes.[4]

The spirit of the Nuremberg Code thus no longer constitutes a distant model to emulate in investigating the interaction between medicine and human rights under military dictatorships in Argentina, Chile, and Uruguay (1973-1989). To make this clear, seven central questions on medical practice under the military regimes will be dealt with in three blocks, as follows:

Section I: 1) Can the direct participation of doctors in torture be proved?
2) Did doctors collaborate with the military regime?
3) Did they participate in the passing on of the infants of "missing" mothers? and
4) Were doctors simply docile fellow travellers of the regimes of terror?
Section II: 5) Did doctors resist the violation of human rights?
6) Are the findings of the commissions set up to investigate ethics within the profession reliable?
Section III: 7) Which (new) attitudes towards recent areas of conflict in medical ethics can be derived from these events?

The events in South America will be analyzed using a new approach designed for the source material. Some of the occurrences can only be understood with the data supplied by *Amnesty International*. Despite all denials by governmental officials, these data have proved conscientious and verifiable *a posteriori*.

The direct participation of doctors in repressive acts of state terrorism - but also in forms of resistance - has led to historically new situations. As is often the case in situations that are hard to imagine in everyday terms, knowledge of these fields of medical activity has remained somewhat fragmentary and anecdotal and seems to be the dubious privilege of chance witnesses and a select number of researchers.[5]

Section I: Towards Unconditional Obedience

The willingness to submit to a repressive system was explicit among several members of the medical profession. Dr. Guido Díaz Paci's opinion on torture, which he expressed to the special commission of the department of ethics of the Doctors' Association of Chile, is especially relevant as he was responsible for political prisoners for over six years as a military doctor.

> I believe, ... that torture represents an extreme form of physical duress and that this physical duress is legitimate when it does not cause any harm... the duress that only causes pain... is the same as the one children experience when they have their ears pulled or are spanked... I believe that psychological duress, such as sleep deprivation or the like, can be allowed...[6]

Torture and Medical Practice

Normally, an activity is culturally recognized as such when it is so named. The Chilean Doctors' Association (CMC: Colegio Médico de Chile) gives the following definition on the topic:

> The supervision of torture from the medical viewpoint includes the ongoing analysis of the ability of the victim to bear the abuse. It also includes the treating of wounds caused by the torture, as well as that the torture not be made public so that the victim remains in the hands of his henchmen.[7]

Torture under medical supervision In Argentina, Dr. Liwski describes the following situation that took place during the "trials of national restructuring":

> Already chained, the first voice that I heard was from someone telling me he was a doctor and informing me about the severity of the bleeding and that I should therefore not attempt to resist... Back then there was a second... utterance by (this Dr.) Vidal about a comment that he had made to one of the torturers, almost literally: "On the third or fourth day of the torture, it must be intensified because by then the acetylcholine starts running out and we know that any attempt to resist at this point is pointless..." This comment... referred to the knowledge of the (physiological) mechanisms that occur in the course of the application of torture... One or two days later, after the torture had been continued and I was informed that I would be tortured together with my then 3 and 6 year-old daughters, Ana and Julieta, Vidal is consulted by the main torturer, commissar Raffo, about the conditions that must be taken into consideration when torturing children. Vidal's answer was very categorical; he said that electrical shocks could be used at a body weight of 25 kilograms upwards.[8]

The report *Truth and Reconciliation* delivers a lot of detailed information about the events in the region of San Antonio, Chile, events which can be considered representative of the general situation in Chile after the coup d'état of 1973:

> Characteristically... the doctors present, also wearing hoods, watched over the torture (so that there would be no fatalities) and treated the worst victims in case of emergency... The report by a humanitarian organization at the end of 1973 and the beginning of 1974 shows a high rate of medical intervention on the inmates of the prison; the rate was five to six times higher than in other prison visited...[9]

In Uruguay, the possible resistance of the prisoners was medically supported:

After being committed to a prison camp, each new inmate was examined by a doctor who then drew up a "complete medical report". This report was handed on to the officers that were responsible for the prisoner. The officers responsible for the interrogation often used this information about already existing health problems to determine the limits of the torture. When the officer knew, for instance, that the prisoner had problems with his heart, the time spent submersed in the "submarine" had to be shortened or replaced by another method. Additionally, the officers sometimes demanded medical examinations during the torture in order to decide whether it should be discontinued...[10]

Specific medicinal tasks in the prison camps During the dictatorships, medicinal tasks in prisons and concentration camps seem to have followed criteria much different than those during times of democracy. In Argentina, this particular attitude towards medicine can be reconstructed using the following statement:

While I was in La Escuelita, I received medical treatment twice. Once during torture when I was still blindfolded, someone examined my heart and lungs with a stethoscope. Then urine samples were taken because one of my kidneys had been damaged. I felt like a animal in a laboratory experiment with a doctor who examined my vital functions but did not look upon me as a human being. Another prisoner told me he knew the doctor. He could see the doctor under his blindfold and had recognized him. I only remember that his last name was German and that he was a doctor in the first division of the marines in Bahía Blanca.[11]

The situation in prisons and other camps in Chile does not seem to have been much different:

Alberto Barraza... stated in his declaration before the tribunal that a doctor had examined him three times during his torture. "After each examination the doctor said, 'Everything seems fine, you can continue the treatment.' It was obviously the same doctor who gave pills three times a day and a bitter drink that tastes of peppermint."

Dr. Mandressi recounted these events for Uruguay in summary fashion to L. Weschler, a journalist for the *New Yorker*:

You must understand that these guys were experts. They were very well educated in the application of methods that caused great pain without leaving behind any physical trace or killing the victim. There were relatively few deaths due to torture in Uruguay. That's because there were normally doctors who took part in the interrogations.[12]

Torture and inhumane treatment on a medical basis Doctors were not only physically present during the various repressive activities, but also seem to have made efforts to perfect their professional services.

Dr. Bloche gives us an example of the professional ambition of this kind of activity for Uruguay:

> A former employee of the prison at Libertad says that the reports of the doctors helped in keeping an eye on the "activities and manner of conduct of the prisoners." "We have learned a lot in the recent past. When we observe very nervous behavior, a lot of talking, too many conversations, we took measures to neutralize (the inmates)... We gave them, for instance, less free time, changed their cells, took away their books, and tightened security. All that reduced their activity because they could never sleep well or rest."[13]

The use of non-therapeutic drugs and psychological techniques In daily parlance, we use the term "therapeutic arsenal" to mean the known and common techniques and medicaments with which disturbances and illnesses are treated. Here, we are concerned with the development of such an arsenal that was not designed for therapeutic goals.

In Chile, several reports are based on the statements of an anesthesiologist of the military who had given drugs to the prisoners. One of the reports reads:

> They took me into a hospital once where a young doctor called.... examined me. She spoke reassuringly: "They have punished you severely. We will take care of you now, don't worry. We're just going to give you a shot to calm you down." They gave me a shot of sodium pentothal, as I later found out...[14]

In such a formal country as Uruguay, it is not surprising that the police ask the courts for permission to use sodium pentothal during interrogations of prisoners, even when this happened in August 1970. Shortly before, the senate of the republic had established a commission to clear up the accusations of torture that apparently were part of the normal practices of the police, even before the coup d'état of 1973. A court doctor who was a witness for the commission stated: "And you want to know whether torture was used? You must be the only Uruguayan who doesn't know that".[15]

Killings by medical means The use of medical knowledge in the killing of prisoners was much less wide-spread. The information this study is based on only takes account of Argentina (in Chile and Uruguay, such practices cannot be ruled out, but there is little solid evidence for it at the present). The report "Nunca más" supplies the following report:

> The three vehicles drove along an unpaved side-street up to the gate in front of the tree-covered square where officer Dr. Bergé (...) was waiting. The

three bodies of the three former rebels, who were still alive at this point, were taken out of the vehicles and thrown on the lawn. The doctor gave each of them two shots of a poisonous red liquid directly into the heart. Two died, but the doctor declared all of them dead.. The priest von Wernich spoke to me about the impression that this event had made on him; he said that what we had done had been necessary, that it had been a patriotic act and that God knew that it was the best thing for the country. Those were his own words...[16]

Harm caused by unpreventable neglect The experiences of the prisoners with medical treatment seems to also be affected by the disrespect of their rights as patients. Dr. Liwski explains what happened when he fell ill as a prisoner:

About 60 or 65 days after I had disappeared, I caught typhoid fever. (Dr.) Vidal was brought into my cell. I could see him directly, and he informed me that the best medicine for this illness was chloramphenicol. Everyone who works in health care knows that (for typhoid fever) long-term treatment with high doses is necessary if the treatment is to be effective... after 48 hours, the chlormphenicol was discontinued. There was hardly any effect (though there was the risk that the bacteria would become resistant to the medicine).[17]

Medical-ethical reflections Now that the majority of Latin American States, including the three countries discussed here, have signed and ratified the Convention against torture, there should not be any more obstacles toward the realization of the postulate "torture and medical practice are contradictory and rule one another out".[18] It can be assumed, however, that the mere formulation of good intentions will not suffice to raise awareness among doctors and the general public; open discussions about what actually happened will be necessary to make a human rights culture out of mere regulations.[19]

Medicine and Law: A Dubious Relationship

There are various areas of medical activity that have attracted the interest of authoritarian regimes and in which only those have been allowed to work who had the full trust of the regime. Court medicine has played an important role here.

In the following, ethical conflict situations will be illustrated in which the interaction between medicine and the law seems problematic.

Autopsies and the practice of "making people disappear" The operations of the court autopsy clinic in Buenos Aires during the dictatorship in Argentina sheds light on the forms of collaboration between court medicine and the system of repression and allows us to understand how a part of the military mechanism of "making the dead disappear" worked. The dead were brought into the autopsy clinic, identified, and then taken away by the military and buried anonymously without informing family members of these events:

> It was always the same procedure: the neighboring streets were cordoned off during the night and army trucks came to the complex and stopped in front of the building. The cargo was dropped off there. Everyone in the neighborhood was too afraid to talk openly about what everyone eventually knew.[20]

False health reports or death certificates The intention behind the changing of diagnoses, the giving of false explanations, or incorrect estimations seems to serve not only the secrecy of the act, as stated above, but also a second, parallel field of activity that has remained unpunished.

In Chile, the cooperation of doctors in state terrorism has been documented as follows:

> Another form of doctor participation in the secrecy of torture is the filling out of false autopsy reports and/or death certificates, a practice that has been corroborated in research by the ethics department.[21]

The death of the Uruguayan doctor Vladimir Roslik shortly after his arrest in 1984 deserves special attention. This death led to the first study by the Doctors' Association on the responsibility of military doctors in cases of human rights violations in Uruguay. It became clear that several doctors who worked for the military had basic difficulties distinguishing between medicinal and military tasks.

In his statement before the ad hoc committee of the *Asociación Médica del Interior* (AMEDRIN), Dr. Eduardo Saíz Pedrini mentioned that the order to carry out three examinations of Dr. Roslik within 24 hours was part of the routine. He claimed not to have heard Dr. Roslik complaining about the torture and that he had also been ordered to carry out the autopsy on Dr. Roslik after his death. In his official autopsy report, he claimed that the death had been caused by "the ceasing of breathing and heartbeat".

With the help of another physician, Dr. Burjel, the family of Dr. Roslik succeeded in getting a second autopsy done which produced clear evidence that he had suffered a violent death at the hands of his tormentors.

The military physician Dr. Eduardo Saíz Pedrini, who had directed the official autopsy of Dr. Roslik, was afterwards excluded from the Doctors' Association in March of 1985 - which did not prevent him from being sent to Sinai the same year as part of the Uruguay contingent of the international peace keeping mission of the UN.[22]

Semantics of collaboration Without wanting to go into conscious or unconscious collaboration, I would like to demonstrate how medical euphemisms are useful in hiding human rights violations. One example of a subtle argumentative strategy is given by Dr. Mautone, then head doctor of anatomic pathology at a military hospital, who gave as causes of death in his reports "acute edema of the lungs" or "acute insufficiency of the lungs and the heart", both of which were "caused by stress" in patients who had obviously died as a consequence of their being tortured. As he put it himself, he left the further definition of the diagnostic word "stress" up to the discretion of the courts.

Medical-ethical reflections The obedient cooperation of medical examiners with the terror regimes deserves special attention, all the more so because many of these doctors still view such practices as common and are thus little given to questioning their actions.

The Appropriation of Descendants

Definition of the problem The handing over of children born to mothers held in prison or "missing" to people who are not related to them at all was a typical occurrence in Argentina's secret prison camps. Estimates are that over 300 children were taken away from their blood relations and given up for adoption in this manner.

Ramón Camps, a high-ranking officer with the Argentinean army, stated in an interview on this issue with the Spanish weekly "Interviú" almost programmatically:

> [I]t wasn't people who disappeared, it was subversive elements. I personally never killed a single child; what I did was hand them over to charity organizations so they could find new parents. The subversive parents raise their children to be subversive. This has to be prevented...[23]

The report by CONADEP includes the names of several doctors who took part in these activities directly:

> As soon as the child was born, the mother was "invited" to write a letter (that invariably stayed in the camp files) to her family members who were to receive the child... We have found out from the commentaries that a list of couples from the marines who couldn't have children were in the navy hospital waiting to be given these children to adopt. A gynecologist from the hospital was responsible for the list.[24]

R. Salguero goes into specifics on the procedure:

> The patients (the imprisoned-vanished mothers) were specially marked by cards with 'N.N' in place of their names.[25]

Scientific searches for stolen progeny The emptiness left behind by the "vanished" generation of parents looking - also through legal channels -

for the children born in prison was filled by the so-called "grandmothers of the Plaza de Mayo". These were the mothers of the "missing", who knew that their grandchildren must have been born in the camps and fought for their return.[26]

- The progress of genetics as a biomedical discipline was invaluable for the identification of these children who were illegally given up for adoption to couples who were close to the regime.
- To determine the identity and relationship of these children, hematological studies of genetic material were carried out using modern methods (blood groups, protein and enzymes of the blood serum, histological compatibility).
- The results of these examinations constitute proof of the determination of both the identity and the relationship and has been taken up in regular cases of the courts.[27]

Medical-ethical reflections There is still a "zone of silence"[28] around many of the children born during the incarceration of their parents. The grandmothers of the Plaza de Mayo have for Argentina a number of clues at their disposal which could be used to continue the search. As it is clear that doctors in Latin America participated in the illegal adoption of children, the powers of the authorities both within and without the profession must be strengthened in order to prevent events from happening again.

Doctors and the philosophy of the military dictators

The special role that doctors played during the dictatorships in South America consists in the participation and resistance that doctors exhibited vis-à-vis these regimes.[29] The extent to which doctors were active not only in their professional areas, but also in the founding and spreading of totalitarian ideas remains an important question.

In this context, the theoretical activity of a Chilean military doctor should be mentioned. This doctor summarized his thoughts on the dealings with the members of Allende's government after it had been toppled by the military. The article was published on 11 October 1973 in the influential newspaper "El Mercurio" under the title "The Unredeemable". He divides the "44% who voted for the Unidad Popular in March 1973" into five groups: extremists; very dangerous and intelligent activists; ideological activists; people who were active in the parties of Unidad Popular; and sympathizers of Unidad Popular. He then suggests special repressive measures designed for such attitudes.[30]

In Uruguay, Dr. Martín Gutiérrez, the head doctor of the prison "Liberdad" and later advisor to the governing junta, made the following clear statements about the situation of the prisoners in the prisoners and barracks:

The war continued in the prisons. Day by day, rule by rule, their stated aim was to cause psychological harm.[31]

On the unconditional loyalty of the doctors to the upper ranks of the military, Dr. Marabotto, also from Uruguay, stated in no unspecific terms:

> The function of the military doctor in every country and under every political regime is to support the commander in technical ways. The commander is ultimately responsible for what is done or not done in his unit; the doctor is a "staff officer" under his command, in other words a medical advisor.[32]

Medical-ethical reflections The dimension of the philosophy of doctors, especially of military doctors under totalitarian regimes, is becoming increasingly important as it is hardly plausible that they acted as puppets of the respective tyrants. Rather, their ideas may have fostered the attitude among military personnel that, say, torture is just another war tactic.

Section II: The Other Side of the Story

This study of medical practice under military regimes in Argentina, Chile, and Uruguay would not be complete if the dimension of active reactions against the totalitarian intentions of these regimes were not paid adequate attention. During that time of suppression, the participation of doctors in activities to uphold ethical responsibility can also be found; people who went beyond the passive resistance and gave meaning to fundamental principles of professional ethics.

Indeed, during the dictatorships there were a number of personal initiatives and ecumenical groups who devoted themselves to the furthering of human rights, for example in Chile:

> One of the doctors who offered aid to torture victims was Dr. Pedro Castillo, a thorax surgeon and member of the American College of Surgeons. During a wave of firings of academics in 1975, Dr. Castillo lost his position as head of the surgical department at the University of Chile. In 1981, he founded the National Commission against Torture... At the beginning of May, agents from the CNI began to keep his house in Santiago under surveillance... (On 27 May he was) arrested at his home and taken to the prison camp in Borgono Street... (Shortly thereafter) the *Vicaría* de Solidaridad and the Chilean human rights commission openly stated that the secret police was infuriated that (he and two other) doctors had taken the state to court on charges of torture. These charges contained detailed accounts of torture chambers of the secret police and confirmed in a few cases the presence of doctors in the chambers... Three weeks after their arrest, the three doctors showed up at the prison in Valparaíso. The military judge on the case allowed two North American

doctors to visit Dr. Castillo and his colleagues. Visibly affected by what had happened to them, they reported that they had been kept in solitary confinement for three weeks, most of the time blindfolded, without any access to their family or to lawyers. One of the Americans later told the press that "they were mostly concerned by the fact that they had been publicly accused of association with terrorist acts. Their professional lives could be destroyed by such accusations." On 1 July 1981, a military court in Valparaíso ruled that there was no evidence that the three doctors had been involved in terrorist organizations and that the accusation of illegal political acts was not in the jurisdiction of the military court anyway. The military judge handed the second accusation over to a civil court, which refused to hear the case and ordered that the men be set free immediately.[33]

There is also the following report on the non-discriminatory treatment of patients in Uruguay:

After an armed conflict between the army and the Tupamaros, I was called to treat the wounded as a surgeon. I determined that Mr. Z., a Tupamaro, had been shot in the chest and that an officer had been scraped on the buttocks by a bullet. I ordered that we begin treatment of Mr. Z. but was told that he could wait as long as there was an officer to be treated. I insisted that the treatment of more severe injuries has medical priority and devoted myself to Mr. Z.[34]

Medical-ethical reflections Even after the return of parliamentary democracy, the horror of the totalitarian phase lives on in the consciousness of those who lived under it. The acknowledgement of acts protecting the principles of medical ethics at the time is important as there were examples of active, daily resistance by doctors in the situations studied.

The Trials Against Doctors under Conditions of Legal Amnesty

Although no juridical procedures were undertaken in the three countries to clear up the personal responsibility of those who participated in torturing, murdering, and abducting of people, it must be emphasized that the doctors' associations have looked for ways to show the borders of professional ethics under military dictatorships. To a larger or smaller extent, professional organizations have shown clearly that the activities of doctors in supporting the state system of repression cannot be viewed as acceptable under any circumstances. The ethical ruling *inter pares* has met with great resonance among the public in the three countries.

In Argentina, a "Health Tribunal on Ethics against Impunity" was held on 3 December 1987. Three doctors who were held directly responsible by many former inmates for torture, kidnapping, and murder were tried *in absentia*. Dr. Diana Kordon based her argument as prosecutor on the given ethical code and stated further:

The first article of the ethical code ratified by the Doctors' Association of the Republic of Argentina in 1955 clearly states: "The doctor must treat the ill with care all the time and respect their *conditio humana*. He shall not use his medical knowledge against the laws of humanity."

She supported her accusation with statements by people who had suffered under state terrorism and had to do directly with the doctors standing trial (cf. the above statements by Dr. Liwski). The prosecutor explained in her opening statement:

> The participation of doctors was necessary for the application of repressive methods. They determined how much torment the prisoners could bear. They directed and oversaw the continuation of torture in order to receive a maximum of information. The most despicable task of these doctors was to proscribe the amount of torture and take part actively in the torture. They also participated in the kidnapping of children born in prison by aiding the imprisoned pregnant women and (then) filling out false reports...[35]

The tribunal unanimously found them guilty of having committed serious ethical mistakes and crimes against humanity. In its final statement, the tribunal called on universities, the academic community, medical associations, and health institutions and authorities to refuse these doctors any access to teaching, research, or practical positions.

Due to its long institutional tradition with legal statutes (declared invalid by the military dictatorship in 1973), Chile's medical association, the Colegio Médico de Chile, began as early as 1983 to rule on ethical conflicts based on political repression shortly after the first inner-association elections in which the military government did not intervene. The research of the committee for ethics drew people's attention because doctors who had collaborated with the repressive regimes were being called to task before an internal court without further ado. Thus, the committee was performing the function of a parallel court that due to its very existence was bringing the blindness of justice to this topic to light and calling on the repressive system to answer for concrete cases.

From 1983 to the present, a large number of cases in which doctors' participation in repression was investigated have been heard outside of courtrooms. Only those cases in which the doctors were found to be directly responsible beyond a doubt were ever made public.[36] In light of this, it is not surprising that the members of the board of the CMC were also persecuted by the military government between 1983 and 1989 and confined as political prisoners for several months.[37]

In Uruguay, there was a similar development in the medical associations, the Federación Médica del Interior (State Medical Association) and the Sindicato Médico del Uruguay (Medical Association of Uruguay). G. Martirena remembers the impetus behind the founding National Commission for Medical Ethics:

Even if this constitutes an affront to the medical establishment in Uruguay, the fact is nonetheless irrefutable that there were doctors who actively or passively participated in the torturing of political prisoners or who violated ethical norms in service to the higher-ups they had sworn allegiance to... In light of these facts, the Seventh National Medical Congress took place in July 1984 - when the dictatorship was still in power in Uruguay... With the votes of all delegated doctors, the National Commission for Medical Ethics was founded.[38]

Shortly after the Commission began its functions, the government passed a resolution signed by then defense minister Dr. Justo M. Alonso Leguísamo in which the commission was incorrectly described as a tribunal:

1. It is forbidden for military doctors to make any sort of statements before ethics tribunals of the Seventh National Medical Congress. The speaker must be informed when any such situation occurs.
2. For the publications and information of the health service of the armed forces, and for the archives. [39]

Despite this ban, the investigations of the ethics commission of court-martial found in the numerous accusations enough violations against professional ethics to form their own opinion.[40]

Medical-ethical reflections It can be argued, especially in light of the official aversion to any form of questioning the time of the dictatorships in all of the three countries, that the actions of the medical associations and organizations were socially and culturally unique. As these ethically motivated acts failed to be imitated by other associations and legal systems, this example sheds light on the conditions of the post-dictatorial years.

Section III: In Lieu of an Epilogue: New Topics of Conflict in Medical Ethics

It can be assumed that the years of the dictatorships included not only the dimension of terror but also the questioning of all areas of social life, which suggests that new challenges for professional ethics arose and/or became apparent during those years. Here, the thesis is that an accentuated sensibility for ethical conflicts exists in the post-dictatorial era. In the course of this section, some areas will be touched upon which serve as the basis for professional ethics and have not yet been culturally dealt with and for which no final solutions have been found. It is, however, important to take the concrete experiences of many doctors during the repression into account in order, for instance, to understand the special sensibility for the living conditions of people who, for whatever reasons, are imprisoned.

Former Torturers and their Psychotherapeutic Treatment

Even if there are no moral scruples in wartime about doctors treating the injured of the opposing army, the psychotherapeutic treatment of active participants of torture is a very touchy subject today in South America.

D. Lagos reports from Argentina about the clinical history of a former torturer shortly after the return of democracy. The patient, who had often been treated for nervous problems in the previous eight years (1978-1986) in Buenos Aires and was then taking part in individual psychotherapy, exhibited symptoms of depression and paranoia. It seemed as though the vow of silence about his activities as a torturer were renewed with each new psychotherapist and that they were not thematized in psychotherapy for that reason. This corresponded with the behavior of the patient towards the therapist: he only wanted him to stop the symptoms. D. Lagos then began reflecting on the behavior of some of the other therapists who in keeping the vow of silence had become accomplices and had only supported his efforts to "nullify the symptoms" and tacitly exculpated him by recognizing him in his role as a patient without going into the clinical history of the fundamental elements of his biography and psychopathology.[41]

Doctors and the Death Penalty

The active participation of doctors in the death penalty is a very timely topic as death by injection can apparently be accepted as a quite aseptic form of execution. The CMC has stated rejection of every attempt to bind doctors to these functions (the death penalty still exists in the penal code of Chile). The CMC's rejection was based on the refusal of Dr. Start (1982) in the United States to carry out the death penalty in Oklahoma by giving a man an intravenous injection.[42] This refusal led to an intensive debate on professional ethics (the Hippocratic Oath explicitly forbids the administering of lethal drugs) and the functions of prison doctors. It is no doubt the merit of the CMC that this form of execution was not taken from the US into a country that otherwise generally belongs to the avant-garde when it comes to taking up such "progressive measures" from Western culture.[43]

Doctors and Hunger Strikes

The professional practice and the ethical conflict of health personnel are the central topics of debate in Uruguay. M. de Pena, M. Jáuregui and G. Mesa[44] analyzed their some 25 years of experience in the field of medical practice:

> In the case of a hunger strike, the participants are healthy and prepared to put their health at risk, even to the point of death, for a higher goal that has nothing to do with their health. Their interests thus conflict with those of the

> doctors... The disregard for this confrontation between the equal "duties" of the two groups can lead to the failure of the treatment...[45]

They side with the declaration by the WMA when they say:

> it is the duty of the doctor to respect the autonomy of the patient. A doctor needs the expressed consent of patients before his knowledge can be put to use to help them...

Ethical Norms for the Medical Treatment of Prisoners

The directors and many members of Chile's Medical Association had, as stated, taken up very close contact with the opposition to the dictatorship and gotten to know the physical conditions in Chile's prisons and the arbitrariness that characterized the relations between guards and inmates. This sensibility led the CMC as early as 1985 to pass a declaration on the medical treatment of prisoners.[46]

Toward Legislation against Crimes against Humanity

The medical organizations in the three countries have not only pushed for the respecting of human rights in medical practice, but also taken initiatives to break through the "zones of denied services and silence" that still are prevalent in legislation. The medical association in Uruguay has proposed legislation on "crimes against humanity" in which all possible crimes that play a role in terror regimes are listed and specific sanctions are suggested. Even if it is not possible to enact this law retroactively, its passing would nonetheless spark the hope that the events of state terrorism truly do belong to the past and that doctors (and other professional groups) will no longer be able to play innocent when human dignity is attacked.

Future directions

Based on all these examples in the areas of medical activities discussed here, it is clear that the systematic representation of concrete events of medically assisted human rights violations can help to open new access routes to a hitherto unknown professional sphere and raise awareness of this knowledge among the public.

Military doctors are mainly responsible for the violations against human rights in South America. Admittedly, these doctors in the three countries did not have unlimited room to act in: individual resistance was often a possibility, and there is nothing to suggest that doctors who held to the Hippocratic Oath were attacked or disadvantaged; some military doctors even stepped down from their positions in order to avoid collision with their own political and ethical principles. Collective resistance came about during the military dictatorships in Chile and Uruguay for one specific purpose: to make the human rights violations committed by doctors public and to foster closer scrutiny.

To find out and understand how doctors were active in and against the system of repression, it can be helpful to gain a better understanding of this period and how people acted back then, but also of how to recognize possible tendencies, even in times of peace.

Notes

This essay in based on the research for my *Habilitation* thesis as a Privatdozent entitled "*Medizinische Ethik und die existentielle Lage von Ärzten unter Bedingungen totalitärer Herrschaft in Südamerika*" at the Medical School at Hamburg University. The complete work (with the results of some field work among doctors in South America) appeared in Spanish in 1995 in Caracas as *Entra la obediencia y la oposicíon. Los médicos y la ética profesional bajo la dictadura militar*; in Germany, it will soon be published under the title *Medizinische Ethik in Krisenzeiten. Ärzte zwischen Gehorsam und Auflehnung unter der Militärdiktatur in Südamerika* by the Nomos Verlag, Baden Baden. An English version is being prepared in London.

1 "According to UNICEF, in Argentina 18,000 children still die within their first year, two-thirds of them of preventable causes." Quote from La Mortalidad Infantil Neonatal, in: Salud, Problema y Debate Vol 4, No 7: 41-3. See also A.E. Fica & F.A. Cabello (1992): Cólera en Latinoamerica: La relación entre salud pública y economía. In: Interciencia. Vol 17, No 5: 276-283

2 International discussions on bioethics are supported by, among others, institutes such as the "Fundación J.M. Mainetti para el progreso de la medicina" in La Plata, Argentina and its publishing division (cf. G.D. Pis (1994): La bioética como fenómino cultural. In. Quirón, Vol 25 No 1: 34-44). Applied research and planning in social medicine, which has a long tradition in South America, was taken up again at universities in Argentina, Chile, and Uruguay after the return of democracy (cf. H. Dúran (1991): La Salud Pública para un nuevo escenario. In: Salud y Cambio. Revista Chilena de Medicina Social. Vol. 3, No 6: 53-4). The human rights dimension has, as mentioned above, found acknowledged access to medical journals (see articles by D. Kordon, G. Martirena, and G. Seelmann in the Journal of Medical Ethics (1991) Vol. 17, Supplement).

3 S. Martirena, G. (1992), "Ética - Médicos y Derechos Humanos" Montevideo and Sindicato Médico del Uruguay (1992), "La ética médica. Normas, códicos y declaraciones internacionales" Montevideo.

4 For instance, a) the Declaration of the World Association of Doctors (AMM: 1948, 1968, and 1983) on the ethical definition of medical practice, b) the Declaration of the General Assembly of the United Nations on Torture and Other Inhumane Treatment (9. XII. 1975), and c) the Declaration of Tokyo (AMM: 1975) on the participation of doctors in torture.

5 The shadow of this period in these three countries is still apparent in many areas of medical practice, and the effect of the terror is still present among those apparently unaffected by it. As a young doctor from Argentina put it, "Although I was only performing my duties as a medical student back then and generally kept out of all discussions, I now realize that I have little recollection of many things from back then, as

though many events that happened in my presence had simply been 'erased'." Personal communication with Dr E. Sánchez at the VI. Symposium "Culture and Psychosocial Situations in Latin America." Hamburg September 1992.

6   F.S. Rivas (1990), Traición a Hipócrates. Médicos en el aparato de la dictadura, Santiago, p. 128.

7   E. Stover (1987), The open secret: Torture and the medical profession in Chile (American Association for the Advancement of Science/AAAS), p. 69.

8   N.I. Liwski: Nunca más: 28 and Declaración ante el Tribunal: 15-16.

9   Report by the National Commission for Truth and Reconciliation: Official unabridged edition, La Nación, 5.3. 1991: 24.

10   M.G. Bloche (1987), Uruguay military physicians: Cogs in a system of state terror (AAAS), p. 6.

11   Statement by Carlos Sanabria, in: E. Stover and E.O. Nightingale (1985), "The Breaking of Bodies and Minds" p. 52-3.

12   Source: L. Weschler(1991), A miracle, a universe. Settling accounts with torturers, New York, p. 126.

13   S. Bloche, ibid, p. 7

14   Report of the CMCH, Stover, ibid: 71.

15   Source: J. Mañana C. (1992), Historia del Sindicato Médico del Uruguay, Montevideo 133-135.

16   Statement by Julio Alberto Emmed before the CONADEP, Court File Nr. 683.

17   Liwski, statement before the tribunal, p. 16.

18   Cf. the Declaration of Tokyo 1975.

19   The Chilean Doctors' Association has adopted the following definitions in its statutes: "The participation of doctors in torture takes place, roughly speaking, in the following manners:

        1.   Analysis of the ability of the victim to bear the torture.

        2.   The supervision of torture and active intervention in cases of complications.

        3.   The passing on of professional knowledge to torturers.

        4.   The falsifying or intentional omission of medical information in health reports or autopsy reports.

        5.   Medical services in the course of torture which are not reported or resisted.

        6.   The direct use of torture by the doctor.

        7.   Keeping such activities secret." See report by the CMCH in Stover, ibid, p. 75.

20   A. Colombo in Madres de Plaza de Mayo o.J.: 10-11.

21   See the report by the CMCH in Stover, ibid, p. 74-75. He makes a point of stressing: "In the case of Alvarez, for example, the department has confirmed several abnormalities in the autopsy report signed by Dr. Exequiel Jiménez Ferry... The case (of Dr. Jiménez) raises serious questions about the extent to which inadequate autopsies have led to miscarriages of justice." Ibid, p. 75.

22   Source: personal communication with Dr. Burjel, Bloche ibid: 7 and Martirena ibid: 29-49.

23   Cf. the protocoll of the ethics tribunal for health against pardons (3.12.1987), p. 20.

24   Nunca más: 303.

25   R. Salguero in: Nunca más: 313.

26   "At the time (1979-81), we began to study scientific terms. Our argumentation was

linear. For instance, gestures are (in our opinion) handed down; there are children who hold their hands exactly like their fathers, who cross their legs just like their mothers, who stand like their grandmothers..." S.M. Herrera and E. Temembaum (1988): Indentidad, despojo y restitución. Buenos Aires, p. 94.

27 Cf. R. Torres M. (1987), La problemática especifica de los niños desaparecidos. In: La desaparición. Crimen contra la humanidad. Asamblea Permantente por los Derechos Humanos, Buenos Aires, p. 137-148.

28 Due to the amount of clinical work on people affected by the state terrorism, Marcelo Viñar writes: "This zone of silence is, however, critical. The un-admittable, says Maurice Blanchot (1984) is not what is not admitted, but when there are no confessions or honest avowals that could uncover it. The un-admittable is hidden in its essence when something pressing or not postpone-able brings it to life because of a mistake or an omission: 'You wouldn't know.'" Source: Violencia social y realidad en psicoanálisis. In: J. Puget and René Kaes (1991): Violencia de estado y psicoanálisis. Buenos Aires.

29 Sociological studies on the conduct of doctors during these serious social changes have yet to be published. "There are, for example, only anecdotes about the activities of the doctors in Chile although they initially took part in the opposition to Allende's government and even welcomed the coup as an adequate solution, only then to go into the fundamental opposition to the dictatorship and have a great influence on the founding of the democratic pact, the *Concertación Democrática*, that comprised the political basis for the fall of dictator Pinochet by the ballet." Personal communication with Dr. Luis González, former chairman of the Doctors' Association and present ambassador of Chile to Belgium.

30 Based on Dr. Schuster's classification (cf. K. Resczcynsky et al., ibid, p. 270), the professional status of many Chilean doctors was redefined: "Three doctors from the United States who had been sent to Chile by the Federation of American Scientists (FAS) in June of 1974 to investigate the claims of human rights violations made by doctors spoke with Dr. Arriagada, director of the national health service SNS (about possible systematic persecutions H.R.). Dr. Arriagada admitted that the military government had ordered directors of hospitals to divide the personnel of the health sector into three categories. Category A was composed of people considered safe and irreplaceable. Category B contained the names of possible activists and the politically active. Category three contained those considered dangerous; they were fired from the SNS, while those on list B were transferred... The visiting doctors were showed a copy of list C containing 1700 names."

31 See Bloche, ibid, p. 6.

32 See the statement by Dr. N. Marabotto before the National Commission for Medical Ethics on 26 October 1986. Source: Martirena, ibid, p. 69.

   * *Solidarity curacy* is the name of a religious organisation that supports people harmed by the dictatorships. H.R.

33 See Stover, ibid. p. 48-50.

34 Personal communication with one of the doctors interviewed during the field research.

35 Ibid.

36 This balanced attitude toward presumed violations of professional ethics as well as possible active participants in crimes against humanity has not only created sympathy in a society that remains torn apart and bitterly needs such points of reference in order to reconstruct its sense of justice and the certainty that the crimes committed have been atoned for and the guilty parties brought to justice. The revenge murder of a doctor found guilty of passively supporting the repression by a extremist group in 1990 must be viewed in this context.

37 Personal communication with Dr. Luis González, former chairman of the CMC.

38   See G. Martirena (1988), Uruguay. La tortura y los médicos, Montevideo, p. 14 and 15.

39   Cf. Resolution Nr. 15.057 from 7 August 1984, published on the same day in Bulletin Nr. 8082 of the Ministry of Defense.

40   The Commission recommended in this context that the approbation of these doctors be withdrawn.

41   See D. Lagos (1988), Professional Ethics - Social Ethics - Mental Health and Impunity. In: D. Kordon et al.: Psychological effects of political repression. Buenos Aires, p. 157-62.

42   The American Medical Association declared in 1982 that no doctor may participate in executions. The discussion was ended when the government decided that the person giving the injection does not have to be a doctor.

43   See Vida médica (1985), Vol. 36, Nr. 3: 75-82.

44   Sources: Lecture before the First International Congress: "Salud psicosocial: Cultura y democracia en América Latina," Asunción, Paraguay, 1992. manuscript, 24 p. and "WMA Declaration on Hunger-Strikers (1991)," in: British Medical Association: Medicine betrayed. The participation of doctors in human rights abuses. London, 1992.

45   In this context, they list possible problem areas in the interaction between health personnel and hunger strikers: "uncritical support of the campaign ('putting on the shoes of the strikers'); doubts about the effectiveness of the (paternalistic attitude)... The surveillance of a regulated hunger strike is thus a preventive act in that the health squad sees to it that the participants in the hunger strike suffer as little harm as possible" and they close with the conclusion that the medical treatment of hunger strikers does not represent a "decision to assist in suicide" (which is punishable by art. 315 of Uruguay's penal code), but rather is an integral part of the medicinal practice in that it is not the "crime of denial of assistance." Ibid.

46   Cf. AI Index: AMR 22/36/86: "Human rights in Chile: The role of the medical profession." September 1986.

Appendix

The Nuremberg Code, 1947

1. The voluntary consent of the human subject is absolutely essential. This means that the person involved should have legal capacity to give consent; should be so situated as to be able to exercise free power of choice, without the intervention of any element of force, fraud, deceit, duress, over-reaching, or other ulterior form of constraint or coercion; and should have sufficient knowledge and comprehension of the elements of the subject matter involved as to enable him to make an understanding and enlightened decision. This latter element requires that before the acceptance of an affirmative decision by the experimental subject there should be made known to him the nature, duration, and purpose of the experiment; the method and means by which it is to be conducted; all inconveniences and hazards reasonably to be expected; and the effects upon his health or person which may possibly come from his participation in the experiment.

    The duty and responsibility for ascertaining the quality of the consent rests upon each individual who initiates, directs, or engages in the experiment. It is a personal duty and responsibility which may not be delegated to another with impunity.

2. The experiment should be such as to yield fruitful results for the good of society, unprocurable by other methods or means of study, and not random and unnecessary in nature.

3. The experiment should be so designed and based on the results of animal experimentation and a knowledge of the natural history of the disease or other problem under study that the anticipated results will justify the performance of the experiment.

4. The experiment should be so conducted as to avoid all unnecessary physical and mental suffering and injury.

5.   No experiment should be conducted where there is an *a priori* reason to believe that death or disabling injury will occur; except, perhaps, in those experiments where the experimental physicians also serve as subjects.

6.   The degree of risk to be taken should never exceed that determined by the humanitarian importance of the problem to be solved by the experiment. Proper preparations should be made and adequate facilities provided to protect the experimental subject against even remote possibilities of injury, disability, or death.

8.   The experiment should be conducted only by scientifically qualified persons. The highest degree of skill and care should be required through all stages of the experiment of those who conduct or engage in the experiment.

9.   During the course of the experiment the human subject should be at liberty to bring the experiment to an end if he has reached the physical or mental state where continuation of the experiment seems to him to be impossible.

10. During the course of the experiment the scientist in charge must be prepared to terminate the experiment at any stage, if he has probable cause to believe, in the exercise of the good faith, superior skill, and careful judgment required of him that a continuation of the experiment is likely to result in injury, disability or death to the experimental subject.

Contributors

Archer, Luís, Ph.D., Professor, Universidade Nova de Lisboa, Lissabon, Portugal

Arnold, Pascal, Dr., Institut du Fédéralisme, Université de Fribourg, Switzerland

Baker, Robert, Ph.D., Professor, Department of Philosophy, Union College, Schenectady, New York, USA

Carson, Ronald A., Ph.D., Professor, Institute for the Medical Humanities, University of Texas Medical Branch at Galveston, Galveston, Texas, USA

Deutsch, Erwin, Dr. Dr. h.c. mult., Professor, Juristisches Seminar, Georg-August-Universität, Göttingen, Germany

Douraki, Thomaïs, Ph.D., Ministry of National Economy, Athens, Greece

Engelhardt, Dietrich von, Dr., Professor, Institut für Medizin- und Wissenschaftsgeschichte, Universität zu Lübeck, Germany

Hermerén, Göran, Dr., Professor, Department of Medical Ethics, Faculty of Medicine, Lund, Sweden

Herranz, Gonzalo, Dr., Professor, Departamento de Bioética, Universidad de Navarra, Pamplona, Spain

Honigman, Paul, Field Fisher Waterhouse, Solicitors, London, United Kingdom

Horner, J. Stuart, Dr., Professor, Beth Shemesh, Samlesbury, United Kingdom

Kanovitch, Bernard, Dr., Professor, Chaire Benjamin Edmond de Rothschild pour l'Ethique Biomédicale, Paris, France

Kimura, Rihito, J.D., Professor, Director, Asian Bioethics Program, Kennedy Institute of Ethics, Washington D.C., USA

Krause, Todd L., Ph.D., J.D., The University of Houston Health Law and Policy Institute, Houston, Texas, USA

Lepicard, Etienne, M.D., Professor, Division of Medical History, The Hebrew University of Hadassah Medical School, Jerusalem, Israel

355

Leven, Karl-Heinz, PD Dr., Institut für Geschichte der Medizin, Albert-Ludwigs-Universität, Freiburg i.br., Germany

Levi, Joel, attorney, Ramat Gan, Israel

Mathieu, Bertrand, Dr., Professor, Faculté de Droit, Dijon, France

Mattéï, Jean-François, Ph.D., Professor, Département de Génétique Médicale, Hôpital de la Timone, Marseille, France

Michaud, Jean, Dr., Professor, Cour de cassation, Paris, France

Moatti, Jean-Paul, Dr., Département de Génétique Médicale, Hôpital de la Timone, Marseille, France

Moulin, Anne-Marie, M.D., Professor, INSERM Unité 158, Hôpital des Enfants Malades, Paris, France

Plantholz, Markus, attorney, Hamburg, Germany

Rauch, Carmen, Dr., Département de Génétique Médicale, Hôpital de la Timone, Marseille, France

Reiter-Theil, Stella, Dr., Dipl.-Psych., Zentrum für Ethik und Recht in der Medizin, Universitätsklinikum der Albert-Ludwigs-Universität, Freiburg i.Br., Germany

Riquelme, Horacio, Dr., Dr., Transkulturelle Psychiatrie, Universität Hamburg, Germany

Rothman, David J., Ph.D., Professor, College of Physicians & Surgeons of Columbia University, New York, USA

Rüttgers, Jürgen, Dr., Bundesminister für Bildung, Wissenschaft, Forschung und Technologie, Bonn, Germany

Spagnolo, Antonio, Dr., Istituto de Bioética, Università Cattolica del Sacro Cuore, Rome, Italy

Sprumont, Dominique, Dr., Professor, Faculté de Droit et des Sciences Economiques, Institut de Droit de la Santé, Université de Neuchâtel, Switzerland

Tröhler, Ulrich, Dr., Ph.D., Professor, Institut für Geschichte der Medizin, Albert-Ludwigs-Universität, Freiburg i.Br., Germany

de Wachter, Maurice A.M., Dr., Professor, Waterloo, Belgium

Wellmer, Hans-Konrat, Dr., Professor, Chefarzt für Chirurgie i.R., Bielefeld, Germany

Winslade, William J., Ph.D., J.D., Professor, Institute for the Medical Humanities, University of Texas Medical Branch at Galveston, Galveston, Texas, USA

Translators